2nd Edition of Health Emergency and Disaster Risk Management (Health-EDRM)

2nd Edition of Health Emergency and Disaster Risk Management (Health-EDRM)

Editors

Emily Ying Yang Chan
Holly Ching Yu Lam

MDPI • Basel • Beijing • Wuhan • Barcelona • Belgrade • Manchester • Tokyo • Cluj • Tianjin

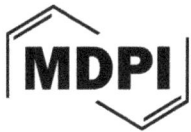

Editors
Emily Ying Yang Chan
Collaborating Centre for Oxford
University and CUHK for
Disaster and Medical
Humanitarian Response
(CCOUC), Faculty of Medicine
The Chinese University
of Hong Kong
Hong Kong

Holly Ching Yu Lam
Genomic and Environmental
Medicine, National Heart and
Lung Institute
Imperial College London
London
United Kingdom

Editorial Office
MDPI
St. Alban-Anlage 66
4052 Basel, Switzerland

This is a reprint of articles from the Special Issue published online in the open access journal *International Journal of Environmental Research and Public Health* (ISSN 1660-4601) (available at: www.mdpi.com/journal/ijerph/special_issues/Health-EDRM-2).

For citation purposes, cite each article independently as indicated on the article page online and as indicated below:

LastName, A.A.; LastName, B.B.; LastName, C.C. Article Title. *Journal Name* **Year**, *Volume Number*, Page Range.

ISBN 978-3-0365-1750-6 (Hbk)
ISBN 978-3-0365-1749-0 (PDF)

© 2021 by the authors. Articles in this book are Open Access and distributed under the Creative Commons Attribution (CC BY) license, which allows users to download, copy and build upon published articles, as long as the author and publisher are properly credited, which ensures maximum dissemination and a wider impact of our publications.

The book as a whole is distributed by MDPI under the terms and conditions of the Creative Commons license CC BY-NC-ND.

Contents

About the Editors vii

Emily Ying Yang Chan and Holly Ching Yu Lam
Research in Health-Emergency and Disaster Risk Management and Its Potential Implications in the Post COVID-19 World
Reprinted from: *International Journal of Environmental Research and Public Health* **2021**, *18*, 2520, doi:10.3390/ijerph18052520 1

Nan Zhang, Boni Su, Pak-To Chan, Te Miao, Peihua Wang and Yuguo Li
Infection Spread and High-Resolution Detection of Close Contact Behaviors
Reprinted from: *International Journal of Environmental Research and Public Health* **2020**, *17*, 1445, doi:10.3390/ijerph17041445 5

Mélissa Généreux, Mathieu Roy, Tracey O'Sullivan and Danielle Maltais
A Salutogenic Approach to Disaster Recovery: The Case of the Lac-Mégantic Rail Disaster
Reprinted from: *International Journal of Environmental Research and Public Health* **2020**, *17*, 1463, doi:10.3390/ijerph17051463 23

Sho Takahashi, Yoshifumi Takagi, Yasuhisa Fukuo, Tetsuaki Arai, Michiko Watari and Hirokazu Tachikawa
Acute Mental Health Needs Duration during Major Disasters: A Phenomenological Experience of Disaster Psychiatric Assistance Teams (DPATs) in Japan
Reprinted from: *International Journal of Environmental Research and Public Health* **2020**, *17*, 1530, doi:10.3390/ijerph17051530 37

Holly Ching Yu Lam, Zhe Huang, Sida Liu, Chunlan Guo, William Bernard Goggins and Emily Ying Yang Chan
Personal Cold Protection Behaviour and Its Associated Factors in 2016/17 Cold Days in Hong Kong: A Two-Year Cohort Telephone Survey Study
Reprinted from: *International Journal of Environmental Research and Public Health* **2020**, *17*, 1672, doi:10.3390/ijerph17051672 49

Maki Umeda, Rie Chiba, Mie Sasaki, Eni Nuraini Agustini and Sonoe Mashino
A Literature Review on Psychosocial Support for Disaster Responders: Qualitative Synthesis with Recommended Actions for Protecting and Promoting the Mental Health of Responders
Reprinted from: *International Journal of Environmental Research and Public Health* **2020**, *17*, 2011, doi:10.3390/ijerph17062011 65

Emily Ying Yang Chan, Zhe Huang, Eugene Siu Kai Lo, Kevin Kei Ching Hung, Eliza Lai Yi Wong and Samuel Yeung Shan Wong
Sociodemographic Predictors of Health Risk Perception, Attitude and Behavior Practices Associated with Health-Emergency Disaster Risk Management for Biological Hazards: The Case of COVID-19 Pandemic in Hong Kong, SAR China
Reprinted from: *International Journal of Environmental Research and Public Health* **2020**, *17*, 3869, doi:10.3390/ijerph17113869 79

Masatsugu Orui, Chihiro Nakayama, Yujiro Kuroda, Nobuaki Moriyama, Hajime Iwasa, Teruko Horiuchi, Takeo Nakayama, Minoru Sugita and Seiji Yasumura
The Association between Utilization of Media Information and Current Health Anxiety Among the Fukushima Daiichi Nuclear Disaster Evacuees
Reprinted from: *International Journal of Environmental Research and Public Health* **2020**, *17*, 3921, doi:10.3390/ijerph17113921 . . . . **97**

Evan Su Wei Shang, Eugene Siu Kai Lo, Zhe Huang, Kevin Kei Ching Hung and Emily Ying Yang Chan
Factors Associated with Urban Risk-Taking Behaviour during 2018 Typhoon Mangkhut: A Cross Sectional Study
Reprinted from: *International Journal of Environmental Research and Public Health* **2020**, *17*, 4150, doi:10.3390/ijerph17114150 . . . . **109**

Junwei Ma, Xiao Liu, Xiaoxu Niu, Yankun Wang, Tao Wen, Junrong Zhang and Zongxing Zou
Forecasting of Landslide Displacement Using a Probability-Scheme Combination Ensemble Prediction Technique
Reprinted from: *International Journal of Environmental Research and Public Health* **2020**, *17*, 4788, doi:10.3390/ijerph17134788 . . . . **119**

Young-Jae Kim, Jeong-Hyung Cho and E-Sack Kim
Differences in Sense of Belonging, Pride, and Mental Health in the Daegu Metropolitan Region due to COVID-19: Comparison between the Presence and Absence of National Disaster Relief Fund
Reprinted from: *International Journal of Environmental Research and Public Health* **2020**, *17*, 4910, doi:10.3390/ijerph17134910 . . . . **143**

Emily Ying Yang Chan, Jean Hee Kim, Eugene Siu Kai Lo, Zhe Huang, Heidi Hung, Kevin Kei Ching Hung, Eliza Lai Yi Wong, Eric Kam Pui Lee, Martin Chi Sang Wong and Samuel Yeung Shan Wong
What Happened to People with Non-Communicable Diseases during COVID-19: Implications of H-EDRM Policies
Reprinted from: *International Journal of Environmental Research and Public Health* **2020**, *17*, 5588, doi:10.3390/ijerph17155588 . . . . **155**

Emily Ying Yang Chan, Tiffany Sze Tung Sham, Tayyab Salim Shahzada, Caroline Dubois, Zhe Huang, Sida Liu, Kevin K.C. Hung, Shelly L.A. Tse, Kin On Kwok, Pui-Hong Chung, Ryoma Kayano and Rajib Shaw
Narrative Review on Health-EDRM Primary Prevention Measures for Vector-Borne Diseases
Reprinted from: *International Journal of Environmental Research and Public Health* **2020**, *17*, 5981, doi:10.3390/ijerph17165981 . . . . **163**

Elizabeth A. Newnham, Peta L. Dzidic, Enrique L.P. Mergelsberg, Bhushan Guragain, Emily Ying Yang Chan, Yoshiharu Kim, Jennifer Leaning, Ryoma Kayano, Michael Wright, Lalindra Kaththiriarchchi, Hiroshi Kato, Tomoko Osawa and Lisa Gibbs
The Asia Pacific Disaster Mental Health Network: Setting a Mental Health Agenda for the Region
Reprinted from: *International Journal of Environmental Research and Public Health* **2020**, *17*, 6144, doi:10.3390/ijerph17176144 . . . . **191**

Nina Lorenzoni, Verena Stühlinger, Harald Stummer and Margit Raich
Long-Term Impact of Disasters on the Public Health System: A Multi-Case Analysis
Reprinted from: *International Journal of Environmental Research and Public Health* **2020**, *17*, 6251, doi:10.3390/ijerph17176251 . . . . **201**

Hsin-I Shih, Tzu-Yuan Chao, Yi-Ting Huang, Yi-Fang Tu, Tzu-Ching Sung, Jung-Der Wang and Chia-Ming Chang
Increased Medical Visits and Mortality among Adults with Cardiovascular Diseases in Severely Affected Areas after Typhoon Morakot
Reprinted from: *International Journal of Environmental Research and Public Health* **2020**, *17*, 6531, doi:10.3390/ijerph17186531 . . . . **217**

Sida Liu, Emily Yang Ying Chan, William Bernard Goggins and Zhe Huang
The Mortality Risk and Socioeconomic Vulnerability Associated with High and Low Temperature in Hong Kong
Reprinted from: *International Journal of Environmental Research and Public Health* **2020**, *17*, 7326, doi:10.3390/ijerph17197326 . . . . **233**

About the Editors

Emily Ying Yang Chan

Emily Y. Y. Chan, MD, SM (Harvard), FFPH (UK) serves as a Professor and Assistant Dean at the Faculty of Medicine, Director of CCOUC and Centre for Global Health (CGH), Chinese University of Hong Kong (CUHK). She is Co-chair of the WHO Thematic Platform for Health Emergency and Disaster Risk Management (Health-EDRM) Research Network and WHO COVID-19 Research Roadmap Social Science working group, a member of the World Meteorological Organization SARS-CoV-2/COVID-19 Task Team and Asia Pacific Science Technology & Academia Advisory Group of the United Nations Office for Disaster Risk Reduction, a Visiting Professor at Oxford University Nuffield Department of Medicine, a Fellow at Harvard University FXB Center, and CEO of the GX Foundation. Her research interests cover disasters and humanitarian medicine, climate change and health, global and planetary health, human health security and Health-EDRM, remote rural health, implementation and translational science, ethnic minority health, injury and violence epidemiology, and primary care.

Holly Ching Yu Lam

Holly Lam (PhD) is an environmental epidemiologist. Having completed her PhD at the Jockey Club School of Public Health and Primary Care, Chinese University of Hong Kong (CUHK), investigating associations between meteorological factors and respiratory hospital admissions in Hong Kong, she worked on environmental health studies in the school and joined the Collaborating Centre for Oxford University and CUHK for Disaster and Medical Humanitarian Response (CCOUC) to work on research projects quantifying exposure–health–outcome associations, assessing risk perceptions and analyzing knowledge–attitude–practice for health-risk reductions in emergencies/disasters. She now works as a Medical Research Council (MRC) Early Career research fellow at the National Heart and Lung Institute, Imperial College London, focusing on environmental exposures and allergic condition associations. Her research interests cover assessing the health effects of ambient exposures and climate change and identifying related prevention strategies.

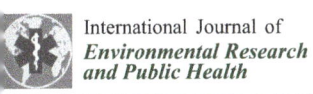

Editorial

Research in Health-Emergency and Disaster Risk Management and Its Potential Implications in the Post COVID-19 World

Emily Ying Yang Chan [1,2,*] and Holly Ching Yu Lam [3]

1. JC School of Public Health and Primary Care, Faculty of Medicine, The Chinese University of Hong Kong, Hong Kong, China
2. Nuffield Department of Medicine, University of Oxford, Oxford OX3 7BN, UK
3. Genomic and Environmental Medicine, National Heart and Lung Institute, Imperial College London, London SW7 2AZ, UK; ching.lam@imperial.ac.uk
* Correspondence: emily.chan@cuhk.edu.hk

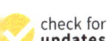

Citation: Chan, E.Y.Y.; Lam, H.C.Y. Research in Health-Emergency and Disaster Risk Management and Its Potential Implications in the Post COVID-19 World. *Int. J. Environ. Res. Public Health* **2021**, *18*, 2520. https://doi.org/10.3390/ijerph18052520

Received: 25 February 2021
Accepted: 2 March 2021
Published: 4 March 2021

Publisher's Note: MDPI stays neutral with regard to jurisdictional claims in published maps and institutional affiliations.

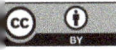

Copyright: © 2021 by the authors. Licensee MDPI, Basel, Switzerland. This article is an open access article distributed under the terms and conditions of the Creative Commons Attribution (CC BY) license (https://creativecommons.org/licenses/by/4.0/).

Health-Emergency Disaster Risk Management (Health-EDRM) is one of the latest academic and global policy paradigms that capture knowledge, research and policy shift from response to preparedness and health risk management in non-emergency times [1]. This concept encompasses risk analyses and interventions, such as accessible early warning systems, timely deployment of relief workers, provision of suitable drugs, and medical equipment to decrease the impact of disasters on people before, during, and after an event(s). The approach emphasizes the investment into disaster health risk reduction efforts which may thereby strengthening health systems and capacity to ensure community health resilience building. Health emergency disaster risk management (Health-EDRM) thus refers to the systematic analysis and management of health risks surrounding emergencies and disasters, and plays an important role in reducing hazards and vulnerability along with extending preparedness, response, and recovery measures [1].

Disasters such as earthquakes, cyclones, floods, heat waves, nuclear accidents, and large-scale pollution incidents cost human lives and incur long-term health and well-being implications. The most vulnerable population subgroups in the majority of the disasters often comprise of extreme ages, remote living areas, and endemic poverty, as well as people with low literacy. However, scientific evidence gaps remain in the published literature regarding health risks patterns and cost-effectiveness Health-EDRM risk reduction strategies to facilitate a more efficient reduction of global disaster risks through global policies and initiatives [2,3]. The first Special Issue of *IJERPH*, published in 2018–2019 with the thematic focus on Health-EDRM included 20 papers that characterized disaster risks, analysed health risk and interventions effectiveness [4]. The 2nd edition (2019–2020) further compiles 16 scientific papers that have been published in 2020. Papers included in this 2nd edition demonstrate the diverse range of health-related disaster and emergency risk management topics and research analyses that evaluate short- and long-term health impacts, associated risk factors, risk assessment methods and tools as well as multidisciplinary research methods related to program evaluation and policy analysis.

With the complexity and interconnectedness of modern living, multidisciplinary research methodologies development is crucial, as it may enhance the assessment of health risks, impacts and promote understanding of health risks, disaster and humanitarian medicine for non-health stakeholders. The study of Zhang et al. [5] shows how multidisciplinary methodologies might be applied to examine communicable disease spread among close-contacts. Ma et al. [6] proposes a landslide risk prediction approach that might be useful to prevent mortality and morbidity in at-risk communities.

In the 21st century, the human health impacts of climate change are expected to be significant globally. In this issue, five studies are published to delineate population health risks that may be associated with climate change in various contexts. The studies examine socio-demographic patterns of self-help and community bottom-up health protection strategies during extreme temperature events [7,8] (Lam et al., Liu et al.) and typhoon/hurricane [9,10] (Shang et al., Shih et al.). In addition, with the global increasing health risks associated with vector-borne diseases as a result of climate abnormalities, [11] Chan et al. present a narrative review paper of the current understanding of primary preventive Health-EDRM measures that might reduce the health risks of vector-borne disease in communities.

Another research article subset published in this edition is related to the evaluation of human health and well-being with man-made/technology-related disasters. In their case study, Genereux et al. [12] analyze how mixed-method-based need assessment might capture potential health risks and needs and subsequently enhance effectiveness and relevance response and recovery of the 2013 Lac-Megantic Rail disaster. The study of Orui et al. [13] finds an association between media information and post nuclear accident health anxiety. The findings of this study may inform policymakers and clinical practitioners about mental and health risk reduction strategies. Based on a mixed-method approach, Lorenzoni et al. [14] examines various long-term implications of disasters on public health system performance, security and health protection.

Psychosocial and mental health risks and impacts are another important research development area of the Health-EDRM. Takahashi et al. and Umeda et al. have examined the acute mental health needs [15] of disaster victims and potentially how to protect and promote the mental risks of responders [16]. Newnham et al. [17] described the activities and strategic plans of a newly established mental health network in Asia Pacific that aims to encourage and build the research agenda of Health-EDRM-related issues in the region.

Among all the major global disasters in 2020, SARS-CoV2, the biological hazard which caused the COVID-19 pandemic, once again showed how health risks may be far-reaching to cause mortality and affect lives in the 21st century. Within a year, the pandemic has accumulated over 110 million cases and 2.5 million deaths [18]. Meanwhile, research and reported experiences in Asia, as the first global region that was hit by the pandemic in early 2020, might be useful to facilitate understanding of health risks and impacts of a new disease of unknown origin. Kim et al. reports on the COVID-19 impact on mental health status of people living in Daegu, South Korea, the community with the 2nd highest rate of COVID-19 beyond Wuhan city PRC China, during the early phase of the pandemic [19]. Chan et al. [20] examines the sociodemographic predictors of health risk perception, attitudes and behavioral practices of the management COVID-19 in a high-density metropolis—HK, China during the first 2 months of the pandemic (6). The same research team also published an article that examines the health risks and situation of people with non-communicable diseases during the pandemic [21].

In the upcoming months, the global research community is expected to receive a significant amount of Health-EDRM research outputs related to the COVID-19 pandemic. With heavy emphasizes on the hierarchy of prevention and adverse disaster risk reduction [22], researchers and policy makers of Health-EDRM should be proactive in the application of the concepts and tools highlighted in the Health-EDRM paradigm and frameworks [23]. Such efforts will improve research effectiveness for strengthening practice and policy making that aim to protect human health and well-being from future epidemics and disasters.

Author Contributions: Writing—Original Draft Preparation, E.Y.Y.C.; Writing—Review & Editing, H.C.Y.L. Both authors have read and agreed to the published version of the manuscript.

Funding: This research received no external funding.

Institutional Review Board Statement: Not applicable.

Informed Consent Statement: Not applicable.

Acknowledgments: Our special thank goes to the Editorial Office and Chi Shing Wong for their facilitation and coordination in this Special Issue in Health-EDRM.

Conflicts of Interest: The authors declare no conflict of interest.

References

1. World Health Organization. *Health Emergency and Disaster Risk Management: Overview*; World Health Organization: Geneva, Switzerland, 2019; ISBN 9789241516181.
2. Chan, E.Y.Y.; Murray, V. What are the health research needs for the Sendai Framework? *Lancet* **2017**, *390*, e35–e36. [CrossRef]
3. Kayano, R.; Chan, E.Y.Y.; Murray, V.; Abrahams, J.; Barber, S.L. WHO thematic platform for health emergency and disaster risk management research network (TPRN): Report of the kobe expert meeting. *Int. J. Environ. Res. Public Health* **2019**, *16*, 1232. [CrossRef] [PubMed]
4. Ying, E.; Chan, Y.; Ching, H.; Lam, Y. *Health-Related Emergency Disaster Risk Management (Health-EDRM)*; MDPI: Basel, Switzerland, 2020; ISBN 9783039363148.
5. Zhang, N.; Su, B.; Chan, P.T.; Miao, T.; Wang, P.; Li, Y. Infection spread and high-resolution detection of close contact behaviors. *Int. J. Environ. Res. Public Health* **2020**, *17*, 1445. [CrossRef] [PubMed]
6. Ma, J.; Liu, X.; Niu, X.; Wang, Y.; Wen, T.; Zhang, J.; Zou, Z. Forecasting of landslide displacement using a probability-scheme combination ensemble prediction technique. *Int. J. Environ. Res. Public Health* **2020**, *17*, 4788. [CrossRef] [PubMed]
7. Lam, H.C.Y.; Huang, Z.; Liu, S.; Guo, C.; Goggins, W.B.; Chan, E.Y.Y. Personal cold protection behaviour and its associated factors in 2016/17 cold days in Hong Kong: A two-year cohort telephone survey study. *Int. J. Environ. Res. Public Health* **2020**, *17*, 1672. [CrossRef] [PubMed]
8. Liu, S.; Chan, E.Y.Y.; Goggins, W.B.; Huang, Z. The mortality risk and socioeconomic vulnerability associated with high and low temperature in Hong Kong. *Int. J. Environ. Res. Public Health* **2020**, *17*, 7326. [CrossRef] [PubMed]
9. Shang, E.S.W.; Lo, E.S.K.; Huang, Z.; Hung, K.K.C.; Chan, E.Y.Y. Factors associated with urban risk-taking behaviour during 2018 typhoon mangkhut: A cross sectional study. *Int. J. Environ. Res. Public Health* **2020**, *17*, 4150. [CrossRef] [PubMed]
10. Shih, H.I.; Chao, T.Y.; Huang, Y.T.; Tu, Y.F.; Sung, T.C.; Wang, J.-D.; Chang, C.M. Increased medical visits and mortality among adults with cardiovascular diseases in severely affected areas after typhoon morakot. *Int. J. Environ. Res. Public Health* **2020**, *17*, 6531. [CrossRef] [PubMed]
11. Chan, E.Y.Y.; Sham, T.S.T.; Shahzada, T.S.; Dubois, C.; Huang, Z.; Liu, S.; Hung, K.K.C.; Tse, S.L.A.; Kwok, K.O.; Chung, P.H.; et al. Narrative review on health-edrm primary prevention measures for vector-borne diseases. *Int. J. Environ. Res. Public Health* **2020**, *17*, 5981. [CrossRef] [PubMed]
12. Généreux, M.; Roy, M.; O'sullivan, T.; Maltais, D. A salutogenic approach to disaster recovery: The case of the lac-mégantic rail disaster. *Int. J. Environ. Res. Public Health* **2020**, *17*, 1463. [CrossRef] [PubMed]
13. Orui, M.; Nakayama, C.; Kuroda, Y.; Moriyama, N.; Iwasa, H.; Horiuchi, T.; Nakayama, T.; Sugita, M.; Yasumura, S. The association between utilization of media information and current health anxiety among the fukushima daiichi nuclear disaster evacuees. *Int. J. Environ. Res. Public Health* **2020**, *17*, 3921. [CrossRef] [PubMed]
14. Lorenzoni, N.; Stühlinger, V.; Stummer, H.; Raich, M. Long-term impact of disasters on the public health system: A multi-case analysis. *Int. J. Environ. Res. Public Health* **2020**, *17*, 6251. [CrossRef] [PubMed]
15. Takahashi, S.; Takagi, Y.; Fukuo, Y.; Arai, T.; Watari, M.; Tachikawa, H. Acute mental health needs duration during major disasters: A phenomenological experience of disaster psychiatric assistance teams (dpats) in japan. *Int. J. Environ. Res. Public Health* **2020**, *17*, 1530. [CrossRef] [PubMed]
16. Umeda, M.; Chiba, R.; Sasaki, M.; Agustini, E.N.; Mashino, S. A literature review on psychosocial support for disaster responders: Qualitative synthesis with recommended actions for protecting and promoting the mental health of responders. *Int. J. Environ. Res. Public Health* **2020**, *17*, 2011. [CrossRef] [PubMed]
17. Newnham, E.A.; Dzidic, P.L.; Mergelsberg, E.L.P.; Guragain, B.; Chan, E.Y.Y.; Kim, Y.; Leaning, J.; Kayano, R.; Wright, M.; Kaththiriarachchi, L.; et al. The asia pacific disaster mental health network: Setting a mental health agenda for the region. *Int. J. Environ. Res. Public Health* **2020**, *17*, 6144. [CrossRef] [PubMed]
18. Johns Hopkins University & Medicine COVID-19 Dashboard by the Center for Systems Science and Engineering (CSSE) at Johns Hopkins University (JHU). Available online: https://coronavirus.jhu.edu/map.html (accessed on 4 March 2021).
19. Kim, Y.J.; Cho, J.H.; Kim, E.S. Differences in sense of belonging, pride, and mental health in the daegu metropolitan region due to COVID-19: Comparison between the presence and absence of national disaster relief fund. *Int. J. Environ. Res. Public Health* **2020**, *17*, 4910. [CrossRef] [PubMed]
20. Chan, E.Y.Y.; Huang, Z.; Lo, E.S.K.; Hung, K.K.C.; Wong, E.L.Y.; Wong, S.Y.S. Sociodemographic predictors of health risk perception, attitude and behavior practices associated with health-emergency disaster risk management for biological hazards: The case of COVID-19 pandemic in Hong Kong, SAR China. *Int. J. Environ. Res. Public Health* **2020**, *17*, 3869. [CrossRef]
21. Chan, E.Y.Y.; Kim, J.H.; Lo, E.S.K.; Huang, Z.; Hung, H.; Hung, K.K.C.; Wong, E.L.Y.; Lee, E.K.P.; Wong, M.C.S.; Wong, S.Y.S. What happened to people with non-communicable diseases during COVID-19: Implications of H-EDRM policies. *Int. J. Environ. Res. Public Health* **2020**, *17*, 5588. [CrossRef] [PubMed]
22. Chan, E.Y.Y.; Shaw, R. *Public Health and Disasters—Health Emergency and Disaster Risk Management in Asia*; Springer: Singapore, 2020.
23. WHO Headquarters and Regional Offices (PAHO, AFRO, EMRO, EURO, SEARO, WPRO). *WHO Guidance on Research Methods for Health and Disaster Risk Management*; World Health Organization: Geneva, Switzerland, 2020.

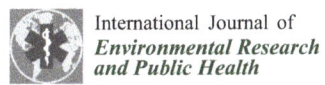

Article

Infection Spread and High-Resolution Detection of Close Contact Behaviors

Nan Zhang [1], Boni Su [2], Pak-To Chan [1], Te Miao [1], Peihua Wang [1] and Yuguo Li [1,*]

[1] Department of Mechanical Engineering, The University of Hong Kong, Pokfulam Road, Hong Kong 999077, China; zhangnan@hku.hk (N.Z.); ptjchan@connect.hku.hk (P.-T.C.); miaote@connect.hku.hk (T.M.); phwang@connect.hku.hk (P.W.)
[2] China Electric Power Planning & Engineering Institute, Beijing 100120, China; bnsu@eppei.com
* Correspondence: liyg@hku.hk; Tel.: +852-96773662

Received: 20 December 2019; Accepted: 20 February 2020; Published: 24 February 2020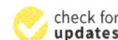

Abstract: Knowledge of human behaviors is important for improving indoor-environment design, building-energy efficiency, and productivity, and for studies of infection spread. However, such data are lacking. In this study, we designed a device for detecting and recording, second by second, the 3D indoor positioning and head and body motions of each graduate student in an office. From more than 400 person hours of data. Students spent 92.2%, 4.1%, 2.9%, and 0.8% of their time in their own office cubicles, other office cubicles, aisles, and areas near public facilities, respectively. They spent 9.7% of time in close contact, and each student averagely had 4.0 close contacts/h. Students spent long time on close contact in the office which may lead to high infection risk. The average interpersonal distance during close contact was 0.81 m. When sitting, students preferred small relative face orientation angle. Pairs of standing students preferred a face-to-face orientation during close contact which means this pattern had a lower infection risk via close contact. Probability of close contact decreased exponentially with the increasing distance between two students' cubicles. Data on human behaviour during close contact is helpful for infection risk analysis and infection control and prevention.

Keywords: infection spread and control; infection risk; human behavior; close contact; sensor-based; indoor environment; indoor positioning; head and body motion; open-plan office

1. Introduction

Indoor human behaviors directly impact on indoor thermal comfort [1], energy efficiency [2], office design [3], and exposure to pollutants (e.g., infectious microbes) [4]. Indoor human behaviors in and between different environments also directly impact on the infection risk [5]. Close contacts are believed to facilitate the spread of many viral respiratory diseases such as influenza [6], SARS [7], MERS [8], and even Ebola [9].

Infection risk via close contact is influenced by interpersonal distance, respiratory activities, and movement of body parts. Interpersonal distance directly affects the risk of virus exposure due to inhalation and deposition, the so-called short-range airborne and large droplet routes, respectively [10]. A threshold distance of close contact less than 1.5 m to 2 m is generally accepted as risky [11–13]. Human respiratory activities such as breathing, talking, and coughing can generate droplets of different numbers and sizes [14–18]. Infectious pathogens are shed and exhaled by the infected during these respiratory activities, and transported by the exhaled air streams, while inhalation of fine droplets and exposure to large droplets are also affected by the inspiratory air streams and body/head/arm movement [19]. Relative face orientation (e.g., face-to-face, face-to-side) and posture are important factors in determining the cross-infection, especially over short distance [20]. Exposure of face-to-back close contact is much smaller than it of face-to-face pattern [21,22]. Posture also important in droplet deposition, for example, droplets deposited on trousers on the thighs of a sitting person should be more than on a standing person.

Very little data exist on indoor close contact behaviors, especially data combining all of the factors mentioned above. Some human behaviors are difficult to accurately monitor with high temporal resolution [11,19]. Electronic sensors such as radiofrequency identification devices (RFIDs) are the most commonly used to collect human contact data. These devices, however, can only detect close contact by taking readings of interpersonal distance every 20 s, and only one-on-one close contact can be detected [23,24]. A temporal resolution of 20 s is not sufficient, as the median value duration of a close contact is 17 s [11]. Moreover, human respiratory activities and movement of body parts (e.g., head and body) cannot be detected by this means. Body movements impact the air flows in a room. To collect close contact data with high temporal resolution, video recordings have been used, which can be processed second-by-second [11,19]. This approach is subject to human error on the part of the video analysts, and also time-consuming.

Office are the most common form of workplace for the most of employees, with open-plan designs widely used [25,26]. In this study, we monitored and analyzed indoor human behaviors in a graduate student office using automatic devices installed on the hats and clothes of the participants. These devices overcome nearly all of the shortcomings mentioned above and automatically collect high-resolution data on indoor human behaviors. The data monitored included the indoor position, head and body motion, and posture of each individual which are important for infectious disease transmission. We collected more than 1,440,000 s of data for 49 students across two days. This study supported data of indoor human behaviors on close contact. From indoor positioning distribution, we can know that which part in the office has higher infection risk. Combining individual inhalation and exhalation patterns with head's and body's motion during close contact, high-precision quantitative risk assessment on infection spread and control could be conducted.

2. Materials and Methods

The experiments were conducted in two close-by Chinese graduate student offices on two consecutive Saturdays. The choice of two nearly identical offices was due to the need of minimising microbial interference, as the experiment also contained another part on surface microbial monitoring, which is not reported in this paper.

2.1. Room Setting

Each room was designed for a maximum of 30 students, i.e., containing 30 cubicles (Figure 1). There were 26 students (13 male and 13 female) in Room 1 on the first experiment day (day 1), and 23 students (12 male and 11 female) in Room 2 on the second experiment day (day 2). A total of 32 students participated in the experiment, and 17 of them in both experiments. Among 32 participants, 27 students were those who worked in the institute and five students were invited by some students who were in the institute. In addition, three pairs of students were romantically involved. We selected these students because they were familiar with the experimental environment, which should minimize any bias caused by environment. The length (12.2 m) and height (2.73 m) of both rooms were the same, and the layouts of the cubicles in the two rooms were symmetrical, see Figure 1.

Each room had a water dispenser and a group of lockers. Only Room 2 had a printer. Each room was divided into six cubicle regions (marked by dotted lines in Figure 1), and students in the same cubicle region were more likely to communicate with each other. All of the students were monitored by 22 video cameras (1080P) from 8:30 a.m. to 9:30 p.m. The indoor temperature during the experimental days, which controlled by central air conditionings, was between 26 and 27 degrees. There were 27 fluorescent tubes on the ceiling of the office to keep the luminance, therefore, combing with the high-resolution cameras, most human behaviors can be captured. Each camera monitored one or two office cubicles, except for two with a global view, one camera for the door, and one camera for the water dispenser.

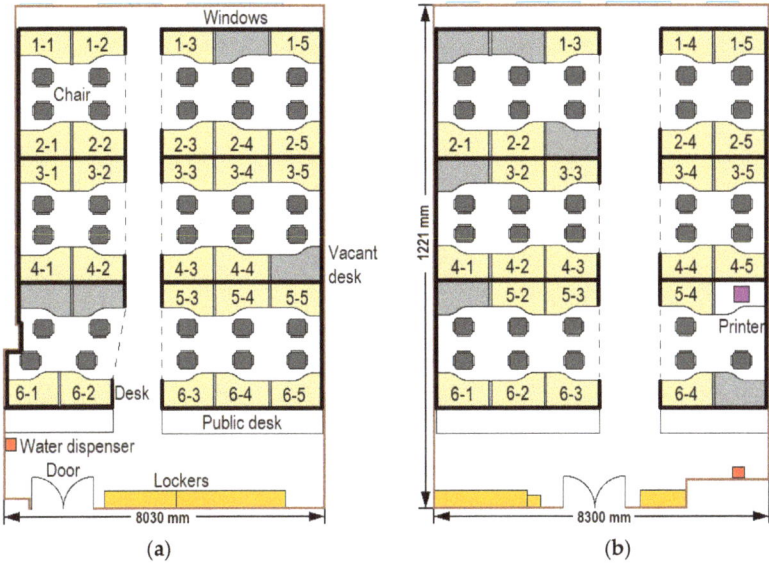

Figure 1. Room settings: (**a**) Room 1; (**b**) Room 2.

2.2. Detection Devices

The sensors we developed are shown in Figure 2a. The sensors for indoor positioning and head motion were installed on the participants' hats, and those for body motion were installed on the chest of a tight shirt. An ultrawide band (UWB) radio real-time location system (RTLS) was applied to obtain the indoor positions of all participants [27,28]. The distance resolution of UWB is within 0.1 m when there is no obstruction. To ensure continuous data transmission, the UWB tag was installed on the top of each hat, and four UWB anchors were installed on the office ceiling. An inertial measurement unit (IMU), which can measure and record the position and motion of the head and body (i.e., rotation), was also installed on the top of each hat and the front of each tight shirt. A microphone was installed on the collar band of the shirt to determine when the participants were talking. To protect privacy, only the sound level was recorded. Adjustable bands on the hat and around the head were used to avoid relative movement between the hat and head. Tight clothing was worn to avoid relative movement between the shirt and body. All of the data recorded during the experiment were saved in a chip. The weight of a device on hats and shirts was 73 g, and the weight of hat with fixed accessories was 159 g. Therefore, each student worn a hat of 232 g on the head and worn a device of 73 g on the shirt. Light weight brings a much smaller impact on human behaviors.

Rotations were recorded in the form of quaternions. To obtain the absolute (relative to the ground) rotation of the head and body, all of the participants underwent calibration after wearing and before taking off the hat and the shirt. During the calibration, the participant stood still and faced the same wall while keeping his/her head and body upright for 10 s. For any IMU (head or body), the quaternions during the calibrations before and after the experiment were denoted as q_{start} and q_{end}, respectively. If the difference between q_{start} and q_{end} was greater than a threshold value (equivalent to 10° rotation), it was probable that the participant had moved the hat or shirt during the experiment, and the data were discarded. Data were also regarded as invalid if the fluctuation of rotation between 10-s calibrations was more than 5°. To eliminate drift errors for all sensors, the quaternions were adjusted from all valid raw data based on spherical linear quaternion interpolation (Equation (1)):

$$q = q_{raw} q_{start}^{-1} \left(q_{start} q_{end}^{-1} \right)^{(t-t_{start})/(t_{end}-t_{start})}, \qquad (1)$$

where t is time, t_{start} and t_{end} are the time of the calibrations before and after the experiment. The steering vectors ($\vec{x_h}, \vec{y_h}, \vec{z_h}$ for head and $\vec{x_b}, \vec{y_b}, \vec{z_b}$ for body, relative to the ground) can be obtained from the quaternions (Figure 2b). Usually, the horizontal rotation of the head relative to the body direction is more important. The relative steering vectors of head to body ($\vec{x_{hb}}, \vec{y_{hb}}$, and $\vec{z_{hb}}$) can be calculated using coordinate transformation (Equation (2)):

$$\begin{bmatrix} \vec{x_{hb}} & \vec{y_{hb}} & \vec{z_{hb}} \end{bmatrix} = \begin{bmatrix} x_{\vec{x_b}} & y_{\vec{x_b}} & 0 \\ x_{\vec{y_b}} & y_{\vec{y_b}} & 0 \\ 0 & 0 & 1 \end{bmatrix} \begin{bmatrix} \vec{y_h} & \vec{y_h} & \vec{z_h} \end{bmatrix}, \tag{2}$$

where $x_{\vec{x_b}}$ and $y_{\vec{x_b}}$ are the components of $\vec{x_b}$ the in x and y directions and $x_{\vec{y_b}}$ and $y_{\vec{y_b}}$ are the components of $\vec{y_b}$ in the x and y directions, respectively. Here, the roll and pitch of the head are relative to the ground; only the yaw of the head is relative to the body. There is no yaw of the body because no relevant reference point on the waist was monitored. Therefore, data on three head motions (yaw, pitch, and roll) and two body motions (pitch and roll) were collected.

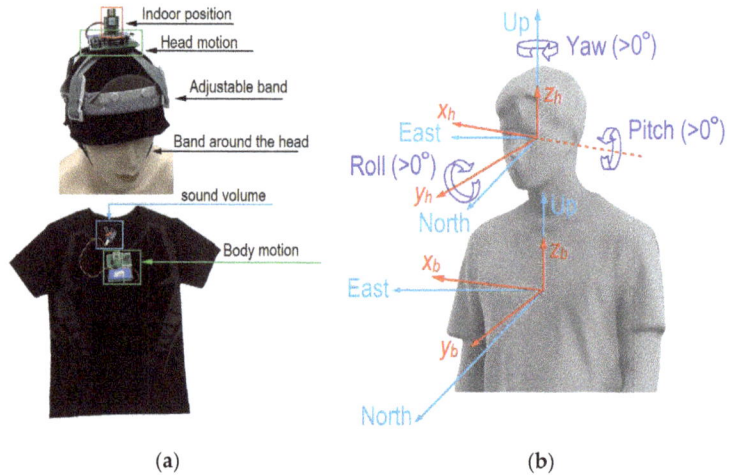

Figure 2. Device design and motions of head and body. (**a**) Device for indoor positioning, and head and body motion detection; (**b**) current and base vectors for head and body.

All of the sensors were calibrated prior to the experiments. We first installed the IMUs on a large plate, and performed specific rotations with different angles (e.g., 45°, 90°, 135°, 180°) in three directions. The IMU was regarded as well-calibrated when the difference between all measured values and real values was less than 2°. The UWB sensors were also calibrated in the experimental rooms before the experiments. We chose five indoor points at which to perform calibration to reduce the error of indoor positioning to no more than 10 cm.

2.3. Close Contact Behavior

As motions relevant to the inhalation/exhalation flows, we considered individual head and upper body motions, human respiratory activities (e.g., coughing, sneezing, and speaking), and the features of relative position (e.g., interpersonal distance and relative face orientation) of two people. The definitions of head and body motions can be found in Zhang et al. [11].

Close contact was defined as any full or partial face-to-face interaction within 2 m [23,29–31]. A face-to-face interaction can occur with or without conversation, including when two individuals read a book or watch a computer screen together. An event was not counted as close contact if the distance between the two students was shorter than 2 m but there was no interaction between them; for example, if two students used their own computers in their own cubicles. If any close contact lasted for more than 1 s, it was counted as a single close contact. If the two students were separated (more than 2 m apart or with no interaction) by more than 1 s, the individual students' close contact behavior (e.g., with another student at that distance) was counted separately. In this study, interpersonal distance was defined as the distance between the sensors on the two participants other than those on their faces. In addition to interpersonal distance, the relative face orientation angle of the two participants was also obtained. This is the angle between the normal of the two students and ranges from 0° to 180° [11].

2.4. Data Processing

During the two experimental days, 1,440,492 s of human behavior data were collected. The first author processed all video episodes second by second, recording all visible close contacts between each pair of students in the office. The collected data include posture (standing, sitting, and squatting), whether two students were in close contact, the identities of those in close contact, and the start and end time of each episode of close contact. The indoor position and head and body motions were monitored by sensors. The indoor position data on *day 1* were unfortunately missed, which means that all of the valid indoor position data were from *day 2*. Out of the 23 participants, 21 had indoor position data during *day 2*, and in total 717,168 s of indoor position data were collected. Among these data, 10,827 s (1.5%) was lost or disrupted, and linear interpolation was used to approximate these data. To maintain the accuracy of all recorded data on head and body motions, we discarded the data for which the difference between two calibrations was more than 10° or the fluctuation during each calibration was more than 5°. After data filtering, 541,200 s of data on head and body motions were valid. Moreover, a total of 1,250,392 s of valid data on sound levels were recorded by the microphones over the two days. All of the results reported below are based on these valid data.

3. Results

3.1. General Human Behavior Data

While indoors, the students spent 5.3% of their time standing, 94.6% sitting, and only 0.1% squatting. We divided the office into functional areas, i.e., occupied office cubicles, vacant office cubicles, aisle, and areas near public facilities (Figure 3a). Figure 3b shows the distribution of indoor positions during *day 2*, where red indicates the highest coverage rate (≥40 times per 25 cm^2). Occupied office cubicles had the highest coverage rate, mainly due to occupation by their owner (Figure 3b). The students spent on average 92.2% of their time staying in their own cubicles. For the remaining 7.8% of the time, the students occupied other places. The results show that they spent most of the latter time in the aisle close to the doorway, the area close to the door, and areas close to the printer and the water dispenser (Figure 3c). Some students had a particularly close relationship with certain others or even a romantic relationship (e.g., boy-/girlfriend), and their office cubicles had a higher probability of being occupied by others. Most vacant office cubicles had a very low occupied percentage. In general, when outside their own cubicle, the students spent 47.9%, 4.5%, 37.4%, and 10.2% of their time in occupied office cubicles, vacant office cubicles, the aisle, and areas near public facilities.

Based on 541,200 valid data of head and body motions, we obtained the general characteristics of these motions for the overall group of students. Figure 4a illustrates the head and body motions. The circle shows the probability distribution of face orientation in the form of a projected half sphere; the reader can imagine that the eyes are located at the center of the sphere. This half sphere is divided into 1296 sectors, each of them 5° × 5°. The top, bottom, left, and right correspond to the participant raising, lowering, left-turning, and right-turning the head by 90°. The center indicates that the student is looking almost exactly forward.

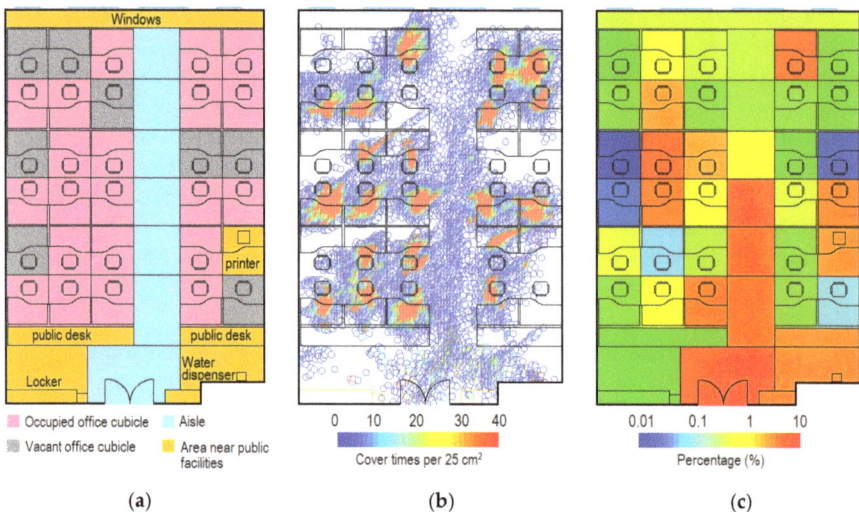

Figure 3. Indoor positioning in Room 2 (*day 2*). (**a**) Functional area; (**b**) Distribution of indoor positions; (**c**) Distribution of indoor positions by functional area during the time spent in other places (i.e., students outside their own cubicles). (Indoor positioning data for students 3-4 and 3-5 were lost).

This provides an intuitive visualization of the students' preferred head motions. In the office, the students preferred to look towards the red and orange grids in the circle (i.e., lower their head), and had a very low probability of raising their head (blue grids). To characterize the head motions, we considered the movement of the head in three directions independently. In the horizontal direction, the average degree of yaw was 4.1°, which means that the students on average slightly turned their head to the right by 4.1°.

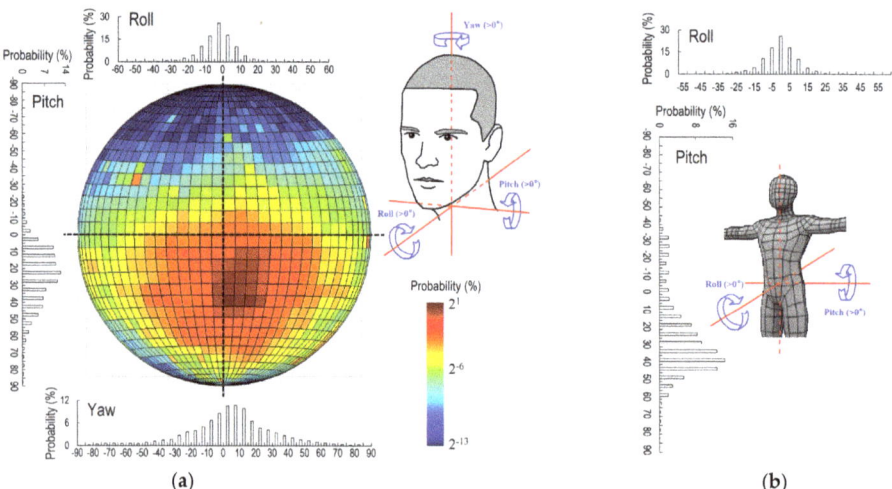

Figure 4. Indoor human behavior in terms of head and body motion. (**a**) Head motion; (**b**) Body motion. (Yaw of head is relative to the body; pitch and roll of head and all body motions are relative to the ground).

The students had almost equal probability of turning their head left and right, i.e., the probability distribution of yaw was symmetric. The average degree of pitch was 23.0°, which means that the students preferred to lower their head by 23.0° on average. Indeed, the head was lowered during 93.5% of indoor time. The students on average tilted (rolled) the head 2.8° to the left. The probability distributions of left and right tilts were almost the same. The students spent 86.1% and 97.4% of time tilting their head within 15° and 30°, respectively.

Figure 4b shows the body motions during indoor time. The students on average lowered their bodies (pitch) by 23.2°, and spent 85.6% of indoor time bending their bodies forward. The average degree of body roll was 3.7°, which means that the students on average slightly tilted their bodies to the right. The probability distribution of roll was almost symmetric. The students spent 86.7% and 98.2% of time tilting their bodies within 15° and 30°, respectively.

Three postures were considered in this study: standing, sitting, and squatting. Here we only analyzed head and body motions during standing and sitting because the students spent very little time squatting (0.1%). Figure 5 lists the probability distributions of head and body motions in three directions for all students during indoor time. The rolling of the head and body showed little difference between standing and sitting postures, and the participants had only a slightly higher probability of bending their head during sitting than during standing. However, the characteristics of yaw and pitch of the head, and pitch of the body, differed by posture. The average angles of head yaw during standing and sitting were −3.0° and 4.5°, respectively. The students on average lowered their heads by 30.9° and 24.1° while standing and sitting, respectively. The pitch of the body was strongly linked to posture. The average angles of pitch of the body during standing and sitting were 21.2° and 24.7°, respectively. However, the students had a higher probability of keeping their body bent forward at a large angle during standing ($\beta_b > 60°$ during 8.1% of the time) than during sitting ($\beta_b > 60°$ during 0.7% of the time). The most common forward-bending angle of the body during standing was between 10° and 15°, while that during sitting was 35° to 40°.

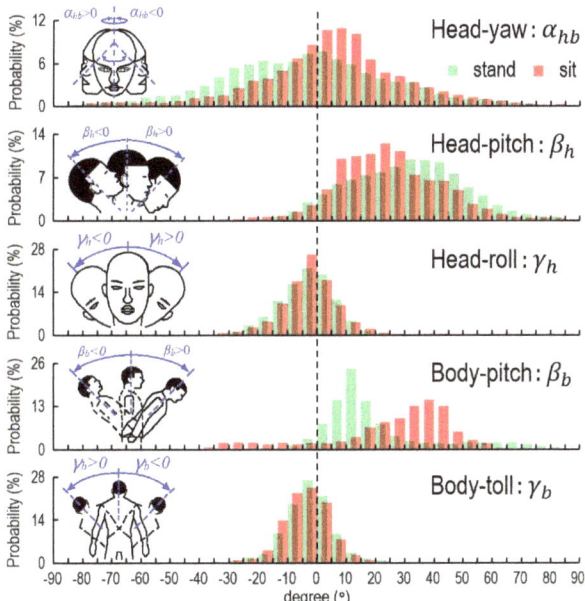

Figure 5. Probability distribution of head and body motions by posture.

3.2. Indoor Behavior During Close Contact

The students spent more than 9.7% of their time in close contact and each student had on average 4.0 close contact episodes per hour. The probability distribution of close contact fitted a log-normal distribution (Figure 6). The average and median durations of close contact were 54.5 and

15 s, respectively. Close contacts with duration between 8 and 16 s had the highest frequency. The durations of 38.2%, 68.8%, and 82.8% of close contacts were no more than 10, 30, and 60 s, respectively. From the microphone data, at least one student was speaking during 68.6% of the time during close contact. One-on-one close contacts accounted for more than 90% of close contact time, while 7.8%, 1.5%, and 0.6% of close contact time involved three, four, and five students simultaneously. Six-student conversations only accounted for 0.06% of close contact time.

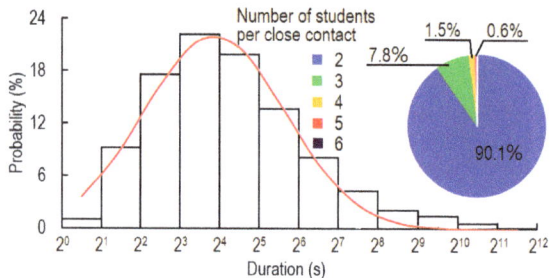

Figure 6. Probability distribution of duration per close contact.

During close contact, 22.9%, 76.3%, and 0.8% of students stood, sat, and squatted, respectively (Table 1). During 59.6% of the close contact time, both students were sitting. The pattern of one standing and one sitting was adopted during 33.5% of the close contact time. The students almost never chatted with each other while one stood and one squatted (0.1% of close contact time).

Table 1. Probability distribution of individual postures and posture pattern of students during close contact.

Description	Posture	Percentage
Individual posture	Sitting	76.3%
	Standing	22.9%
	Squatting	0.8%
Posture pattern	Sitting-sitting	59.6%
	Sitting-standing	33.5%
	Standing-standing	5.6%
	Sitting-squatting	1.2%
	Others	0.1%

Figure 7 shows the characteristics of close contact. As can be seen, 68.2% of the close contacts were between students in the same region, and most were between adjacent students. Only 13.2% of the close contacts were between students in remote regions (Figure 7a). Influenced by the circulation of people, students near the aisle and the door had a higher probability of being contacted (Figure 7b). From Figure 7c, the greater the distance between the office cubicles of two students was, the lower was the probability of a close contact. The average cubicle distance between two students for close contact was 1.25 areas (for the area distribution refer to Figure 3a), and 77.2% of close contacts occurred between two students with a cubicle distance of no more than three areas. The student who had the closest contacts had 50.5 episodes per hour (Figure 7d). On average each student had 4.0 close contact episodes per hour, and no one had zero close contacts during either day. During the two days, 12.2% (total pairs of contact: 141; possible pairs of contact: 1156 = 26 × 25 + 23 × 22) of all possible pairs of students had close contact. Each pair of students had close contact on average 11.3 times per day, and the pair with the highest frequency of close contacts had 100 episodes per day (Figure 7e). As shown in Figure 7f, 22.4%, 40.8%, 59.2%, and 85.7% of the students spent no more than 1%, 5%, 10%, and 20% of their time in close contacts, respectively. The most sociable student spent 34% of her indoor time in close contact. The average and median ratios of close contact time to total indoor time were 9.7% and 6.4%, respectively. During the two days, the students had close contacts with an average of 8.4 and 4.2 students, respectively. The most sociable student had close contacts with 10 and 20 students during *day 1* and *day 2*, respectively (Figure 7g).

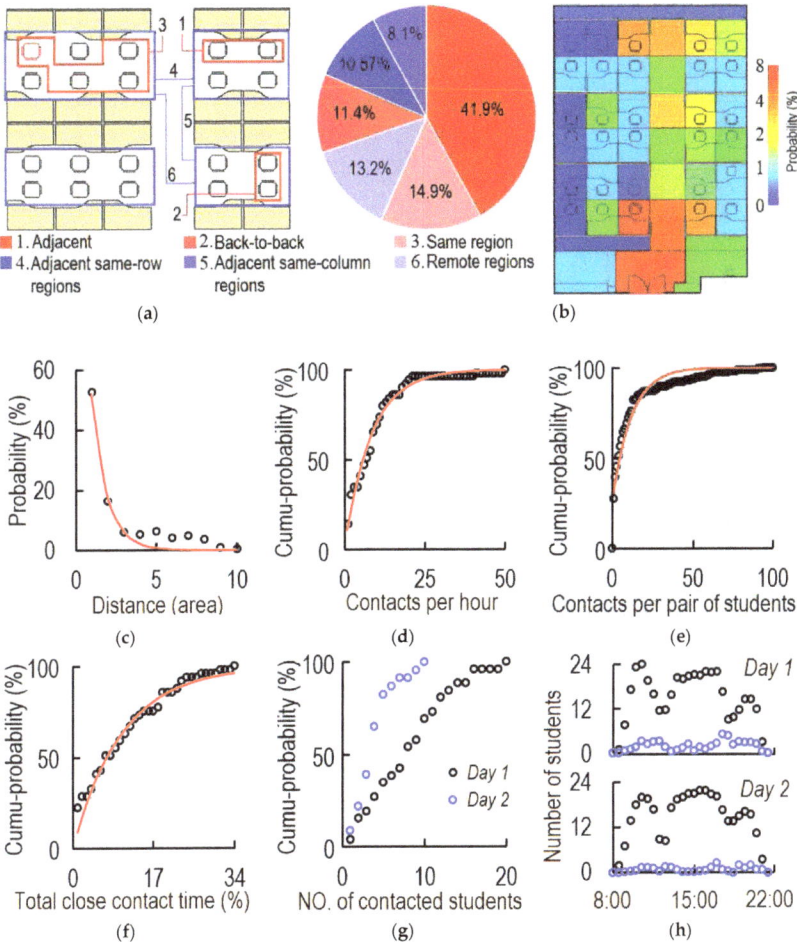

Figure 7. Characteristics of close contact. (**a**) Probability distribution by relative position of students' office cubicles (same region means two students are in the same region but not adjacent or back to back; percentage shows the episodes of close contact occurred in different relative positions); (**b**) Probability of area occupancy by area during close contact between remote students (students in different regions). The colour bar shows the ln values; (**c**) Probability distribution by distance between work cubicles of two students (distance is calculated as number of functional areas between cubicles of the two students, as illustrated in Figure 3a. For example, distance = 1 for adjacent or back-to-back office cubicles, and distance = 5 between *cubicles* 2-2 and 3-2 (see Figures 1b and 3a)); (**d**) Cumulative probability distribution by frequency of close contact (episodes/hour); (**e**) Cumulative probability distribution by total episodes of close contact per day between each pair of participants (episodes/day); (**f**) Cumulative probability distribution by ratio of close contact time to total indoor time (%); (**g**) Cumulative probability distribution by number of contacted students per day; and (**h**) Distribution of number of students who stayed in the room and had close contact during *day 1* and *day 2* (black and blue points are total number of indoor students and total number of students in close contact, respectively).

From Figure 7h, the times of day with the most students in the office were between 9:30 and 11:30 and between 13:00 and 17:30. The peak frequency of close contact was between 11:00 and 12:30 and after 16:00.

Figure 8 shows the interpersonal distance by posture and gender. The average interpersonal distance during close contact was 0.81 m. The average interpersonal distances between sitting-sitting, standing-standing, and standing-sitting students were 0.74 m, 0.93 m, and 0.88 m, respectively. There were three peaks of interpersonal distance during close contact between two students who were sitting. As shown in Figure 8a, the first peak (0.1–0.3 m) was caused by pairs of participants with a very close relationship (e.g., boy-/girlfriend), the second peak (0.6–0.7 m) was caused by pairs of students who sat back-to-back, and the third peak (1.1–1.2 m) corresponded to the distance between two adjacent students. The probability distributions of interpersonal distance for sitting-standing students and standing-standing students accorded with log-normal distributions, and the most frequent interpersonal distances were 0.5 and 0.7 m, respectively. As 60% of close contact was between two sitting students, the overall probability distribution of interpersonal distance (black line) was similar to that of two sitting students.

From Figure 8b, 21.4%, 22.8%, 38.1%, and 17.7% of close contacts were between two male students (M-M), two female students (F-F), a male and a female student (non-couple) (M-F_NC), and couples (M-F_C). The contact rates (ratios of actual relationships with close contact to total possible relationships) for M-M, M-F, and F-F were 15.7%, 25.9%, and 10.3%, respectively. The average episodes of close contact per day between each pair of M-M, M-F_NC, M-F_C, and F-F who had contact with each other were 6.9, 8.2, 70.5, and 12.1, respectively. The average durations per close contact between each pair of M-M, M-F_NC, M-F_C, and F-F were 68.3, 48.7, 53.6, and 58.5 s, respectively. The average interpersonal distances during close contact between these four groups were 0.88 m, 0.70 m, 0.96 m, and 0.71 m, respectively. There was no interpersonal distance shorter than 0.2 m during close contact between two male students. Two female students preferred close contact at a short distance (0.1–0.4 m). Students of different genders (non-couple) had two peaks of interpersonal distance, which were related to their seating position. Couples had a normal distribution of interpersonal distance, and preferred distances between 0.4 and 0.6 m.

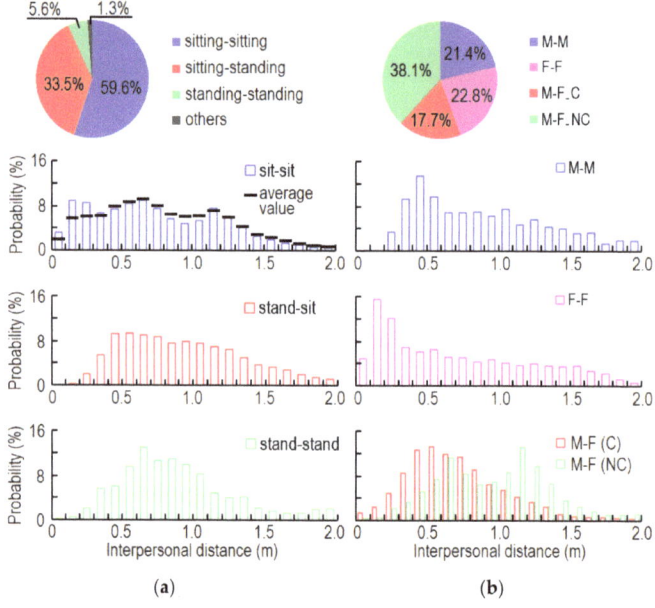

Figure 8. Probability distribution of interpersonal distance by: (**a**) Posture; (**b**) Gender.

There were three major posture patterns during close contacts in the office: sitting-sitting (both students sitting), standing-standing (both students standing), and sitting-standing (one student sitting, the other standing). The head and body motions of students and relative face orientation angles between students under different patterns of posture during close contact are shown in Figure 9. When two students were both standing or sitting, they preferred to look slightly downward. The average pitch angles of the head under sitting-sitting and standing-standing were 14.7° and 20.1°, respectively (Figure 9a,b). The average pitch angles of the body under these two conditions were 24.3° and 17.8°, respectively. However, under the sitting-standing condition (Figure 9c), the eye direction of the standing student was much lower than that of the sitting student.

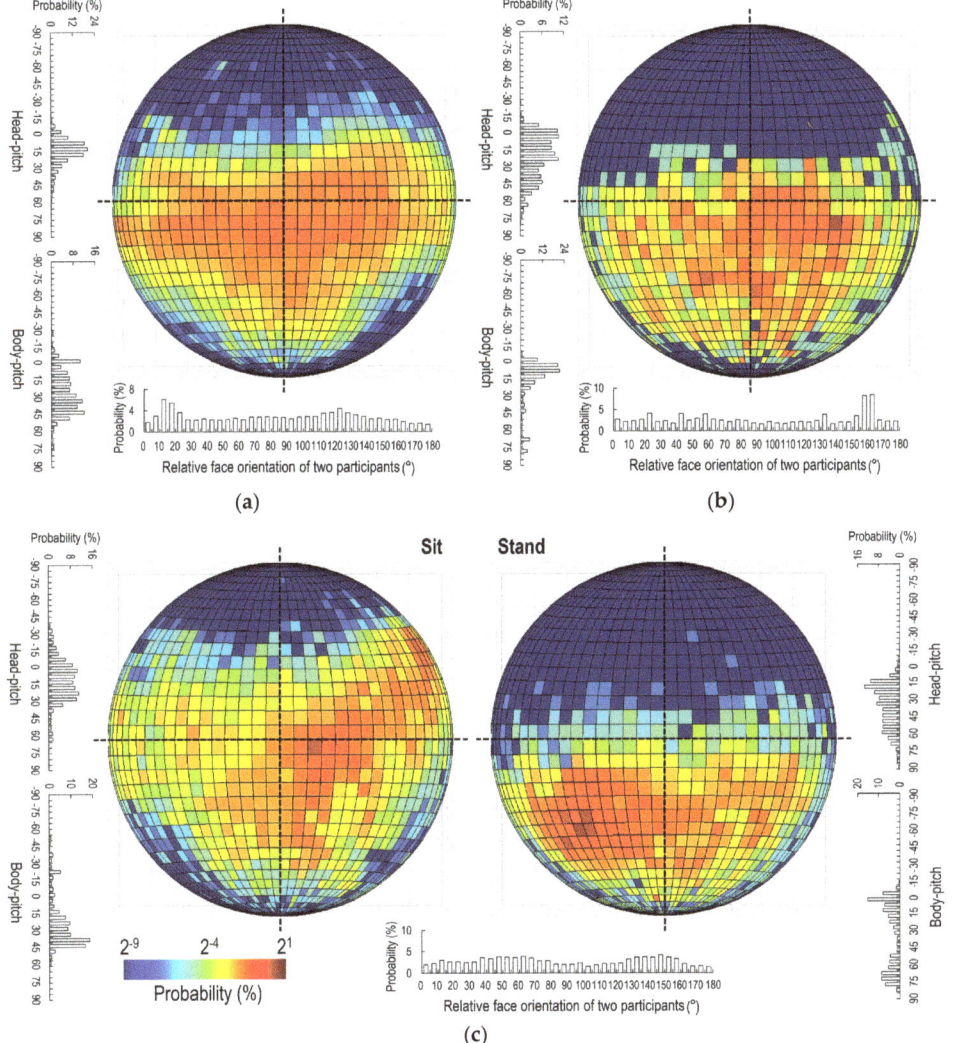

Figure 9. Head and body motions during close contact by posture of the two students: (**a**) Sitting-sitting; (**b**) Standing-standing; (**c**) Sitting-standing. (The circle shows the face orientation of the student; see Figure 4a).

The average pitch angles of the head of the sitting and the standing students in a sitting-standing pattern were 11.3° and 34.0°, respectively, and the average pitch angles of the body were 22.2° and 33.9°, respectively. The relatively low probability of looking downward for the sitting student implies that the standing student was usually located at the side of the sitting student rather than face-to-face. Standing students had a very high probability of facing downward.

Two sitting students had a high probability of only a slight relative angle of face orientation (5° to 25°) during close contact, which means that they usually faced in similar directions. Two standing students preferred face-to-face close contact with a relative face orientation angle between 150° and 170°. There was no obvious preference regarding relative face orientation angle under the sitting-standing pattern.

4. Discussion

4.1. Automatically Collected Indoor Human Behavior

In this study, we provided the first comprehensive dataset combining the indoor position, head and body motions, and posture of students at the same time which are helpful for infection risk assessment via close contact route. Indoor human behavior is strongly dependent on the type of indoor environment. In a hospital ward, patients usually lie in their beds, while health care workers walk between rooms and beds [32]. In an aircraft cabin or a cruise ship, passengers usually sit in their seats, while crew members walk through the aisle to provide service and food [33–35]. Both passengers in an aircraft cabin or a cruise ship and students in an office spend most of their time in their own seats or in aisles. Children in nurseries have been found to spend more time standing than sitting during indoor free-play time [36]. In a primary school, pupils have been found to spend 2.1 times more time sitting than standing during school hours [37]. However, in this study of a graduate student office, the students spent 94.6% of their time sitting. Therefore, people may tend to prefer sitting with increasing age, although the type of environment is also highly influential.

Close contact is an important activity in daily life, and also plays a critical role in infectious disease transmission. The duration of close contacts directly determines the exposure to viruses. Many researchers have reported the distribution of the duration of close contact (Figure 10) in different types of indoor environment. However, RFIDs or wireless sensors can only detect close contacts at intervals of 20 s [24,31,38–41], an insufficient temporal resolution for close contacts, which have a median duration of only 17 s. Although video observations can reach a temporal resolution of 1 s [11], the subjectivity of video analysts and the huge workload are two major shortcomings. As summarised in Figure 10, all types of indoor environment show similar values of the cumulative probability distribution (CDF) of the duration of close contacts. Brief close contacts (<20 s) are dominant, and prolonged close contacts (>300 s) are rare. Conferences and museums have a higher rate of long close contacts, while in hospitals and congress buildings shorter close contacts are more common. In a video observation study of a graduate student office, the average and median duration of close contact were 53.8 s and 17 s [11], respectively. Our study, meanwhile, found the average and median duration to be 54.5 s and 15 s, respectively.

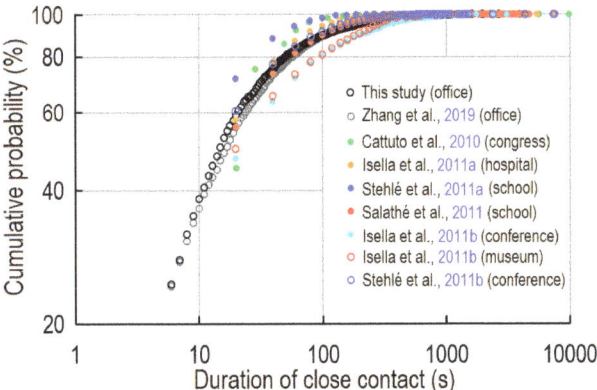

Figure 10. Cumulative probability distribution (CDF) of duration per close contact.

4.2. Close Contact Behavior

We collected and analyzed three types of data during close contact: indoor position, head and body motion/movement, and posture. These three factors are important to infectious disease transmission. Indoor position can help calculating the interpersonal distance of people during close contact. The infection risk decreases sharply with the increase of the interpersonal distance [12,20,42,43]. Posture, and head and body movement influence the body plume during close contact. For example, short-range exposure can be affected strongly by body plumes [44]. Frequent movement of the head and body during conversation can change not only the orientations of the exhaled/inhaled airflows, but also the patterns of body convective flows and the thermal plume. The exhaled airflows of two people also interact with and affect each other [12]. Various gestures involving small movements of the hands, palms, legs, eyebrows and other small-scale facial features may not significantly affect the body plume or exhaled flows [45,46]. Posture also important in droplet deposition. For example, more droplets may deposit on thighs of a sitting person if he/she talks with an infected. People have high probability to touch their thighs and legs with the frequency of more than 30 times per hour [19]. It may lead to a high infection risk because people also have high touch frequency on mucous membranes [47]. Relative face orientation is a critical factor for exposure during close contact, and it could be calculated by body and head motion. Previous studies found that the exposure during face-to-face close contact is the most, followed by face-to-side pattern, while face-to-back pattern had the lowest exposure [21,22].

As no such data on indoor human behavior in an office had previously been published, we mainly compared the sensor-collected data from this study with those of our previous experiment based on video observation [11] (Table 2). As head and body motions cannot easily be recorded using observation methods, the accuracy is difficult to guarantee. This may be the cause of the disagreements between the results in Table 2. In addition, in our previous experiment, all participants were students whose cubicles were in the studied office. In this study, however, some students were from the next room and some were invited into the office under study by students who worked there. Therefore, the various relationship networks may have caused the difference in the characteristics of close contact and of indoor human behaviors during close contact.

Table 2. Comparison of indoor human behaviors during close contact in a graduate student office between the previous observation study and the present sensor-based study.

Parameter.	Description	OB [1]	SB [2]	Parameter	Description	OB [1]	SB [2]
Individual posture	Sitting	59.5%	76.3%	Average ID [3]		0.67 m	0.81 m
	Standing	40.4%	22.9%	ID by gender	M-M	0.66 m	0.88 m
	Squatting	0.1%	0.8%		F-F	0.55 m	0.70 m
Posture pattern of two students	Sit-sit	34.3%	59.6%		M-F (NC)	0.79 m	0.96 m
	Sit-stand	46.2%	33.5%		M-F (C)	0.58 m	0.71 m
	Stand-stand	18.3%	5.6%	ID by posture	Sit-sit	0.59 m	0.74 m
	Others	1.2%	1.3%		Sit-stand	0.72 m	0.88 m
Number of students per close contact	2	87.5%	90.1%		Stand-stand	0.70 m	0.93 m
	3	11.1%	7.8%	Head/body motion	Head (yaw)	0.9°	2.3°
	4	1.2%	1.5%		Head (pitch)	10.3°	17.9°
	5	0.1%	0.6%		Body (pitch)	10.6°	25.3°
	≥6	<0.1%	<0.1%		Body (bend)	0.1°	3.7°

[1] Observation study: all data obtained through observation of video tapes by video analysts.11 [2] Sensor-based study (this study): all data obtained by sensor detection. [3] ID: interpersonal distance.

Our previous experiment showed that students spent 9.9% of their time in close contact interactions, while in this study that percentage was 9.7% ± 8.8%. The probability distributions of the students' posture during close contact differed between the two experiments, although sitting was always the most common posture, followed by standing. Almost none of the students had close contact when squatting. Sitting-sitting and sitting-standing were the most common posture patterns during close contact. In this study, the sitting-sitting pattern was much more dominant than in the previous experiment because all students chose their office cubicles before the experiment. Students with the closest relationships sat next to each other, and could chat without standing up or walking. During both experiments, one-on-one close contact accounted for almost 90% of all close contacts. The number of participants per close contacts depends on the type of indoor environment. For example, more people will participate in a close contact in a group discussion, while one-on-one close contact is very highly probable in a doctor's consulting room.

Preferred interpersonal distances differ by culture, ethnicity, relationship, personal habits, age, gender, and ambient environment [48]. Closer interpersonal distance means higher virus inhalation which increases infection risk via close contact route [42]. The average personal distances for acquaintances and intimately close persons in China are 83.6 and 57.6 cm, respectively [49]. However, there is no clear definition of interpersonal distance. Our previous study defined the interpersonal distance as that between two mouths, while this study defined it as the distance between two sensors worn on the top of the head. The previous study showed the average interpersonal distance in the office to be 0.67 m. In this study, the average interpersonal distance (0.81 m) was larger because of the different definitions of this parameter. Both experiments found the same effect of gender on interpersonal distance: two female students adopted the shortest distance while students of different genders (non-couples) were farthest apart. As an office is a public area, intimate couples do not interact at such close distance as they would otherwise. Posture also influences the interpersonal distance. Both experiments showed that two sitting students had the shortest interpersonal distance. In this study, more than 50% of close contacts were between adjacent or back-to-back students, and the probability distribution of interpersonal distance was strongly influenced by their cubicle positions. A compact indoor design would lead to shorter interpersonal distance during close contact.

The circulation of people around the office strongly influenced the probability of close contacts. Students at long distances apart had low probability of contact with each other. Therefore, a linear office cubicle design would lead to a lower close contact frequency compared with a matrix design because of longer average distance. People are generally disinclined to make close contact with someone a long distance away if there is no critical information to communicate. In this study, most close contacts were between students sitting in the same region because students with good relationships had chosen to sit together. Most students in this office were acquaintances, and had high probability of a brief close contact when encountering each other. Therefore, the students near the aisles, especially those near the door, had a high close-contact frequency with remote students (Figure 7b) as a result of office circulation. There was no close contact between 88% of the possible pairs of students (connection rate = 12%). In general, this value is strongly related to the level of intimacy between people indoors. For example, the connection rate tends to be very high in a home, but low in public environments such as conference rooms and aircraft cabins. This may explain why homes have a higher infection risk than other environments during an infectious outbreak [29].

This sensor-based study recorded higher pitch values of the head and body, which showed that students preferred to lower their head and lean their body forward. When sitting, they were usually looking at a computer monitor (mostly laptop computers) or reading a book from a desk, and therefore both the torso and head leaned forward. Over the long term, such a sitting posture may lead to a high prevalence of kyphosis among students [50]. Research has also showed that tilting the head forward by 15° places about 27 pounds of force on the neck [51]. This increases to 40 pounds at 30°, 49 pounds at 45°, and 60 pounds at 60° [51]. The damage caused by untreated 'text neck' can be of similar severity to occupational overuse syndrome or repetitive stress/strain injury. The office management team could be encouraged to educate their workers and provide ergonomic office equipment such as laptop stands to promote proper posture.

In simulations of infectious disease transmission via the close contact route, face to face is the most common orientation assumed, and all heads are assumed to be at the same height [12,20]. However, in our analysis, the students spent relatively little of their close contact time in a face-to-face position. Staring at the same screen, reading the same paper, or chatting without making eye contact were also common. Before this study, no data had been published on the percentage of time spent speaking during close contact. We found that students in close contact on average spent 68.6% of their time speaking. Studies have shown that talking for 5 min can generate the same number of droplet nuclei as a cough, i.e., some 3000 droplet nuclei [10], and speaking usually involves prolonged exhalation [52]. Our data may provide a reference for the simulation of infectious disease transmission via speaking during close contact. Moreover, combined with indoor surface touching behaviors [19], a comprehensive simulation of infection spread in an office considering the long-range airborne, fomite, and close contact routes could be performed [29]. The results would provide support for infection risk analysis on a large scale such as a city [5,53].

4.3. Limitations

This study has several limitations. The presence of the cameras might have had a psychological impact on the students' behaviors. The experimental hats and shirts showed slight relative movement when the participants moved their heads and bodies. Although we discarded some data with very large fluctuations, some error remained (resolution: 5°). Still, this error was much smaller than that of observation methods. Another limitation is that the interpersonal distance was defined as the distance between two sensors installed on the top of the experimental hats rather than between two mouths or noses. The interpersonal distances obtained in this study were longer than those between two mouths/noses, which are normally used to simulate close contact between two persons. Our experiment collected more than 1440,000 s of indoor data and more than 139,000 s of close contact data over 2 days. This data volume is large, but still insufficient to represent all indoor human behaviors in graduate student offices. Moreover, the close contact behaviors presents the characteristics in the office with around 25 students. Building type and total indoor population will influence the human behaviors.

5. Conclusions

Students spent long time on close contact (9.7%) in the office, which may explain the importance of the close contact route for many respiratory infections. The probability of close contact decreased exponentially with the increasing distance between two students' cubicles. Therefore, students who sit closer to the infected student, have much higher infection risk via close contact route than students who sit further. Comparing with pairs of sitting students, pairs of standing students had lower infection risk via close contact route because they did not prefer a face-to-face talk. The fact that standing students much preferred lower their head and body than sitting students may lead to a shorter distance of exhalation jet than we thought.

Author Contributions: Conceptualization, N.Z., Y.L. and P.W.; methodology, N.Z., B.S. AND P.W.; software, B.S.; formal analysis, N.Z. and P.-T.C.; investigation, N.Z., P.-T.C., T.M., B.S. and P.W.; resources, N.Z.; data curation, N.Z. and Y.L.; writing—original draft preparation, N.Z.; writing—review and editing, N.Z., Y.L., P.-T.C., T.M., B.S. and P.W.; visualization, B.S. and P.-T.C.; supervision, Y.L.; project administration, Y.L.; funding acquisition, Y.L. All authors have read and agreed to the published version of the manuscript.

Funding: This research was funded by a General Research Fund provided by the Research Grants Council of Hong Kong, grant number 17202719; a Collaborative Research Fund provided by the Research Grants Council of Hong Kong, grant number C7025-16G; an HKU ZIRI seed fund, grant number 04004.

Conflicts of Interest: The authors declare no conflict of interest.

References

1. Li, D.; Menassa, C.C.; Kamat, V.R. Non-intrusive interpretation of human thermal comfort through analysis of facial infrared thermography. *Energy Build.* **2018**, *176*, 246–261. [CrossRef]
2. Bornemann, B.; Sohre, A.; Burger, P. Future governance of individual energy consumption behavior change—A framework for reflexive designs. *Energy Res. Soc. Sci.* **2018**, *35*, 140–151. [CrossRef]
3. Bodin Danielsson, C.; Theorell, T. Office employees' perception of workspace contribution: A gender and office design perspective. *Environ. Behav.* **2019**, *51*, 995–1026. [CrossRef]
4. Waits, A.; Emelyanova, A.; Oksanen, A.; Abass, K.; Rautio, A. Human infectious diseases and the changing climate in the Arctic. *Environ. Int.* **2018**, *121*, 703–713. [CrossRef] [PubMed]
5. Zhang, N.; Huang, H.; Su, B.; Ma, X.; Li, Y. A human behavior integrated hierarchical model of airborne disease transmission in a large city. *Build. Environ.* **2018**, *127*, 211–220. [CrossRef]
6. Turgeon, N.; Hamelin, M.È.; Verreault, D.; Lévesque, A.; Rhéaume, C.; Carbonneau, J.; Checkmahomed, L.; Girard, M.; Boivin, G.; Duchaine, C. Design and validation with influenza A virus of an aerosol transmission chamber for ferrets. *Int. J. Environ. Res. Public Health* **2019**, *16*, 609. [CrossRef]
7. Lee, K.M.; Jung, K. Factors influencing the response to infectious diseases: Focusing on the case of SARS and MERS in South Korea. *Int. J. Environ. Res. Public Health* **2019**, *16*, 1432. [CrossRef]
8. Weber, D.J.; Rutala, W.A.; Fischer, W.A.; Kanamori, H.; Sickbert-Bennett, E.E. Emerging infectious diseases: Focus on infection control issues for novel coronaviruses (Severe Acute Respiratory Syndrome-CoV and Middle East Respiratory Syndrome-CoV), hemorrhagic fever viruses (Lassa and Ebola), and highly pathogenic avian influenza viruses, A (H5N1) and A (H7N9). *Am. J. Infect. Control* **2016**, *44*, e91–e100.
9. Umar, A.A.; Sheshi, M.A.; Abubakar, A.A. Knowledge and practice of Ebola virus disease preventive measures among health workers in a tertiary hospital in Northern Nigeria. *Arch. Med. Surg.* **2018**, *3*, 1–5. [CrossRef]
10. Xie, X.; Li, Y.; Chwang, A.T.; Ho, P.L.; Seto, W.H. How far droplets can move in indoor environments—Revisiting the Wells evaporation-falling curve. *Indoor Air* **2007**, *17*, 211–225. [CrossRef]
11. Zhang, N.; Tang, J.W.; Li, Y. Human behavior during close contact in a graduate student office. *Indoor Air* **2019**, *29*, 577–590. [CrossRef] [PubMed]
12. Liu, L.; Li, Y.; Nielsen, P.V.; Jensen, R.L. Short-range airborne transmission of expiratory droplets between two people. *Indoor Air* **2017**, *27*, 452–462. [CrossRef] [PubMed]
13. Wei, J.; Li, Y. Enhanced spread of expiratory droplets by turbulence in a cough jet. *Build. Environ.* **2015**, *93*, 86–96. [CrossRef]

14. Duguid, J.P. The size and the duration of air-carriage of respiratory droplets and droplet-nuclei. *Epidemiol. Infect.* **1946**, *44*, 471–479. [CrossRef]
15. Loudon, R.G.; Roberts, R.M. Relation between the airborne diameters of respiratory droplets and the diameter of the stains left after recovery. *Nature* **1967**, *213*, 95–96. [CrossRef]
16. Chao, C.Y.H.; Wan, M.P.; Morawska, L.; Johnson, G.R.; Ristovski, Z.D.; Hargreaves, M.; Mengersen, K.; Corbett, S.; Li, Y.; Xie, X.; et al. Characterization of expiration air jets and droplet size distributions immediately at the mouth opening. *J. Aerosol Sci.* **2009**, *40*, 122–133. [CrossRef]
17. Fabian, P.; McDevitt, J.J.; DeHaan, W.H.; Fang, R.O.P.; Cowling, B.J.; Chan, K.H. Influenza virus in human exhaled breath: An observational study. *PLoS ONE* **2008**, *3*, e2691. [CrossRef]
18. Xie, X.; Li, Y.; Sun, H.; Liu, L. Exhaled droplets due to talking and coughing. *J. R. Soc. Interface* **2009**, *6*, S703. [CrossRef]
19. Zhang, N.; Li, Y.; Huang, H. Surface touch and its network growth in a graduate student office. *Indoor Air* **2018**, *28*, 963–972. [CrossRef]
20. Ai, Z.T.; Melikov, A.K. Airborne spread of expiratory droplet nuclei between the occupants of indoor environments: A review. *Indoor Air* **2018**, *28*, 500–524. [CrossRef]
21. Pantelic, J.; Tham, K.W.; Licina, D. Effectiveness of a personalized ventilation system in reducing personal exposure against directly released simulated cough droplets. *Indoor Air* **2015**, *25*, 683–693. [CrossRef] [PubMed]
22. Olmedo, I.; Nielsen, P.V.; Ruiz de Adana, M.; Jensen, R.L.; Grzelecki, P. Distribution of exhaled contaminants and personal exposure in a room using three different air distribution strategies. *Indoor Air* **2012**, *22*, 64–76. [CrossRef] [PubMed]
23. Cattuto, C.; Van den Broeck, W.; Barrat, A.; Colizza, V.; Pinton, J.F.; Vespignani, A. Dynamics of person-to-person interactions from distributed RFID sensor networks. *PLoS ONE* **2010**, *5*, e11596. [CrossRef] [PubMed]
24. Vanhems, P.; Barrat, A.; Cattuto, C.; Pinton, J.F.; Khanafer, N.; Régis, C.; Kim, B.-A.; Comte, B.; Voirin, N. Estimating potential infection transmission routes in hospital wards using wearable proximity sensors. *PLoS ONE* **2013**, *8*, e73970. [CrossRef]
25. Di Blasio, S.; Shtrepi, L.; Puglisi, G.E.; Astolfi, A. A cross-sectional survey on the impact of irrelevant speech noise on annoyance, mental health and well-being, performance and occupants' behavior in shared and open-plan offices. *Int. J. Environ. Res. Public Health* **2019**, *16*, 280. [CrossRef]
26. Davis, M.C.; Leach, D.J.; Clegg, C.W. Breaking out of open-plan: Extending social interference theory through an evaluation of contemporary offices. *Environ. Behav.* **2019**. [CrossRef]
27. Martinez-Millana, A.; Lizondo, A.; Gatta, R.; Vera, S.; Salcedo, V.T.; Fernandez-Llatas, C. Process mining dashboard in operating rooms: Analysis of staff expectations with analytic hierarchy process. *Int. J. Environ. Res. Public Health* **2019**, *16*, 199. [CrossRef]
28. Alarifi, A.; Al-Salman, A.; Alsaleh, M.; Alnafessah, A.; Al-Hadhrami, S.; Al-Ammar, M.A.; Al-Khalifa, H. Ultra wideband indoor positioning technologies: Analysis and recent advances. *Sensors* **2016**, *16*, 707. [CrossRef]
29. Zhang, N.; Li, Y. Transmission of influenza A in a student office based on realistic person-to-person contact and surface touch behavior. *Int. J. Environ. Res. Public Health* **2018**, *15*, 1699. [CrossRef]
30. Hornbeck, T.; Naylor, D.; Segre, A.M.; Thomas, G.; Herman, T.; Polgreen, P.M. Using sensor networks to study the effect of peripatetic healthcare workers on the spread of hospital-associated infections. *J. Infect. Dis.* **2012**, *206*, 1549–1557. [CrossRef]
31. Isella, L.; Romano, M.; Barrat, A.; Cattuto, C.; Colizza, V.; Van den Broeck, W.; Gesualdo, F.; Pandolfi, E.; Ravà, L.; Rizzo, C.; et al. Close encounters in a pediatric ward: Measuring face-to-face proximity and mixing patterns with wearable sensors. *PLoS ONE* **2011**, *6*, e17144. [CrossRef] [PubMed]
32. Hang, J.; Li, Y.; Jin, R. The influence of human walking on the flow and airborne transmission in a six-bed isolation room: Tracer gas simulation. *Build. Environ.* **2014**, *77*, 119–134. [CrossRef]
33. Lei, H.; Li, Y.; Xiao, S.; Lin, C.H.; Norris, S.L.; Wei, D.; Hu, Z.; Ji, S.; Norris, S.L. Routes of transmission of influenza A H1N1, SARS CoV, and norovirus in air cabin: Comparative analyzes. *Indoor Air* **2018**, *28*, 394–403. [CrossRef] [PubMed]
34. Xiao, S.; Li, Y.; Lei, H.; Lin, C.H.; Norris, S.L.; Yang, X.; Zhao, P. Characterizing dynamic transmission of contaminants on a surface touch network. *Build. Environ.* **2018**, *129*, 107–116. [CrossRef]

35. Zhang, N.; Miao, R.; Huang, H.; Chan, E.Y.Y. Contact infection of infectious disease onboard a cruise ship. *Sci. Rep.* **2016**, *6*, 38790. [CrossRef]
36. Fees, B.S.; Fischer, E.; Haar, S.; Crowe, L.K. Toddler activity intensity during indoor free-play: Stand and watch. *J. Nutr. Educ. Behav.* **2015**, *47*, 170–175. [CrossRef]
37. Aminian, S.; Hinckson, E.A.; Stewart, T. Modifying the classroom environment to increase standing and reduce sitting. *Build. Res. Informat.* **2015**, *43*, 631–645. [CrossRef]
38. Isella, L.; Stehlé, J.; Barrat, A.; Cattuto, C.; Pinton, J.F.; Van den Broeck, W. What's in a crowd? Analysis of face-to-face behavioral networks. *J. Theor. Biol.* **2011**, *271*, 166–180. [CrossRef]
39. Salathé, M.; Kazandjieva, M.; Lee, J.W.; Levis, P.; Feldman, M.W.; Jones, J.H. A high-resolution human contact network for infectious disease transmission. *Proc. Natl. Acad. Sci. USA* **2010**, *107*, 22020–22025. [CrossRef]
40. Stehlé, J.; Voirin, N.; Barrat, A.; Cattuto, C.; Isella, L.; Pinton, J.F.; Quaggiotto, M.; Broeck, W.V.D.; Regis, C.; Lina, B.; et al. High-resolution measurements of face-to-face contact patterns in a primary school. *PLoS ONE* **2011**, *6*, e23176. [CrossRef]
41. Stehlé, J.; Voirin, N.; Barrat, A.; Cattuto, C.; Colizza, V.; Isella, L.; Régis, C.; Pinton, J.-F.; Khanafer, N.; Broeck, W.V.D.; et al. Simulation of an SEIR infectious disease model on the dynamic contact network of conference attendees. *BMC Med.* **2011**, *9*, 87. [CrossRef] [PubMed]
42. Villafruela, J.M.; Olmedo, I.; San José, J.F. Influence of human breathing modes on airborne cross infection risk. *Build. Environ.* **2016**, *106*, 340–351. [CrossRef]
43. Olmedo, I.; Nielsen, P.V.; Ruiz de Adana, M.; Jensen, R.L. The risk of airborne cross-infection in a room with vertical low-velocity ventilation. *Indoor Air* **2013**, *23*, 62–73. [CrossRef] [PubMed]
44. Murakami, S.; Kato, S.; Zeng, J. Combined simulation of airflow, radiation and moisture transport for heat release from a human body. *Build. Environ.* **2000**, *35*, 489–500. [CrossRef]
45. Pease, A. *Body Language: How to Read others' Thoughts by Their Gestures*; Sheldon Press: London, UK, 1988.
46. Rim, D.; Novoselac, A. Transport of particulate and gaseous pollutants in the vicinity of a human body. *Build. Environ.* **2009**, *44*, 1840–1849. [CrossRef]
47. Nicas, M.; Best, D. A study quantifying the hand-to-face contact rate and its potential application to predicting respiratory tract infection. *J. Occup. Environ. Hyg.* **2008**, *5*, 347–352. [CrossRef]
48. Heshka, S.; Nelson, Y. Interpersonal speaking distance as a function of age, sex, and relationship. *Sociometry* **1972**, *35*, 491–498. [CrossRef]
49. Sorokowska, A.; Sorokowski, P.; Hilpert, P.; Cantarero, K.; Frackowiak, T.; Ahmadi, K. Preferred interpersonal distances: A global comparison. *J. Cross Cult. Psychol.* **2017**, *48*, 577–592. [CrossRef]
50. Mirbagheri, S.S.; Rahmani-Rasa, A.; Farmani, F.; Amini, P.; Nikoo, M.R. Evaluating kyphosis and lordosis in students by using a flexible ruler and their relationship with severity and frequency of thoracic and lumbar pain. *Asian Spine J.* **2015**, *9*, 416. [CrossRef]
51. Neupane, S.; Ali, U.; Mathew, A. Text neck syndrome-systematic review. *Imp. J. Interdiscip. Res.* **2017**, *3*, 141–148.
52. McFarland, D.H. Respiratory markers of conversational interaction. *J. Speech Lang. Hear. Res.* **2001**, *44*, 128–143. [CrossRef]
53. Zhang, N.; Huang, H.; Duarte, M.; Zhang, J. Dynamic population flow based risk analysis of infectious disease propagation in a metropolis. *Environ. Int.* **2016**, *94*, 369–379. [CrossRef] [PubMed]

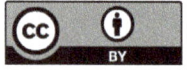

© 2020 by the authors. Licensee MDPI, Basel, Switzerland. This article is an open access article distributed under the terms and conditions of the Creative Commons Attribution (CC BY) license (http://creativecommons.org/licenses/by/4.0/).

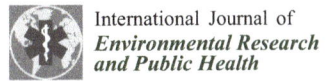

Article

A Salutogenic Approach to Disaster Recovery: The Case of the Lac-Mégantic Rail Disaster

Mélissa Généreux [1,2,*], Mathieu Roy [1,3], Tracey O'Sullivan [4] and Danielle Maltais [5]

1. Faculty of Medicine and Health Sciences, Université de Sherbrooke, Sherbrooke, QC J1H5N4, Canada
2. Eastern Townships Public Health Department, Sherbrooke, QC J1H1R3, Canada
3. Health Technology and Social Services Assessment Unit, Eastern Townships Integrated University Health and Social Services Centre, Sherbrooke, QC J1H 4C4, Canada; Mathieu.roy7@usherbrooke.ca
4. Interdisciplinary School of Health Sciences, Faculty of Health Sciences, University of Ottawa, Ottawa, ON K1N 6N5, Canada; tosulliv@uottawa.ca
5. Department of Human and Social Sciences, Université du Québec à Chicoutimi, Saguenay, QC G7H2B1, Canada; Danielle_Maltais@uqac.ca
* Correspondence: Melissa.genereux@usherbrooke.ca

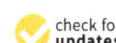

Received: 29 January 2020; Accepted: 20 February 2020; Published: 25 February 2020

Abstract: In July 2013, a train carrying crude oil derailed in Lac-Mégantic (Canada). This disaster provoked a major fire, 47 deaths, the destruction of 44 buildings, a massive evacuation, and an unparalleled oil spill. Since 2013, Public Health has undertaken several actions to address this challenging situation, using both quantitative and qualitative methods. Community-based surveys were conducted in Lac-Mégantic in 2014, 2015 and 2018. The first two surveys showed persistent and widespread health needs. Inspired by a salutogenic approach, Public Health has shifted its focus from health protection to health promotion. In 2016, a Day of Reflection was organized during which a map of community assets and an action plan for the community recovery were co-constructed with local stakeholders. The creation of an Outreach Team is an important outcome of this collective reflection. This team aims to enhance resilience and adaptive capacity. Several promising initiatives arose from the action plan—all of which greatly contributed to mobilize the community. Interestingly, the 2018 survey suggests that the situation is now evolving positively. This case study stresses the importance of recognizing community members as assets, rather than victims, and seeking a better balance between health protection and health promotion approaches.

Keywords: disaster; psychosocial impacts; community resilience

1. Motivation

1.1. The Lac-Mégantic Train Derailment Disaster

On 6 July 2013, in the middle of the night, a train carrying crude oil derailed in the heart of Lac-Mégantic (Quebec, QC, Canada). This small town, situated on a lakeshore in the Estrie region of the province, has a population of 6000 residents.

The train, with no engineer at the controls, spontaneously rolled downhill from its night stop location 11 kilometres away, toward the town of Lac-Mégantic. With a relatively constant downhill slope, the train's descent accelerated to almost 100 kph by the time the locomotives encountered a sharp curve in downtown Lac-Mégantic and most of the trailing cars derailed. As they derailed, 63 tank cars ruptured and escaping crude oil ignited, leading to a succession of powerful explosions and a major conflagration. The fire spread rapidly to nearby structures, destroying 44 buildings. The derailment, the explosions and the subsequent fire resulted in 47 deaths and necessitated mass evacuation of 2000 persons, equivalent to one-third of the town's population.

With the coupling of human suffering and environmental degradation, the Lac-Mégantic derailment caused serious psychosocial and economic consequences, including the relocation of many families forced to leave their homes, loss of many jobs, and closure of many local businesses for weeks before relocating elsewhere in town [1]. Given the impact of this technological disaster, the involvement of public health personnel and resources was critical throughout the emergency response operations. The Public Health Department (PHD) for the Estrie region responded immediately to provide direct services needed to protect the citizens of Lac-Mégantic and on-site responders from several health hazards. The priority at that time was to assess, communicate, and manage immediate risks to public health associated with exposure to chemical, physical and biological agents [1].

In the face of disasters, it is important to recognize that the operational domain of public health in affected communities extends beyond health protection and disease prevention to include promotion of health and well-being. It is with this in mind that Estrie PHD, in collaboration with researchers in the field of psychosocial recovery, conducted a population health survey entitled "Enquête de santé populationnelle estrienne" (ESPE) in 2014. Unknowingly, this was the first of a long series of promising initiatives to mobilize the local community in this post-disaster landscape.

1.2. The Salutogenic Approach

The approach and orientation of the Theory of Salutogenesis are now well established in health sciences and used in various health promotion settings and contexts [2]. Unlike traditional preventive approaches aimed at identifying risk factors, limitations or diseases, asset-based approaches are used to identify factors fostering well-being, resources, or abilities [3]. According to the scientific literature, a greater stock of health assets empowers individuals and communities and helps to improve health and well-being. This is true both directly (i.e., health assets are associated with better health outcomes [4]) and indirectly (i.e., health assets moderate the relationships between a disadvantaged social position and negative health outcomes [5,6]). Examining the role of salutogenic factors in disaster contexts, however, needs further exploration as the field of health emergency and disaster risk management places much more focus on hazards, risks factors, vulnerability, and short- and long-term adverse health outcomes.

1.3. Objectives

Through the case of the Lac-Mégantic train derailment tragedy, we aim to discuss how salutogenesis can be used as a relevant and complementary framework in disaster settings, and how it can be incorporated into post-disaster recovery strategies to promote resilience. More specifically, the objectives of this case study are to: (1) describe the salutogenic approach applied to the Lac-Mégantic train derailment, (2) present the long-term psychosocial outcomes of this disaster, and (3) discuss some benefits observed from applying a salutogenic approach in a post-disaster landscape.

2. Approach

2.1. Quantitative Approach in Addressing a Challenging Environment

Any collective trauma, including technological or natural disasters, is likely to lead to adverse health impacts among survivors and the wider community. Due to the experience of extensive stress and loss, people exposed to large-scale disasters like the Lac-Mégantic train derailment are subject to long-term adverse outcomes [1]. There is now a solid evidence base for the substantial effects of such a tragic event on psychological health in directly affected communities, which may persist over time in the absence of adequate support. Interestingly, disasters may also result in positive psychological outcomes in some exposed persons [7–12].

Among actions that can be performed by public health agencies to bring support to local communities following disasters, monitoring long-term psychosocial outcomes (both positive and negative ones) is certainly relevant. Monitoring helps tailor interventions aimed at supporting affected individuals and communities, by promoting their resilience and recovery processes. The Estrie PHD, in close collaboration with the "Université du Québec à Chicoutimi" (UQAC) and the "University of Sherbrooke", has therefore spent the first years following the event tracking the health needs and assets of those living in the Granit area using repeated cross-sectional community-based surveys.

In 2014, one year following the rail disaster in Lac-Mégantic, the PHD conducted a first health survey using a community-based random sample of 811 adults from the Granit area and additional 8000 adults residing elsewhere in the Estrie region. This representative sample responded to a telephone or web survey covering a variety of physical and psychological health outcomes. The second phase of the ESPE was carried out in the fall of 2015 and sought to better understand the local population's health and well-being, along with its possible link to the July 2013 railway disaster. In total, 1600 adults were recruited randomly in 2015 to take part in this large-scale telephone survey. These included 800 from the Granit area, and 800 from elsewhere in the Estrie region. In the fall of 2018, a third, similar, survey was conducted and is referred to as phase 3. Each of these three studies is composed of a separate sample of adults residing in the Granit area or elsewhere in Estrie; the original sample of participants was not monitored across time. While an additional study was conducted in 2016 by UQAC, a different sampling strategy was used; therefore, it is not used for comparison with the other surveys [13,14].

The adults who agreed to participate in these studies were asked to answer an anonymous questionnaire, which took approximately 30 min to complete. A number of questions were identical across all three surveys, allowing for the comparability of results over time (years 1 to 5 following the tragedy). Various psychosocial outcomes were examined, including adverse effects of disasters (e.g., psychological distress, depressive episodes, signs of post-traumatic stress, diagnosed anxiety or mood disorders, social worker or psychologist consultation, anxiolytic drug use, alcohol abuse), but also positive ones (e.g., resilience, positive mental health, sense of coherence, sense of community belonging, social support). The following outcomes, all self-reported, were examined in at least one of the three cross-sectional surveys. These outcomes have been described more thoroughly elsewhere [8,15].

Deficit-based outcomes: Perception of fair or poor general health, excessive drinking episodes (at least once a week), finding most of the days stressful, psychological distress in the past month, based on the 6 item Kessler Scale (K6, ≥ 7; [16]), signs of post-traumatic stress in the last week (specific to the train derailment) based on the 15 item Impact of Event Scale (score ≥ 26 [17,18]), diagnosed anxiety disorders, diagnosed mood disorders, social worker or psychologist consultation in the past year, and perception of insecurity in the neighbourhood.

Asset-based outcomes: Resilience in the past month, based on the 10 item Connor–Davidson resilience scale (score ≥ 30; [19]), positive mental health, in the past month, based on the 14 item Mental Health Continuum-Short Form questionnaire [20,21], sense of community belonging, sense of coherence, based on the short version (3 items) of the sense of coherence (score ≥ 5; [22]), social support, based on the Multidimensional Scale of Perceived Support (score ≥ 69; [23]).

2.2. Qualitative Approach in Addressing a Challenging Environment

The release of the ESPE 2015 data (i.e., in February 2016) stimulated the emergence of health promotion and advocacy interventions for the local population in Lac-Mégantic. Given the magnitude of the tragedy, it was necessary to take a step back to understand the situation in relation to the normal process of community recovery. It was in this context that in March 2016, the Estrie PHD intensified its work with community partners, first by organizing a day of collective reflection. The purpose of this initiative was to work together to gain understanding of the situation and reverse the cycle. During this day, no fewer than 50 key actors (decision makers, stakeholders, citizens and experts) gathered. The reflection day was divided into two parts: (1) conference and workshops on resilience and lessons learned from the past and (2) conference and workshops on levers for long-term recovery and priorities for the future.

A defining moment during the Day of Reflection occurred during an asset-mapping activity through which participants were invited to construct together an historical timeline that traces key milestones in recovery of their community and to recognize the progress made (Figure 1). More precisely, they were first divided in subgroups, where they had to highlight good moves, or successful interventions and initiatives implemented by local partners and citizens since the tragedy. Then, subgroups had to share their respective thoughts to the larger group in order to collectively construct the timeline. By doing so, the large group was able to identify a wide and diversified range of local assets, including physical, cultural, economic, social and spiritual ones, that all created positive effects on the community.

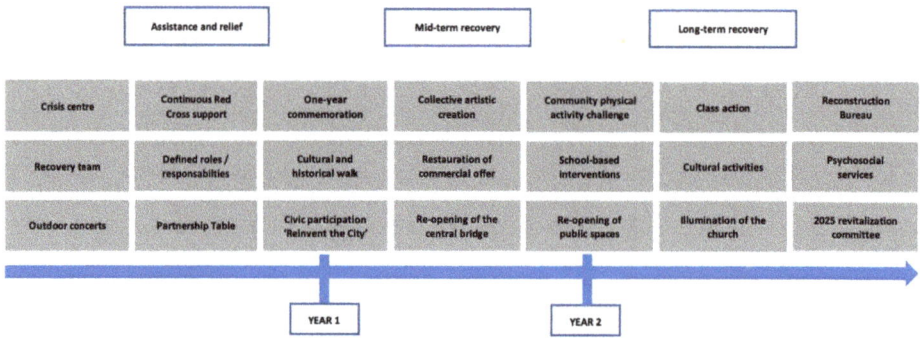

Figure 1. Historical timeline tracing key milestones in recovery of Lac-Mégantic community (March 2016).

Throughout the Day of Reflection, a common vision of the desired future emerged and priorities for action and research were identified, leading to the co-construction of what would become the "Plan for the Recovery and Development of a Healthy Community in Lac-Mégantic and the Granit area". This plan pursues the following objectives:

1. Maintain and adapt psychosocial services to the needs of individuals and the community (outreach services),
2. Stay connected with the community, and
3. Promote community involvement.

In the weeks following the elaboration of the plan (i.e., April 2016), PHD advocated for additional funding to support its implementation. In June 2016, the "Ministère de la Santé et des Services sociaux" and the Canadian Red Cross announced substantial investments that would serve as financial levers to implement the adopted action plan. The ESPE data was an important contribution supporting an informed decision, based on understanding of the long-term psychosocial impacts of the tragedy.

In sum, holding such a Day of Reflection, which brought together key players from the community, contributed to the development of a common vision of solutions and the transmission of a clear, coherent and positive message to decision-makers and the community.

> "Building a project together is really motivating. Especially since everyone feels involved: from citizens to elected officials. It was a very inspiring day!" —A participant of the collective reflection day.

This positive experience supports existing knowledge that beyond traditional surveys, qualitative methods are valuable for listening to, learning from, and engaging local partners and high-risk citizens. Through inclusive and empowering approaches, public health practitioners and researchers can better integrate members of the community as assets rather than victims and take into considerations their capacities in addition to their needs [24].

3. Results

3.1. Observations from the Community-Based Surveys (Quantitative Approach)

3.1.1. The First Years Following the Disaster

In 2014, some differences were observed in the prevalence of deficit-based and asset-based psychosocial outcomes as a function of residential location (Lac-Mégantic, elsewhere in the Granit area, or elsewhere in the Estrie region) (Table 1). Many of these "psychosocial gradients" were stronger in 2015 [15]. Anxiety disorders, for instance, were twice as high in Lac-Mégantic residents as in other residents of the Estrie region in 2015 (14.1% vs. 7.2%, $p = 0.003$). In the same vein, adults in Lac-Mégantic, as opposed to those living elsewhere in the Estrie region, were less likely to report a high level of resilience in 2015 (47.8% vs. 63.3%, $p < 0.0005$), while this was not the case the year before. Similar observations were made for optimal mental health.

Significant time trends from year one to year two post-disaster were also observed. While most psychosocial outcomes did not show any statistically significant improvement among adults, the use of psychosocial services decreased by half among adults residing in Lac-Mégantic between 2014 and 2015 [15].

Some deficit-based (e.g., post-traumatic stress) and asset-based outcomes (e.g., sense of coherence) were only examined as from 2015 (Table 2). Findings from the second wave revealed seven in ten adults in Lac-Mégantic showed moderate to severe signs of post-traumatic stress two years after the disaster. On another note, a strong sense of coherence was observed among 48.2% of adults residing in Lac-Mégantic, regardless of residential location, and this proportion was significantly lower than that observed elsewhere in the Estrie region (61.1%). These findings suggest that the stock of health assets can weaken with time among people directly impacted by a disaster, especially in the absence of adequate support and services [8].

Table 1. Deficit- and asset-based outcomes among a community-based sample of adults according to residential location, two years and five years post-disaster (e.g., Lac-Mégantic train derailment, 6 July 2013), Estrie region, 2014 and 2015.

	2014				2015			
	Lac-Mégantic	Granit (Elsewhere)	Estrie (Elsewhere)	p Value	Lac-Mégantic	Granit (Elsewhere)	Estrie (Elsewhere)	p Value
	n = 240	n = 571	n = 7926		n = 261	n = 539	n = 800	
Deficit-based outcomes								
Perception of fair/poor general health	13.0%	13.9%	12.9%	0.763	19.3%	9.7% (-)	9.6% (-)	<0.0005
Excessive drinking (≥1 episode/week)	10.5%	10.4%	10.2%	0.976	14.6%	13.3%	10.1%	0.087
Finding most of the days stressful	19.6%	21.2%	21.2%	0.862	24.9%	18.2%	22.2%	0.063
Psychological distress	28.9%	30.4%	23.8%	0.001	34.1%	23.2% (-)	22.1%	<0.0005
Anxiety disorder diagnosed by a physician	10.1%	7.0%	6.4%	0.080	14.1%	8.2%	7.2%	0.003
Mood disorder diagnosed by a physician	7.2%	5.5%	5.9%	0.621	9.4%	5.3%	6.6%	0.100
Social worker or psychologist consultation	26.9%	10.2%	10.3%	<0.0005	15.5% (-)	11.9%	11.7%	0.240
Perception of insecurity in the neighbourhood	8.2%	2.0%	2.5%	<0.0005	13.2%	2.8%	1.4%	<0.0005
Asset-based outcomes								
High level of resilience	55.9%	53.2%	56.0%	0.428	47.8%	55.8%	63.3% (+)	<0.0005
Optimal mental health	50.6%	47.0%	49.4%	0.504	44.5%	53.1% (+)	55.1% (+)	0.014
Strong sense of belonging to the community	80.5%	67.3%	55.9%	<0.0005	79.1%	78.2% (+)	67.0% (+)	<0.0005

3.1.2. Long-Term Trends in Psychosocial Outcomes Following the Disaster

Given the increased efforts to support recovery in Lac-Mégantic in recent years, has there been any progress in terms of psychosocial outcomes? With regards to all the data collected from our three surveys, major findings emerge. First, the adverse psychosocial impacts observed in the years following the Lac-Mégantic rail tragedy in 2013 seem to be receding. For example, after reaching a peak in 2015, the proportions of adults reporting an anxiety disorder diagnosed by a doctor stabilized in 2018 in Lac-Mégantic. On the other hand, these proportions increased significantly elsewhere in Estrie from 2014 to 2018. In other words, the gap that had developed between Lac-Mégantic and the rest of Estrie in the first two years after the tragedy is no longer, in many respects [25].

Second, there was still a very high prevalence of signs of post-traumatic stress in 2018 (71.9%). Despite a gradual adaptation of citizens to the losses and stressors experienced during and after the 2013 tragedy, the local community has been deeply affected by the traumatic event and its aftermath. These markers could persist for many years, despite an outward appearance of adaptive functioning of individuals and their community. Finally, protective factors are increasingly observed in Lac-Mégantic, particularly social support and sense of belonging to the community that were especially strong in 2018 [25]. These factors may act as powerful moderators of the adverse effects of primary and secondary stressors typically arising from large-scale disasters.

Table 2. Deficit- and asset-based outcomes among a community-based sample of adults according to residential location, two years and five years post-disaster (e.g., Lac-Mégantic train derailment, 6 July 2013), Estrie region, 2015 and 2018.

	2015				2018			
	Lac-Mégantic	Granit (Elsewhere)	Estrie (Elsewhere)	p Value	Lac-Mégantic	Granit (Elsewhere)	Estrie (Elsewhere)	p Value
	n = 261	n = 539	n = 800		n = 244	n = 564	n = 8022	
Deficit-based outcomes								
Perception of fair/poor general health	19.3%	9.7%	9.6%	<0.0005	11.3% (−)	12.3%	10.0%	0.196
Excessive drinking (≥1 episode/week)	14.6%	13.3%	10.1%	0.087	9.8%	9.3% (−)	7.6% (−)	0.177
Finding most of the days stressful	24.9%	18.2%	22.2%	0.063	23.8%	17.5%	20.3%	0.101
Psychological distress	34.1%	23.2%	22.1%	<0.0005	32.9%	26.5%	28.9% (+)	0.198
Moderate or severe post-traumatic stress	66.6%	35.1%	6.7%	<0.0005	71.9%	34.7%	N/A	<0.0005
Anxiety disorder diagnosed by a physician	14.1%	8.2%	7.2%	0.003	11.3%	8.4%	9.0%	0.351
Mood disorder diagnosed by a physician	9.4%	5.3%	6.6%	0.100	8.6%	5.5%	6.8%	0.252
Perception of insecurity in the neighbourhood	13.2%	2.8%	1.4%	<0.0005	3.2% (−)	1.5%	2.1%	0.238
Asset-based outcomes								
Strong sense of coherence	48.2%	47.9%	61.1%	<0.0005	46.6%	51.3%	54.8% (−)	0.039
Strong sense of belonging to the community	79.1%	78.2%	67.0%	<0.0005	81.8%	66.7% (−)	56.4% (−)	<0.0005
High level of social support	58.7%	67.9%	67.2%	0.033	67.6%	63.7%	67.3%	0.460

(+): Significant increase from 2015 to 2018. (−): Significant decrease from 2015 to 2018.

3.2. Observations from the Field (Qualitative Approach)

3.2.1. The Outreach Team

Following the day of reflection, in 2016, Estrie PHD created a permanent community Outreach Team in Lac-Mégantic. Located outside formal clinical settings (i.e., in the downtown area), this multidisciplinary team has focused on bringing psychosocial services closer to the population.

Four full-time professionals (two social workers, one outreach worker and two community organizers), and two part-time professionals (a kinesiologist and a nutritionist) comprise the team.

The following principles guided the entire Lac-Mégantic outreach initiative: global health, prevention, scientific rigour, a strengths-based approach, empowerment, inter-organizational and intersectoral collaboration, and inclusion. Citizen participation and community development were at the heart of this approach. A wide range of services are offered, ranging from daily interactions with citizens and local organizations (in the form of psychosocial support, response to service requests, rapid detection and response to emerging needs, collaboration with the organization of activities, etc.) to involvement in various projects emerging from the action plan [25].

3.2.2. Promising Initiatives to Mobilize the Local Community

The EnRiCH (Enhancing Resilience and Capacity for Health) Community Resilience Framework for High-Risk Populations [24] inspired the strategies developed within this community to promote community resilience, health and well-being [26,27]. Based on qualitative research conducted in five Canadian communities and a review of scientific literature, this framework provides an asset-based integrated upstream and downstream approach to disaster risk. With the development and use of adaptive capacities as a central element, it advocates three pillars and four areas of intervention, as described in Table 3, all in a cultural context and working with the complexity specific to disasters.

Table 3. EnRiCH Framework components.

Components	Description
Adaptation capacity	Flexibility in changing environments
Mainstay	
Empowerment	Power to activate forces
Collaboration	Relationship with a common vision
Innovation	Emerging new practices
Fields of intervention	
Awareness and information	Collective sharing and learning
Strengths-based management	Mapping and linking forces
Upstream leadership	Proactive resource investing
Social connectivity	People and group networking
Complexity	Dynamic, non-linear context
Culture	Local community context

Source [24].

In line with this reference framework, several promising initiatives have been implemented in recent years within the Lac-Mégantic community to activate community resilience, social cohesion and citizen participation in a post-disaster setting. Committed to keeping track of local innovations and sharing them in formats that are suitable for both experts and practitioners, a synthesis of some of these promising initiatives has been produced and updated on an annual basis by the Outreach Team since 2017 [28]. These initiatives (e.g., social animation, Photovoice, Greeters, walking club) all contributed significantly to empowering citizens and mobilizing the community of Lac-Mégantic and surrounding areas. These initiatives also appear to have had a positive impact on the mental health and well-being of the citizens of this community.

As is generally known, organizing community projects or collective events, increasing opportunities to become involved as citizens, as well as other elements that strengthen social capital, contribute to building resilience in a post-disaster context. The data collected in this regard from 800 adults in MRC du Granit in the framework of ESPE 2018 provides additional support for this knowledge (Figure 2 [25]).

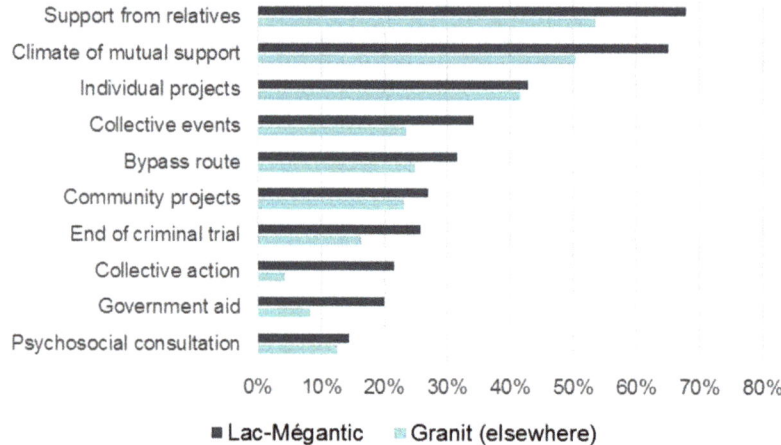

Figure 2. Elements that have significantly improved personal well-being over the past 12 months, "Enquête de santé populationnelle estrienne" (ESPE) 2018 (Granit area, 800 adults).

Photovoice

In 2017, in collaboration with the University of Ottawa EnRiCH research team and PHD of Estrie, the citizens of Lac-Mégantic took part in a Photovoice Initiative to map the assets of their community and develop a positive campaign and vision for the community looking forward to 2025. Over a 6 month, period the Lac-Megantic Photovoice Group met monthly to take photos of community assets and ideas to support their vision for the community. They met to discuss their photos with the group and share their ideas around issues that matter to them. The Lac-Mégantic Photovoice Group planned and hosted two exhibitions to facilitate knowledge mobilization and foster dialogue with decision-makers in Lac-Mégantic and Ottawa, including local and federal politicians. The Photovoice Initiative was highlighted as an inspirational example of community engagement in resilience initiatives in a report by the World Health Organization [29].

"We could express our sadness, our emotions openly because we were welcomed, without criticism. At first it was quite emotional, but over the meetings, this overflow was transformed into something lighter. It did me good. It made a big difference." —A participant of the Photovoice Initiative.

Ephemeral Place

The population is struggling to reclaim the downtown area of Lac-Mégantic, which was largely destroyed during the railway tragedy of 2013. Being under reconstruction, this new place, full of meaning and memories, is a constant reminder of loss. At the same time, there is a desire among citizens to get involved and to revitalize their living environment. In 2018, Ephemeral Place in the heart of the city was created in response to this desire; it is a space to promote social activities, networking and gatherings. This outdoor venue, under the responsibility of the Outreach Team, encourages the involvement of citizens of all ages and all horizons to foster social participation. Since these are temporary installations, it is an opportunity to experiment with concepts or ideas, while creating positive experiences. Through its free and varied leisure activities offered to citizens (5 to 7 with musicians, barbecues, outdoor film screening with popcorn, laughter yoga, intergenerational karaoke, etc.) and its unique approach, Ephemeral Place undeniably supports the long-term recovery of the Lac-Mégantic community [30].

Lessons Learned from a Citizen's Perspective

Inspired from a similar initiative following the bushfires which swept across Victoria, Australia, in 2009 [31], the idea behind this project was to collect statements from people who experienced the tragedy through one-on-one and/or group interviews and to identify overriding themes. Driven by the Outreach Team, this initiative provided a voice and brought together people who wished to contribute in this way, naming what could be changed or improved as a way of managing future disasters. Through their experience, citizens could make recommendations to the different bodies with which they interacted during the rail tragedy of July 2013 but also during the months and years that followed it. A semi-structured interview guide was developed, based on the CHAMPSS Functional Capabilities Framework [32]. The acronym stands for the following categories of functional capabilities: Communication, Awareness, Mobility/Transportation, Psychosocial, Self-Care and Daily Tasks, and Safety and Security. Approximately 12 interviews were conducted with citizens that would not have been reached otherwise, in order to make their voice heard. Data collected through these interviews was then pooled and analyzed to draw emerging themes that were sent to participants for a further validation. By being inclusive and recognizing the various experience lived, this project gave citizens a different opportunity to contribute following the tragedy. All this led to the writing of a document sharing post-disaster good practices, according to the perspectives of citizens with a unique field expertise in the matter. This document could then be submitted to the bodies concerned, upon approval from the group.

4. Recommendations

To our knowledge, this study is among the first to report how a salutogenic approach can contribute to improve health and well-being in the aftermath of a disaster. Only few studies used positive approaches in such type of setting. Leadbeater and colleagues [33] described how community leadership facilitated the social recovery process in the community of Strathewen (Australia), following the 2009 Victorian bushfires. Van Kessel [34], for its part, explained how promoting resilience mitigated impact on mental health after the 2010/11 Victorian floods and the 2009 Victorian bushfires. It is noteworthy that a recent systematic review highlighted a gap in the evidence relating to specific interventions targeting the resilience of adults who have experienced a disaster. Authors from this review call for more studies exploring the ability of interventions to build the intrinsic capacity of a community to adapt to disasters [35]. Despite the paucity of "real-world research" and knowledge on effective asset-based approaches in a post-disaster landscape, many theoretical or conceptual papers support the key role of community resilience in promoting population health in such settings [36–42].

In our case study, the objective was to discuss how a salutogenic approach was used to help the community of Lac-Mégantic in its recovery from a profound tragedy. Our various community-based surveys, combined with continuous on-the-ground presence of the PHD, have provided situational awareness about how the psychosocial impacts resulting from the 2013 rail tragedy decreased over time. Although this tragedy has left its mark, the local community is gradually adapting to its new reality. The asset-based approach used in recovery seems to have contributed to this "new reality" and emphasizes the importance of social capital to activate individual and community resilience in post-disaster contexts.

Many lessons have been identified from this unique and informative experience. First, long-term monitoring of psychosocial impacts through repeated community-based surveys is relevant, if not essential. Such surveys serve as powerful tools for health promotion initiatives and advocacy on behalf of the local population. Such survey support priority setting (e.g., targeting most at-risk populations) and promote risk-informed decision making.

Second, the voices of various groups, including those at heightened-risk, should be heard to take account of their specific needs and capacities. It is important to take time to listen and learn from citizens and consider all members of the community as assets rather than victims. This is critical to promote concrete social measures and psychosocial support tailored to their needs.

Third, regardless of the extent of the problems observed in the field, public health must seek a balance between a health protection (focused on hazards and risk factors) and health promotion (focused on protective factors, local strengths and resources).

Fourth, public health practitioners, academics and leaders must collaborate closely with local organizations and citizen groups. This is fundamental for a successful recovery. Putting citizens at the heart of all considerations helps to make sense out of a chaotic situation and contribute to the recovery of the community.

Fifth, public health organizations should capitalize on existing knowledge to develop and apply strategies and interventions in a post-disaster context. As part of their recovery operations, they should also share their own knowledge and experiences (e.g., lessons learned, tools and resources).

Finally, this rich experience in Granit over the last six years enabled us to identify three key success factors in supporting the psychosocial recovery and social reconstruction following a disaster:

1. Acknowledge the strengths of the community and promote citizen participation;
2. A strong political commitment is essential to support the community through preventive actions, upstream of problems;
3. A public health team must have the resources to be able to support the development and implementation of these actions.

5. Conclusions

This case study gives a concrete example of how asset-based approaches can be fruitful for enhancing community resilience and improving the health and well-being of a community in a post-disaster landscape. The positive evolution of the psychosocial situation in Lac-Mégantic, assessed both quantitatively and qualitatively, demonstrates the importance of developing a common understanding of risks and working together in finding solutions.

6. Future Work

Let us recall the importance of understanding, preventing and reducing psychosocial risks in the months and years following a disaster, whether natural, technological or intentional. In any case, concerted action to promote community resilience is required during, after, and ideally before the occurrence of such an event. As advocated by the United Nations, we must move from a disaster management logic to a risk management logic associated with these events, in partnership—rather than in silos—for the good of the community [43].

Disaster risk reduction, which is closely associated with climate change adaptation (due to the increasing number and intensity of recent disasters), is a pressing field of action for decision-makers, practitioners and researchers to promote health and well-being of communities and to increase their resilience for coping with multi-origin hazards.

While much is known about interventions targeting health needs following disasters (i.e., deficit-based models), less is known about what could foster resilience. Our case study was limited to a very simple design (e.g., post-disaster cross-sectional surveys and field observations). In order to generate stronger evidence-base intervention, future work in this research field should be based on high-quality studies (i.e., randomized or prospective cohort studies).

Author Contributions: Conceptualization, M.G.; methodology, M.G., M.R., T.O., and D.M.; formal analysis, M.G.; writing—original draft preparation, M.G., M.R., T.O., and D.M.; Writing—review and editing, M.G., M.R., T.O., and D.M. All authors have read and agreed to the published version of the manuscript.

Funding: This research received no external funding.

Acknowledgments: The authors wish to acknowledge the financial support of the "Ministère de la Santé et des Services sociaux" and the Canadian Red Cross for the implementation of the Outreach Team and the multiple initiatives to mobilize the local community in a post-disaster landscape.

Conflicts of Interest: The authors declare no conflict of interest.

References

1. Généreux, M.; Petit, G.; Maltais, D.; Roy, M.; Simard, R.; Boivin, S.; Shultz, J.M.; Pinsonneault, L. The public health response during and after the Lac-Mégantic train derailment tragedy: A case study. *Disaster Health* **2015**, *3–4*, 1–8. [CrossRef] [PubMed]
2. Mittelmark, M.; Sagy, S.; Eriksson, M.; Bauer, G.F.; Pelikan, J.M.; Lindstrom, B.; Espnes, G.A. *The Handbook of Salutogenesis*; Springer International: Geneve, Switzerland, 2017.
3. Van Bortel, T.; Wickramasinghe, N.D.; Morgan, A.; Martin, S. Health assets in a global context: A systematic review of the literature. *BMJ Open* **2019**, *9*, e023810. [CrossRef] [PubMed]
4. Lindstrom, B.; Eriksson, M. *The Hitchhiker's Guide to Salutogenesis: Salutogenic Pathways to Health Promotion*; Tuokinprint Oy: Helsinki, Finland, 2010.
5. Levasseur, M.; Roy, M.; Michallet, B.; St-Hilaire, F.; Maltais, D.; Généreux, M. Resilience, community belonging and social participation among community-dwelling older women and men: Results from the Eastern Townships Population Health Survey. *Arch. Phys. Med. Rehab.* **2017**, *98*, 2422–2432. [CrossRef] [PubMed]
6. Roy, M.; Levasseur, M.; Doré, I.; St-Hilaire, F.; Michallet, B.; Couturier, Y.; Maltais, D.; Lindström, B.; Généreux, M. Looking for capacities rather than vulnerabilities: The moderating role of health assets on the association between adverse social position and health outcomes. *Prev. Med. J.* **2018**, *110*, 93–99. [CrossRef] [PubMed]
7. Généreux, M.; Maltais, D. *Three Years after the Tragedy: How the Le Granit Community is Coping*; Bulletin Vision Santé Publique. Centre Intégré Universitaire de Santé et de Services Sociaux de l'Estrie—Centre Hospitalier Universitaire de Sherbrooke: Sherbrooke, QC, Canada, 2017.
8. Kretzmann, J.; Mcknight, J. *Building Communities from the Inside out: A Path towards Building and Mobilising a Community's Assets*; Institute for Policy Research: Evanston, IL, USA, 1993.
9. Galea, S. The long-term health consequences of disasters and mass traumas. *Can. Med. Assoc. J.* **2007**, *176*, 1293–1294. [CrossRef] [PubMed]
10. Goldman, E.S.; Galea, S. Mental Health Consequences of Disasters. *Annu. Rev. Public Health* **2014**, *35*, 169–183. [CrossRef]
11. Maltais, D.; Lachance, L.; Brassard, A.; Dubois, M. Soutien social perçu, stratégies d'adaptation et état de santé psychologique post-désastre de victimes d'un désastre. *Sci. Soc. St.* **2005**, *23*, 5–38.
12. Maltais, D.; Lansard, A.-L.; Roy, M.; Généreux, M.; Fortin, G.; Cherblanc, J.; Bergeron-Leclerc, C.; Pouliot, E.C. Post-Disaster Health Status of Train Derailment Victims with Post-Traumatic Growth. *Australas J. Disaster Trauma Stud.* in press.
13. Maltais, D.; Tremblay, A.J.; Labra, O.; Fortin, G.; Généreux, M.; Roy, M.; Lansard, A.L. Seniors' who experiences the Lac-Mégantic train derailment tragedy: What are the consequences on physical and mental health? *Gerontol. Geriatr. Med.* **2019**, *5*, 1–10. [CrossRef]
14. Maltais, D.; Lavoie-Trudeau, É.; Labra, O.; Généreux, M.; Roy, M.; Lansard, A.L.; Fortin, G. Medium-Term Effects of a Train Derailment on the Physical and Psychological Health of Men. *Am. J. Men's Health* **2019**, *13*, 1–14. [CrossRef]
15. Généreux, M.; Maltais, D.; Petit, G.; Roy, M. Monitoring adverse psychosocial outcomes one and two years after the Lac-Mégantic train derailment tragedy (Eastern Townships, Quebec, Canada). *Prehosp. Disaster Med.* **2019**, *34*, 251–259. [CrossRef] [PubMed]
16. Kessler, R.C.; Barker, P.R.; Colpe, L.J.; Epstein, J.F.; Gfroerer, J.C.; Hiripi, E.; Howes, M.J.; Normand, S.L.; Manderscheid, R.W.; Walters, E.E.; et al. Screening for serious mental illness in the general population with the K6 screening scale: Results from the WHO World Mental Health (WMH) Survey Initiative. *Arch. Gen. Psychiatr.* **2003**, *60*, 184–189. [CrossRef] [PubMed]
17. Horowitz, M.J.; Wilner, N.; Alvarez, W. The impact of event scale: A measure of subjective stress. *Psychosom. Med.* **1979**, *41*, 209–218. [CrossRef]
18. Sundin, E.C.; Horowitz, M.J. Impact of Event Scale: Psychometric properties. *Br. J. Psychiatr.* **2002**, *180*, 205–209. [CrossRef] [PubMed]
19. Connor, K.M.; Davidson, J.R.T. Development of a new resilience scale: The Connor-Davidson Resilience Scale (CD-RISC). *J. Depress. Anxiety* **2003**, *18*, 71–82. [CrossRef] [PubMed]

20. Keyes, C.L.M. Mental illness and/or mental health? Investigating axioms of the complete state model of health. *J. Consult. Clin. Psychol.* **2005**, *73*, 539–548. [CrossRef]
21. Keyes, C.L.M. The mental health continuum: From languishing to flourishing in life. *J. Health Soc. Behav.* **2002**, *43*, 207–222. [CrossRef]
22. Lundberg, O.; Nyström Peck, M. A simplified way of measuring sense of coherence: Experiences from a population survey in Sweden. *Eur. J. Public Health* **1995**, *5*, 56–59. [CrossRef]
23. Zimet, G.D.; Dahlem, N.W.; Zimet, S.G.; Farley, G.K. The Multidimensional Scale of Perceived Social Support. *J. Person. Assess.* **1988**, *52*, 30–41. [CrossRef]
24. O'Sullivan, T.L.; Kuziemsky, C.E.; Corneil, W.; Lemyre, L.; Franco, Z. The EnRiCH community resilience framework for high-risk populations. *PLoS Curr. Disasters* **2014**, *6*, 1–19. [CrossRef]
25. Généreux, M.; Maltais, D. *Social Reconstruction of the Lac-Mégantic Community Following the Tragedy: Assessment of the First Six Years*; Bulletin Vision Santé Publique. Centre Intégré Universitaire de Santé et de Services Sociaux de l'Estrie—Centre Hospitalier Universitaire de Sherbrooke: Sherbrooke, QC, Canada, 2019.
26. Généreux, M.; Petit, G.; Roy, M.; Maltais, D.; O'Sullivan, T. The "Lac-Mégantic tragedy" seen through the lens of The EnRiCH Community Resilience Framework for High-Risk Populations. *Can. J. Public Health* **2018**, *109*, 261–267. [CrossRef] [PubMed]
27. Généreux, M.; Petit, G.; Lac-Mégantic Community Outreach Team; O'Sullivan, T. Part 5: Public health approach to supporting resilience in Lac-Mégantic: The EnRiCH Framework. In *Health 2020 Priority Area Four: Creating Supportive Environments and Resilient Communities. A Compendium of Inspirational Examples*; Ziglio, E., Ed.; World Health Organization: Geneva, Switzerland, 2018; pp. 156–162.
28. Généreux, M.; Schluter, P.J.; Takahashi, S.; Usami, S.; Mashino, S.; Kayano, R.; Kim, Y. Psychosocial Management Before, During, and After Emergencies and Disasters-Results from the Kobe Expert Meeting. *Int. J. Environ. Res. Public Health* **2019**, *16*, 1309. [CrossRef] [PubMed]
29. The Lac-Mégantic Photovoice Group; Nault-Horvath, E.; Maillet, M.; Stewart, C.; Petit, G.; O'Sullivan, T. Use of Photovoice as a Tool to Support Community Resilience in Lac-Mégantic. In *Health 2020 Priority Area Four: Creating Supportive Environments and Resilient Communities. A Compendium of Inspirational Examples*; Ziglio, E., Ed.; World Health Organization: Geneva, Switzerland, 2018; pp. 163–168.
30. Généreux, M.; The Outreach Team. *Promising Initiatives to Mobilize the Local Community in a Post-Disaster Landscape*; Centre Intégré Universitaire de Santé et de Services Sociaux de l'Estrie—Centre Hospitalier Universitaire de Sherbrooke: Sherbrooke, QC, Canada, 2018; 48p.
31. McAllan, C.; McAllan, V.; McEntee, K.; Gale, W.; Taylor, D.; Wood, J.; Thompson, T.; Elder, J.; Mutsaers, K.; Leeson, W. *Lessons Learned by Community Recovery Committees of the 2009 Victorian Bushfires. Advice We Offer to Communities Impacted by Disaster*; Cube Management Solutions: Victoria, Australia, 2011; 22p.
32. O'Sullivan, T.; Toal-Sullivan, D.; Charles, K.; Corneil, W.; Bourgoin, M. *Community Resilience Through a Functional Capabilities Lens: The CHAMPSS Framework*; University of Ottawa: Ottawa, ON, Canada, 2013; 18p.
33. Leadbeater, A. Community leadership in disaster recovery: A case study. *Austr. J. Emerg. Manag.* **2013**, *26*, 41–47.
34. Van Kessel, G.B.; Gibbs, L.; MacDougall, C. Strategies to enhance resilience post-natural disaster: A qualitative study of experiences with Australian floods and fires. *J. Public Health* **2014**, *37*, 328–336. [CrossRef] [PubMed]
35. Van Kessel, G.B.; MacDougall, C.; Gibbs, L. Resilience–rhetoric to reality: A systematic review of intervention studies after disasters. *Disaster Med. Public Health Prep.* **2014**, *8*, 452–460. [CrossRef] [PubMed]
36. Abramson, D.M.; Grattan, L.M.; Mayer, B.; Colten, C.E.; Arosemena, F.A.; Bedimo-Rung, A.; Lichtveld, M. The resilience activation framework: A conceptual model of how access to social resources promotes adaptation and rapid recovery in post-disaster settings. *J. Behav. Health Serv. Res.* **2015**, *42*, 42–57. [CrossRef]
37. Castelden, M.; McKee, M.; Murray, V.; Leonardi, G. Resilience thinking in health protection. *J. Public Health* **2011**, *33*, 369–377. [CrossRef]
38. Gibbs, L.; Harms, L.; Howell-Meurs, S.; Block, K.; Lusher, D.; Richardson, J.; MacDougall, C.; Waters, E. Community wellbeing: Applications for a disaster context. *Austr. J. Emerg. Manag.* **2015**, *30*, 20–24.
39. Jackson, S.F.; Fazal, N.; Gravel, G.; Papowitz, H. Evidence for the value of health promotion interventions in natural disaster management. *Health Promot. Int.* **2017**, *32*, 1057–1066. [CrossRef]
40. Aiena, B.J.; Buchanan, E.M.; Veronica Smith, C.; Schulenberg, S.E. Meaning, resilience, and traumatic stress after the deepwater horizon oil spill: A study of Mississippi coastal residents seeking mental health services. *J. Clin. Psychol.* **2016**, *72*, 1264–1278. [CrossRef]

41. Greene, G.; Paranjothy, S.; Palmer, S.R. Resilience and vulnerability to the psychological harm from flooding: The role of social cohesion. *Am. J. Public Health* **2017**, *105*, 1792–1795. [CrossRef] [PubMed]
42. Karlin, N.J.; Marrow, S.; Weil, J.; Baum, S.; Spencer, T.S. Social support, mood, and resiliency following a Peruvian natural disaster. *J. Loss Trauma* **2012**, *17*, 470–488. [CrossRef]
43. United Nations. *Sendai Framework for Disaster Risk Reduction 2015–2030*; United Nations Office for Disaster Risk Reduction: Geneva, Switzerland, 2015.

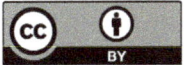

© 2020 by the authors. Licensee MDPI, Basel, Switzerland. This article is an open access article distributed under the terms and conditions of the Creative Commons Attribution (CC BY) license (http://creativecommons.org/licenses/by/4.0/).

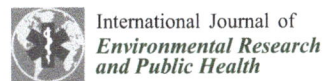

Article

Acute Mental Health Needs Duration during Major Disasters: A Phenomenological Experience of Disaster Psychiatric Assistance Teams (DPATs) in Japan

Sho Takahashi [1,2,*], Yoshifumi Takagi [3], Yasuhisa Fukuo [4,5], Tetsuaki Arai [6], Michiko Watari [4] and Hirokazu Tachikawa [1,2]

1. Department of Disaster and Community Psychiatry, Faculty of Medicine, University of Tsukuba; Tsukuba, Ibaraki 305-8577, Japan; tachikawa@md.tsukuba.ac.jp
2. Department of Community and Disaster Assistance, Ibaraki Prefectural Medical Center of Psychiatry, Asahi-machi, Kasama, Ibaraki 309-1717, Japan
3. Nihon Fukushi University, Okuda, Mihama-cho, Chita-gun, Aichi 470-3295, Japan; cch61030@gmail.com
4. DPAT secretariat, commissioned by the Ministry of Health, Labor and Welfare, Kasumigaseki Chiyoda-ku, Tokyo 100-8916, Japan; josukef3@gmail.com (Y.F.); watari@dpat.jp (M.W.)
5. Kanagawa Psychiatric Center, Serigaya, Konan Ward, Yokohama, Kanagawa 233-0006, Japan
6. Department of Psychiatry, Division of Clinical Medicine, Faculty of Medicine, University of Tsukuba, Tsukuba, Ibaraki 305-8577, Japan; 4632tetsu@md.tsukuba.ac.jp
* Correspondence: takahashi.sho.fn@u.tsukuba.ac.jp; Tel.: 81-29-853-3057

Received: 25 December 2019; Accepted: 24 February 2020; Published: 27 February 2020

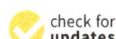

Abstract: Background: How long acute mental health needs continue after the disaster are problems which must be addressed in the treatment of victims. The aim of this study is to determine victims' needs by examining activity data from Disaster Psychiatric Assistance Teams (DPATs) in Japan. Methods: Data from four disasters were extracted from the disaster mental health information support system (DMHISS) database, and the transition of the number of consultations and the activity period were examined. Results: Common to all four disasters, the number of consultations increased rapidly from 0–2 days, reaching a peak within about a week. The partial correlation coefficient between the number of days of activity and the maximum number of victims showed significance. The number of victims and days of activity can be used to obtain a regression curve. Conclusions: This is the first report to reveal that mental health needs are the greatest in the hyper-acute stage, and the need for consultation and the duration of needs depends on the number of victims.

Keywords: disaster; Kumamoto earthquake; DMHISS; disaster psychiatry; Japan; acute mental health needs; duration of activity; DPAT (Disaster Psychiatric Assistance Team)

1. Introduction

In recent years, the question of how to respond to psychiatric disorders, as well as psychological problems, that arise among disaster victims has become a significant challenge. Many investigative studies have shown that the incidence of disorders such as post-traumatic stress disorder (PTSD) and depression increase markedly after disasters [1]. The criteria for PTSD require that the person was exposed to actual or threatened death, serious injury, or sexual violence [2]. There is a relationship between PTSD and disaster response. It is also known that psychosocial problems that accompany disasters, such as poverty, community breakdown, and the exacerbation of pre-existing psychiatric disorders, have long-term effects on the well-being of victims. Furthermore, existing psychiatric hospitals and health centers in disaster areas lose functionality during disasters and become unable to adequately undertake their consultations and diagnostic functions.

Following recent disasters around the world, such as Hurricane Katrina, the 9/11 terrorist attacks, and major earthquakes, postdisaster mental health services (MHS) have been organized and various kinds of mental health support have been provided [3]. The Inter-Agency Standing Committee (IASC), a nongovernmental organization (NGO), established a set of guidelines in 2007 on how mental health support should be conducted during disasters. These guidelines position mental health support for disaster areas within the broader context of psychosocial support, to create a system of combined mental health services and psychosocial support services (MHPSS), with interventions divided into four levels of specialized services, namely, focused specialized services, nonspecialized support, community and family support, and basic services and security [4]. Concerning specialized services, the guidelines state that interventions by specialists in psychiatry or psychology are necessary, but that due to the diverse social and cultural backgrounds of people in disaster areas, it is not possible to provide guidelines with regard to the specific services to be offered or the types of organized activities to be carried out.

Japan has been significantly affected by disasters, with one quarter of global disasters having occurred there in recent decades [5]. In the Hanshin-Awaji Earthquake of 1995, many people suffered from PTSD, and a psychiatric aid station was established to provide assistance. This led to a broader awareness of the need for psychological support for disaster victims. The 2011 East Japan Earthquake caused many people to suffer from PTSD due to the tsunami, along with the considerable stress suffered by those living in evacuation shelters. In response, several organizations and institutions, such as universities with psychiatry departments, academic associations, and NGOs organized disaster medical services [6], involving the creation of mental health care (*kokoro no care* in Japanese) teams, which carried out support work in the disaster areas. However, a lack of coordination among the teams, as well as their varied composition, led to confusion when providing assistance. There were also tragic cases in which patients in psychiatric hospitals were left behind during evacuation procedures immediately after the disaster, and who died because they could not be brought to the evacuation sites.

Drawing on these experiences, the DMAT system was modified to take into account specific psychiatric needs, and officially approved disaster psychiatric assistance teams (DPATs), which are dispatched to provide mental health support services to people in disaster areas, were established in 2013. The Ministry of Health, Labor, and Welfare (MHLW) determined the definition and role of a DPAT, set up a DPAT head office in Tokyo, and established DPATs in each prefecture and in designated cities in Japan. Since then, the number of teams across the country has gradually increased to 374 in 2017. Meanwhile, the support activities of DPATs have expanded as various disasters have occurred, such as volcanic eruptions, landslides, floods, and earthquakes. We found no other reports of such teams that have been organized to respond to mental health needs in acute phases of disasters in such a specialized and sophisticated manner.

However, clear guidelines have still not been determined for DPATs concerning the scale of activities to be carried out and at what point the work should be concluded. Because *kokoro no care* team that was active before the creation of DPATs focused primarily on mid- to long-term psychological support, data cannot be obtained that would contribute to the development of practical guidelines for acute phase activities. In relation to DPATs, a disaster mental health information support system (DMHISS) and an online database where all teams document their consultation activities have been established and are used in support activities, and it is now possible to do comparative studies using shared disaster support activity data. Therefore, we have examined data on support activities from multiple disasters that have occurred since the creation of DPATs. The aims of this study were to consider: (1) the scope of mental health needs in the acute phase of disasters, (2) whether organized MHS composed of specialists is necessary, and (3) the scale and time period necessary for the activities of acute-phase MHS.

2. Materials and Methods

2.1. Subject of Investigation

The period of investigation extended from 2013, when the DPAT system was first created, until 2016. The subject of investigation concerned the activity reports of DPATs, as well as daily reports from the DMHISS database, in relation to four disasters where support activities were conducted during that period, namely, the eruption of Mount Ontake (2014), the Hiroshima landslides (2014), the Kanto-Tohoku torrential rains (2015), and the Kumamoto earthquake (2016).

In the 2012fiscal year, the Toshiba Solutions Corporation was commissioned by the MHLW to develop a disaster mental health information support center. This resulted in the creation of the DMHISS, an online information system that aims to consolidate the activity logs of MHS and contribute to support that is appropriate for the needs of specific disaster areas. It came into nationwide operation in March 2013.

The functions of the DMHISS are divided to cover: (1) a normal period (prior registration of support teams), (2) an initial response period (coordination of support teams to be dispatched), (3) an activity period (collection of activity logs), and (4) a postactivity period (processing and analysis of activity logs). To facilitate these functions, an activity log collection tool allows data to be divided into microdata to record individual consultation trends and to record the daily activity logs of each DPAT team.

Items to be entered into the activity logs include team information (for example, team name, affiliation, and dispatch period) and type of support (for example, the results of processed data). Before and after its period of activity, each DPAT team enters its activity records into the DMHISS microdata sheet and the daily activity log. As a result, information concerning the people receiving consultations and details about the support activities of that day can be shared in real time between the disaster area itself, the base headquarters, the coordination headquarters, and the DPAT head office, thus making it possible to acquire detailed information about the activities of each DPAT [7].

2.2. Methods of Investigation

The definition of a DPAT, the structure of the organization, and an overview of its activities are first set out, followed with an explanation of the methods of investigation.

2.2.1. The Definition of a DPAT, the Structure of the Organization, and an Overview of Its Activities

A DPAT is a psychiatric team that has received specialized training for disaster management, which enables it to be dispatched to disaster areas. Additionally, DPATs are organized according to the administrative districts responsible for responding to disasters.

The main activities of a DPAT are: (1) responding directly or indirectly to the psychological problems experienced by residents in a disaster area at evacuation shelters, (2) coordination of the transport of patients from psychiatric hospitals whose functionality has been affected by the disaster, and (3) support for disaster relief workers. When DPATs are called into action, they move quickly to the disaster area or accident site, i.e., within 48 h, and in coordination with government agencies, fire departments, police departments, and defense forces, they conduct support activities for up to several months until there is no further need (Figure 1). A DPAT team consists of five people (composed of one psychiatrist, two nurses, and two logistics personnel for administrative work). Each team is dispatched to a site to conduct support activities for approximately one week. A reconnaissance team arrives in the disaster area within 48 h, sets up a DPAT coordination headquarters, coordinates with DMATs, coordinates the dispatched teams, and provides initial services at evacuation shelters. After that, the regional DPATs that follow continue the support activities in one-week rotations (Figure 2). The DPATs engage with the disaster countermeasure headquarters operating at the prefectural level, as well as with appropriate authorities at the health center and evacuation shelter levels, and at the level of each team, and coordinate with the DMATs to determine a plan for conducting support activities.

Under the direction of each DPAT headquarters, each DPAT can carry out its support activities at evacuation shelters and elsewhere in a coordinated and integrated fashion (Figure 3). Under the instructions of the disaster coordinator, DPATs also coordinate with medical teams such as DMATs, while medical teams coordinate with police, fire departments, and defense forces; health workers coordinate with health care centers.

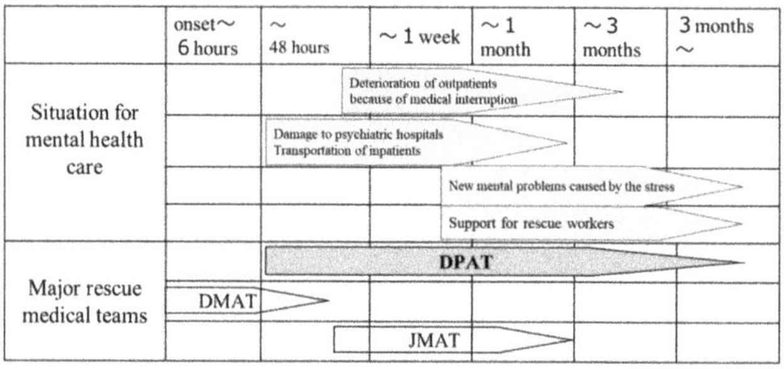

	onset~ 6 hours	~ 48 hours	~ 1 week	~ 1 month	~ 3 months	3 months ~
Situation for mental health care			Deterioration of outpatients because of medical interruption			
		Damage to psychiatric hospitals Transportation of inpatients				
				New mental problems caused by the stress		
			Support for rescue workers			
			DPAT			
Major rescue medical teams		DMAT				
			JMAT			

Figure 1. Postdisaster mental health care needs and DPAT dispatch periods. JMAT: Japan medical association team, DMAT; Disaster medical assistance team, DPAT; Disaster psychiatric assistance team.

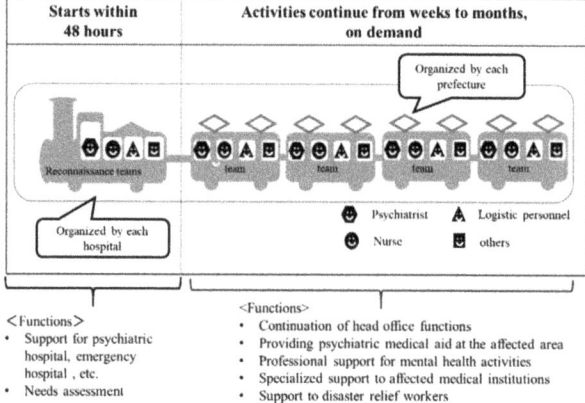

Figure 2. The roles of the reconnaissance Disaster Psychiatric Assistance Team (DPAT) and subsequent DPAT teams.

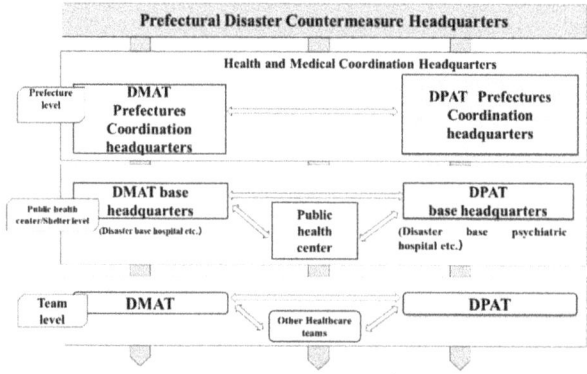

Figure 3. The Disaster Medical Assistance Team (DMAT) operational system.

DPATs arrive slightly later than DMATs, entering the disaster area within 48 h, and continue their activities for longer than DMATs, depending on the scale of the disaster. The timeline of their activities remains unspecified. DPAT: Disaster Psychiatric Assistance Team; DMAT: Disaster Medical Assistance Team; JMAT: Japanese Medical Association Team.

The reconnaissance team enters the disaster area within 48 h, establishes a headquarters, provides support for affected psychiatric hospitals and other health care institutions as required, and conducts need assessments for the disaster area. The subsequent teams provide services such as mental health care assistance, psychological support, and support for disaster relief workers in the affected area. These subsequent teams operate on a rotational basis.

DPATs engage with the disaster countermeasure headquarters at the prefectural level, with appropriate authorities at the health center and evacuation shelter levels, and at the team level with other teams, and collaborate with DMATs to determine a plan for support activities. Under the direction of the DPAT headquarters, each DPAT team carries out its support activities at evacuation shelters and elsewhere in a coordinated and integrated fashion.

2.2.2. Methods of Investigation

First, we summarized the damage situation and DPAT activities in relation to the four aforementioned disasters based on activity reports.

Next, we extracted data from the DMHISS database for these disasters, and created a data set for the daily reports. Following this, we aggregated the information on the dispatch and support structures for each disaster area, changes over time in the number of consultations provided, the number of teams engaged in support activities, and the duration of the period of activity. Furthermore, we divided the dispatch and support structures into four models as proposed by Katō et al. [8]: (a) an outside support model, wherein multiple support workers come from outside the disaster area to provide assistance; (b) a supervision model, wherein outside support workers serve as supervisors, but the support activities are carried out by local staff; (c) a local collaboration model within the region, wherein local organizations such as mental health and welfare centers take the lead in providing support, and; (d) a general support model, wherein mental health is incorporated into ordinary health care services.

We also estimated the duration period of activity for DPATs. At the time of estimation, we supplemented our data with data concerning the support provided by mental health care (*kokoro no kea*) teams before the creation of the DPAT system in relation to the Sayō-chō floods, the Niigata Chūetsu earthquake, the Hanshin-Awaji earthquake, and the East Japan earthquake, as derived from studies published in various documents such as the Cabinet Office's White Papers on Disaster Management and interviews conducted in each disaster area.

Concerning ethical considerations, we used only anonymous aggregated data from the DMHISS and publicly available documents for this study. This study was carried out with the approval of the Japan Psychiatric Hospitals Association Ethics Committee (approval number 161110-01).

3. Results

3.1. Comparison of Dispatch Systems for the Four Disasters

We compared the characteristics of the four disasters and the DPAT dispatch systems (Table 1). The disasters were of diverse types, comprising a volcanic eruption, flood disasters, and an earthquake. Although the number of casualties varied, in terms of damage conditions in relation to the number of people evacuated, the numbers of casualties steadily increased, from low numbers with the volcanic eruption, then rising for the flood disasters, and peaking with the earthquake.

Table 1. Aggregated data on damage situations and DPAT activities for the four disasters.

	Mt. Ontake Eruption	Hiroshima Landslides	Jōsō Floods	Kumamoto Earthquake
Onset date	2014/9/27	2014/8/20	2015/9/9	2016/4/14
Type of disaster	Eruption	Flood	Flood	Earthquake
Maximum evacuees	-	2354	6223	183,882
The number of dead	58	74	2	267
Model (early phase)	c	b	b	a
Model (middle and long term)	-	c	c	b
DPATs dispatch period (days)	6	23	27	90
Total number of DPATs	3	43	28	1242
Total number of consulting cases	12	106	139	2125
Sex (male/female/unknown)	5/7/0	43/63/0	58/70/11	717/1357/51

a–d: due to Models of disaster assistance [8]. Models of disaster assistance. (a) Outside support model: in which many support personnel come from outside the disaster area and provide support. (b) Supervision model: in which external support personnel act as supervisors, with support activities undertaken by regional staff. (c) Local collaboration model: in which the staff of mental health welfare centers mainly comprise locals. (d) General support model: in which mental health support is incorporated into ordinary health care services.

In the acute phase, DPAT dispatch and support operated in accordance with the local collaboration model within the region for the Mount Ontake disaster, the supervision model for the Hiroshima and Kanto-Tohoku disasters, and the outside support model for Kumamoto disaster; that is, the greater the scale of the disaster, the more outside support it required. In the mid- to long-term period, Hiroshima and Jōsō moved to a local collaboration model within the region, while Kumamoto transitioned to a supervision model. The period for which teams were dispatched varied a great deal, from 6 days to 3 months. In terms of the total number of teams dispatched, Mount Ontake had the smallest number of teams dispatched, i.e., three teams, while Kumamoto had the highest number, with 1242 teams taking part in support activities. In terms of the number of consultations, there were a total of only 12 for Mount Ontake, but over 100 each for Hiroshima and Jōsō, and 2125 for Kumamoto. In other words, the greater the scale of the disaster and the greater the number of evacuees, the greater the number of teams that were dispatched, and the longer the period of support activity.

3.2. Changes over Time in the Number of Consultations in the Four Disaster Areas

Next, we compared changes over time for the number of support consultations in each of the four disasters.

Figure 4 shows the changes in the number of consultations over time for three localized disasters, i.e., Mount Ontake, Hiroshima, and Jōsō. In the case of the eruption of Mount Ontake, the period of assistance lasted only four days, since many of the victims were people who had come from other prefectures for sightseeing and who were sent back to their home regions after four days of assistance. For the Hiroshima landslides, the number of consultations per day peaked on the 4th day, and on the 12th day after the flooding. After these days, the number of consultations gradually decreased, reaching 0 after approximately 1 month. For the Jōsō floods, the highest number of consultations occurred on the 1st day, at 27, then hovered in the 10–20 range for the next 3 days, after which it decreased to 7 consultations on the 16th and 20th days, before converging to 0 after approximately 1 month.

The vertical axis shows the number of consultations per day, while the horizontal axis shows the number of days following the disaster. The lines of the graph represent the changes in the number of consultations over time for each disaster.

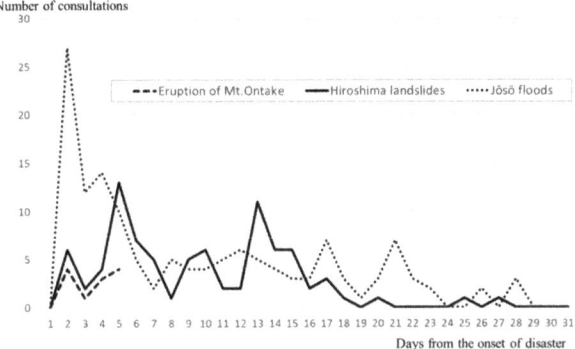

Figure 4. Changes over time in the number of consultations per day for the Mount Ontake eruption, the Hiroshima landslides, and the Jōsō floods.

Figure 5 shows the changes in the number of consultations over time for the Kumamoto earthquake. Immediately after the earthquake, patients were moved out of psychiatric hospitals that were at risk of collapsing, so support consultations at evacuation shelters essentially started on the 5th day. There were 66 consultations on the 6th day after the earthquake, with the number peaking on the 8th day, with 101 consultations. After that, the number of consultations decreased with fluctuations, but there were still more than 20 consultations on the 45th day. Two months after the earthquake, the number finally decreased to 15, and assistance continued with fluctuations before concluding after a total of 2–3 months.

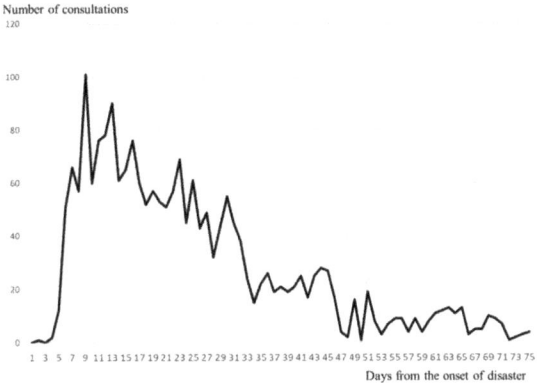

Figure 5. Change over time in the correspondence count per day for the Kumamoto earthquake.

The vertical axis shows the number of consultations per day, while the horizontal axis shows the number of days following the disaster.

For all four disasters, the number of consultations started to increase substantially on days 0–2, and reached a peak within approximately 1 week (1–8 days); the larger the scale of the disaster, the longer it took for the number of consultations to converge to 0. Especially in Kumamoto, the scale of the disaster was significantly greater than for the other three disasters, and the number of consultations also showed greater multimodal variation.

3.3. Estimation of the Period of DPAT Support from the Scale of the Disaster

In order to quantitatively consider the relationship between the scale of the disaster and the duration period of support, we also investigated the duration of the support period, the maximum number of evacuees, the number of dead, and the number of buildings damaged for other large-scale disasters in Japan, and compared the results (Table 2). An investigation of the partial correlation for each index showed that the partial correlation coefficient between the number of days of assistance and the maximum number of evacuees was significantly high, at 0.97 ($p < 0.001$).

Table 2. The number of DMS activity days and major indicators of damages in large-scale disasters.

Name of Disaster	Team Activity Days	Maximum Number of Evacuees	The Number of Dead	Number of Houses Damage
Sayō-chō Floods	22	2219	20	1790
Hiroshima landslides	27	2257	58	4559
Jōsō Floods	32	10,390	2	8327
Niigata Prefecture Chuetsu Earthquake	60	76,615	68	123,664
Kumamoto Earthquake	75	183,882	50	206,148
Great Hanshin-Awaji Earthquake	120	307,022	6400	256,312
Great East Japan Earthquake	120	409,146	15,735	1,137,785
Partial correlation coefficient (R2) with team activity days	-	0.97	−0.01	−0.57

A scatter plot detailing the number of evacuees and the number of days of assistance, where the number of evacuees is x and the number of days of assistance is y, yielded a regressive curve of $y = 0.0002x + 29.797$ ($R2 = 0.95$) (Figure 6).

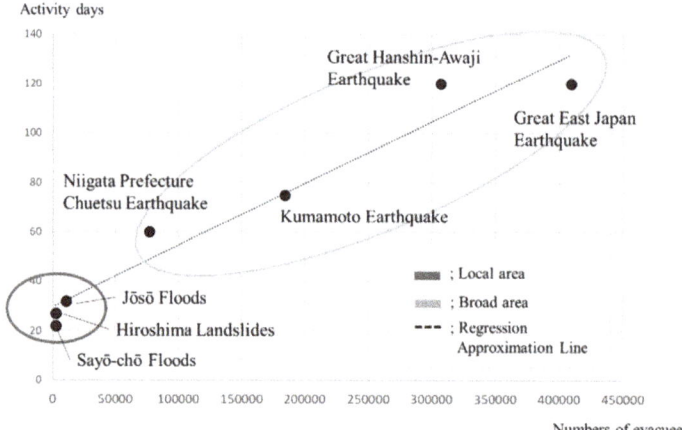

Figure 6. Plot of the team activity days and the maximum number of evacuees.

Figure 6 plots the disasters on a scatter diagram, where the vertical axis represents the team activity period (number of days) and the horizontal axis represents the maximum number of evacuees (number of people). The dotted line represents the regression line, the numerical formula represents the regression line formula and the regression coefficient, and the ellipses show the concentrations of localized disasters (Sayō-chō, Hiroshima, and Jōsō) and large-scale disasters (Niigata, Kumamoto, Hanshin-Awaji, and East Japan).

4. Discussion

Using mainly DPAT activity data, this study elucidated the need for mental health care in the acute phase of a disaster, the systems necessary to provide it, and criteria for determining the duration of team activity. This study is novel, not only because it provides an outline of the assistance activities of DPATs for the first time using real-time and objective data, but also in the sense that it has determined indices not seen in reports thus far to relate mental health needs in the acute phase of a disaster, the duration period of activities typically carried out in MHS in the acute phase, and the scale of the disaster.

In the section below, we provide a summary and interpretation of the results of the investigation.

4.1. The Role of DPATs Nationally and Internationally

In the MHPSS teams that existed prior to the DPAT system, mental health needs in the acute phase were not gauged, there was not a clear chain of command, and there was no training for support workers, so various problems tended to arise and were less effectively addressed in disaster areas. It would appear, when considering that in the Jōsō floods the DPATs successfully conducted assistance activities in coordination with the Japan Red Cross, and that in the Kumamoto earthquake, patients were successfully transported in a safe and organized manner, that the DPAT system has proved itself, in comparison to the MHPSS, to be a useful disaster mental health service in Japan, especially in the acute phase.

In the United States, under the assistance of the Federal Emergency Management Agency (FEMA) [9], the administrative agencies of each state have jurisdiction over various disaster support activities. However, although various psychological first aid (PFA) guidelines have been established, there are no specialized and standardized teams for disaster psychiatry. For example, mass shooting episodes have increased in recent decades with crisis response teams, which is not for disasters [10]. In Thailand, the Department of Mental Health established a mental health crisis assessment and treatment team (MCATT) system in 2012 [11]. A MCATT comprises a team of specialists including psychiatrists, doctors, psychiatric nurses, nurses, psychologists, and social workers, to provide assistance to disaster victims; it works in coordination with medical emergency response teams, disaster medical assistance teams, and surveillance rapid response teams. According to official requirements, ministries must configure subdistrict or state-level MCATTs with at least one team in each regional hospital (HEALTH, 2018). In South Korea, Korean disaster psychiatric assistance teams (K-DPATs) have begun activities [12] based on the DPAT system in Japan. However, any results concerning the activities of these teams remain unreported.

Compared with these other international MHPSS systems, a unique characteristic of the DPAT system is that standardized teams, centered around a psychiatrist and which have received specialized training, carry out organized mental health care activities starting from the ultra-acute phase after a disaster. Through sharing the results of DPAT activities both in- and out- side of Japan, this system has the potential to become a leading model in disaster mental health care.

4.2. Mental Health Care Needs in the Acute Phase of a Disaster

The number of consultations increased immediately after the disaster, reaching a peak in the ultra-acute to acute phase (ranging from 2 to 7 days), regardless of the disaster. Since psychological reactions result from the physical danger experienced immediately following a disaster, and since the most common conditions that arise in a disaster such as PTSD and depression are diagnosed after a certain period of observation, there has been a conventional general belief that mental health support may best be carried out after the acute phase. However, the results of this study have shown that mental health care needs are highest in the ultra-acute phase, so it is necessary for DPATs to do everything they can during this period. Based on the results of the responses to the four disasters, we also noted that consultation needs depended heavily on factors related to the scale of the disaster, such as the number of evacuees. For DPAT activities henceforth, it would be advisable to conduct overall preparation and training to provide swift and large-scale assistance starting from the ultra-acute phase and proportionate to the number of evacuees.

4.3. The Duration Period of DPAT Activities

The required duration period of DPAT activities can be determined by the time it takes for a local area's mental health and welfare system to recover. However, opinions vary as to what constitutes "recovery", and DPATs have struggled from their inception with the question of when to conclude their activities. Based on the regression equation for the two-dimensional scatter plot, $y = 0.0002x + 29.797$, with approximately one month as the y-intercept, we estimate that the recovery period increased by two days for each 10,000-maximum number of evacuees. Further, the same formula suggested that disasters should be considered separately, as both localized disasters, wherein assistance activities may last no more than one month, and disasters that occurred over a wide area, wherein assistance activities may last more than two months, had recovery times which were substantially influenced by the number of evacuees. The use of this kind of predictive formula for determining the duration period of activity has not been reported by DMSs working elsewhere. Furthermore, considering that in the mid- to long-term effects, the support model tended to change to a close collaboration model within the affected region, the basic period of DPAT support should perhaps be set at 1 month as a standard, and a method for smoothly transferring responsibilities back to the local mental health and welfare system should be considered. Furthermore, the periods of time following a disaster are usually divided into the immediate aftermath (ultra-acute phase), the acute phase, the middle phase, and the recovery phase (the long-term), but the number of days comprising each period has not been clearly defined. Considering our results, we suggest that, to facilitate recovery management, the time periods may be defined as an ultra-acute phase lasting 1–2 weeks, an acute phase lasting 1 month, and a mid- to long-term phase for subsequent engagement. As acute-phase mental health care assistance activities by DPATs and other forms of assistance continue to expand in the future, the predictive formula and its interpretation developed in this study should provide practical guidance for recovery interventions.

4.4. Limitations of this Study

This study had various limitations. Only a limited amount of data could be obtained concerning disasters, and there was a lack of prior relevant research. We searched the literature for intervention and comparative studies, but could not find any matches. Also, there was no study like this, so comparisons could not be made. There are only 12 literature publications, but there are few comparable studies, which was a difficult point. A search of past disaster dispatched psychiatric teams for all years showed no results. Few countries have done this, and few have reported on their activities; that is why there are few cited references. Therefore, we think that this paper has novel points.

More data on disasters should be accumulated. Also, the analysis concerning the duration period of activity included recent major disasters, but the MHPSS system was responsible for the mid- to long-term recovery period in relation to support activities conducted following the Hanshin-Awaji Earthquake and the East Japan Earthquake; hence, strictly speaking, its activities cannot be compared with those of the DPATs. In future, further data should be accumulated to aid in the undertaking of more precise analyses.

5. Conclusions

1. We compared activity data from four disasters where DPATs had provided support.
2. We discovered that mental health care needs were greatest in the ultra-acute phase following a disaster.
3. We discovered that the duration of the activity period was 1 month for localized disasters, or longer for disasters covering a wide area, depending on the number of evacuees.
4. It is necessary to accumulate more cases and examples to ensure more precise analyses.

Author Contributions: Conceptualization, S.T. and H.T.; Methodology, S.T. and H.T.; Software, S.T. and Y.F.; Validation, T.A. and H.T.; Formal analysis, S.T. and H.T.; Investigation, S.T., Y.T. and H.T.; Resources, M.W.; Data curation, S.T., Y.T. and Y.F.; Writing—original draft preparation, S.T.; Writing—review and editing, S.T. and H.T.; Visualization, Y.F.; Supervision, T.A. and H.T.; Project administration, S.T., H.T. and M.W.; Funding acquisition, M.W. All authors have read and agree to the published version of the manuscript.

Funding: This paper comprises a part of "A Study on Enhancing the Functionality of Disaster Psychiatric Assistance Teams (DPATs)" that received support from the fiscal year 2016 Ministry of Health, Labor and Welfare

Scientific Research Fund (Integrated Research on Policy for People with Disabilities (Mental Illness Division)) (Issue number:H28-psychiatry-common-005).

Acknowledgments: We would like to express our sincerest sympathy to those struck by disaster, and once again to express our gratitude to everyone on the DPAT teams who have taken part in support activities from the acute phase to the mid- to long-term phase after a disaster.

Conflicts of Interest: The authors declare no conflict of interest.

References

1. Weisaeth, L. Disaster, Risk and preventive intervention. In *Handbook of Studies on Preventive Psychiatry*; Raphael, B., Burrows, G., Eds.; Elsevier: Amsterdam, The Netherlands, 1995; pp. 301–332.
2. American Psychiatric Association. *Diagnostic and Statistical Manual of Mental Disorders*, 5th ed.; American Psychiatric Publishing: Arlington, VA, USA, 2013; pp. 271–280.
3. Rodriguez, J.J.; Kohn, R. Use of mental health services among disaster survivors. *Curr. Opin. Psychiatry* **2008**, *21*, 370–378. [CrossRef]
4. Iasc Guidelines on Mental Health and Psychosocial Support in Emergency Settings: Inter-Agency Standing Committee. Available online: Https://www.who.int/mental_health/emergencies/guidelines_iasc_mental_health_psychosocial_june_2007.pdf (accessed on 23 December 2019).
5. Cabinet Office, Goverment of Japan. Disaster management in Japan. Available online: http://www.bousai.go.jp/kaigirep/hakusho/h22/bousai2010/html/honbun/2b_1s_1_01.htm (accessed on 23 December 2019).
6. Knouss, R.F. National disaster medical system. *Public Health Rep.* **2001**, *116*, 49–52. [CrossRef]
7. Fukuo, Y.; Tachikawa, H.; Takahashi, S.; Takagi, Y.; Yoshida, W.; Komi, M.; Arai, T.; Watari, M. An activity report of Disaster Psychiatric Assistant Team (DPAT) in the 2016 Kumamoto Earthquake: Special reference to the statistical data from Disaster Mental Health Information Support System (DMHISS). *J. Jpn. Emerg. Psychiatry* **2018**, *21*, 86–94.
8. Kato, H. Progress of Disaster Psychiatry in Japan. *Clin. Psychiatry* **2006**, *48*, 231–239.
9. Federal Emergency Management Agency (FEMA). National Incident Management System. Available online: http://www.fema.gov/national-incident-management-system (accessed on 23 December 2019).
10. Lowe, S.R.; Galea, S. The Mental Health Consequences of Mass Shootings. *Trauma Violence Abuse* **2017**, *18*, 62–82. [CrossRef] [PubMed]
11. Department of Mental Health MoPH, Thailand. Mental Health Crisis Assessment and Treatment Team: MCATT. Available online: http://www.skph.go.th/newskph/Doc_file/ManualMCATT2018.pdf (accessed on 23 December 2019).
12. Jo, S.J.; Na, K.S.; Park, J.E.; Lee, M.S. Decision Making Regarding Key Elements of Korean Disaster Psychiatric Assistance Teams Using the Analytic Hierarchy Process. *Psychiatry Investig.* **2018**, *15*, 663–669. [CrossRef] [PubMed]

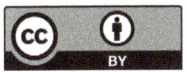

© 2020 by the authors. Licensee MDPI, Basel, Switzerland. This article is an open access article distributed under the terms and conditions of the Creative Commons Attribution (CC BY) license (http://creativecommons.org/licenses/by/4.0/).

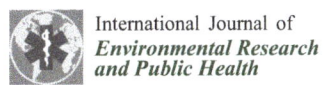

Article

Personal Cold Protection Behaviour and Its Associated Factors in 2016/17 Cold Days in Hong Kong: A Two-Year Cohort Telephone Survey Study

Holly Ching Yu Lam [1,2,3], Zhe Huang [2,3], Sida Liu [2,3], Chunlan Guo [2,3], William Bernard Goggins [3] and Emily Ying Yang Chan [2,3,4,*]

1. National Heart and Lung Institute, Imperial College London, Emmanuel Kaye Building, London SW3 6LR, UK; ching.lam@imperial.ac.uk
2. Collaborating Centre for Oxford University and CUHK for Disaster and Medical Humanitarian Response (CCOUC), Faculty of Medicine, The Chinese University of Hong Kong, Shatin, Hong Kong SAR, China; huangzhe@cuhk.edu.hk (Z.H.); kevin.liu@cuhk.edu.hk (S.L.); theresachunlanguo@gmail.com (C.G.)
3. Jockey Club School of Public Health and Primary Care, Chinese University of Hong Kong, New Territories, Hong Kong, China; wgoggins@cuhk.edu.hk
4. Nuffield Department of Medicine, University of Oxford, Oxford OX3 7LF, UK
* Correspondence: emily.chan@cuhk.edu.hk; Tel.: +852-2252-8411

Received: 7 January 2020; Accepted: 29 February 2020; Published: 4 March 2020

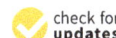

Abstract: *Background:* Despite larger health burdens attributed to cold than heat, few studies have examined personal cold protection behaviours (PCPB). This study examined PCPB during cold waves and identified the associated factors in a subtropical city for those without central heating system. *Methods*: A cohort telephone survey was conducted in Hong Kong during a colder cold wave (2016) and a warmer cold wave (2017) among adults (≥15). Socio-demographic information, risk perception, self-reported adverse health effects and patterns of PCPB during cold waves were collected. Associated factors of PCPB in 2017 were identified using multiple logistic regression. *Results:* The cohort included 429 subjects. PCPB uptake rates were higher during the colder cold wave ($p < 0.0005$) except for ensuring indoor ventilation. Of the vulnerable groups, 63.7% had low self-perceived health risks. High risk perception, experience of adverse health effects during the 2016 cold wave, females and older groups were positive associated factors of PCPB in 2017 ($p < 0.05$). *Conclusions:* PCPB changed with self-risk perception. However vulnerable groups commonly underestimated their own risk. Indoor ventilation may be a concern during cold days in settings that are less prepared for cold weather. Targeted awareness-raising promotion for vulnerable groups and practical strategies for ensuring indoor ventilation are needed.

Keywords: cold; personal health protective behaviour; associated factors; risk perception; subtropical city

1. Introduction

Low ambient temperatures are associated with adverse health effects such as hypothermia and higher risk of cardiovascular diseases, respiratory diseases and infectious diseases globally [1–5]. The elderly, people with illnesses and outdoor workers are more vulnerable during conditions of extreme temperatures [3]. In warmer regions, although winters may be considered milder than in colder regions, due to the less appropriate housing design for low temperatures and acclimatization [4], effects of unusual low temperature might increase mortality and morbidity. Previous studies have shown that populations residing in lower latitudes were more vulnerable to cold temperature [5] and had higher threshold temperatures at which cold effects began to be observed [1]. Adverse health effects related to low temperatures and cold waves have been reported in subtropical regions including Hong Kong, Guangzhou, China, Taiwan and Brisbane, Australia [4,6–13].

As highlighted in the Sendai Framework [14], understanding risks and enhancing preparedness are priorities to support bottom up risk reduction and resilience in communities. Despite the scientific evidence showing the adverse health effects of extreme low temperatures [1,15,16], studies examining personal cold protection behaviours (PCPB) are rare [17]. Several studies focusing on heat protective measures and associated factors have been published, probably due to raising concerns about increasing global temperature [18–22]. Studies from temperate regions have shown socio-demographic factors such as sex and economic status were associated with the uptake of personal protection measures against extreme temperatures [17,18]. In the United Kingdom (UK), females and people with higher income were more likely to apply personal heat protection measures during heat waves [18]. A European study also found females were more likely to wear more outdoor clothes on cold days but the insulation of clothes was poorer than those of males [17].

Risk perception is another important determinant of health behaviours [23,24] Studies from the UK [19], China [20] and Pakistan [21] have reported positive associations between risk perception and protective behaviour against high temperatures. Vulnerable groups, however, had been reported more likely to underestimate their health risks during extreme high temperatures [25]. A focus group study from New York City, United States, found that seniors and people with fair or poor health conditions were not aware of their own risk during hot days [22].

Despite the expected increase in number of hot days and average temperature [26], cold effects on human health are, however, still more severe than the effects of heat and should not be neglected [1,4]. Individual cold protection behaviour, risk perception and other potential associated factors, such as experience of adverse health effects in previous cold waves and socio-demographic factors, are mostly unknown and make the formulation of evidence-based cold-related health protection policy and promotion challenging.

This two-year telephone survey cohort study, conducted immediately after an extreme cold wave in 2016 and a regular cold wave in 2017: (1) explored the perceived health risks and risk perception accuracy at low temperatures; (2) examined the pattern of PCPB; and (3) identified the associated characteristics of PCPB in a subtropical city. The results of this study will support the facilitation of drafting health protection strategy to reduce avoidable health risk during cold waves in warmer regions.

2. Materials and Methods

2.1. Study Period

In Hong Kong, there is no clear definition of a cold wave. The Hong Kong Observatory takes into consideration multiple meteorological parameters and issues a cold weather warning signal when cold weather may incur harm to the public. In this study, cold waves are defined as periods when cold weather warning signals were issued by the Hong Kong Observatory.

This is a two-year telephone survey-based cohort study. Two telephone surveys were conducted, during February of 2016 and March of 2017, one week after the cold weather warning signals were issued by the Hong Kong Observatory on 21–27 January 2016 and 23–27 February 2017, respectively. The surveys were conducted shortly after the cold waves to reduce recall bias. The 2016 survey was completed in eight days while the 2017 survey was finished in eleven days. The cold wave in 2016 was severe and 24 January 2016 was the coldest day in Hong Kong since 1957. The average daily mean temperature during the 2016 cold wave was 10.6 °C (average daily mean temperature in January in 1981, 2010: 16.3 °C). The 2017 cold wave was relatively milder in intensity. The average daily mean temperature within the study cold wave period was 14.8 °C (average daily mean temperature in February in 1981, 2010: 16.8 °C).

Sampling and Subject Recruitment

A random digit dialling approach was used to select households from a full list of landline telephone numbers in Hong Kong and the last birthday method, inviting the household member with birthday closest to the interview date, was used to select Cantonese speaking subjects ≥ 15 years old for the baseline survey in 2016. Quota sampling was adopted to match the population characteristics in terms of age-group, gender and residential districts in the Hong Kong SAR Census in 2011 (2016 Census information was not available at the time of the baseline study). The baseline sample size of 1000 was based on being able to estimate the percentage of people applying a particular cold protection measure with maximum margin of error of 3.5% at a 95% confidence level. Phone calls were made in the evening on weekdays and throughout the day on weekends to minimize bias based on employment status. Oral consent had been sought from each participant at the beginning of the surveys. The study was conducted in accordance with the Declaration of Helsinki and the protocol was approved by the Survey and Behavioural Research Ethics Board, The Chinese University of Hong Kong.

2.2. Variables

Socio-demographic characteristics, self-report history of chronic diseases (conditions that require medical treatment for more than six months), health risk perceptions of cold weather, self-reported health outcomes and protection behaviour patterns within the study period were collected in the survey. Based on the health guidelines provided by the Hong Kong Observatory [27], four personal cold protection measures, which included 'putting on more clothes', 'avoid staying in windy areas', 'use of heating equipment' and 'ensuring adequate indoor ventilation', were studied. The possible biological associations between the four behaviours and human health are shown in Table 1. Details of questionnaire design and phone call algorithm for the 2016 data have been published elsewhere [28]. Follow-up surveys were conducted with the same cohort and using same questions after the 2017 cold wave.

Table 1. Biological association between personal cold protective behaviours and health outcomes.

Protective Measure	Linkage with Human Health	Related Health Benefits from Literature	Personal Characteristics Associated with the Behaviour from Literature
Wearing More clothes	Prevent heat loss through insulation and resistance to evaporation, wind and water. Inner layer to control body temperature and humidity, middle layer for insulation and outer layer to protect against the outer environment [29].	Control heat loss, insulate current temperature and reduce discomfort due to cold injury and hypothermia. Increase manual working performance. High moisture absorbing material can keep the skin dry even when sweating. Ventilating garments prevent post-chilling effect when the wet garment is drying [29].	Elderly people in the UK with problems such as thyroid, poor circulation, anaemia and heart irregularities wore more clothes. To supplement appliance to keep warm [30], Japanese female cooperative workers were more likely to wear one or more items of clothing [31].
Avoid Windy Areas	Protect wind chills from reducing skin temperature through rapid evaporation, especially when weather is overcast. [32]	Reduce the risk of hip fractures, incidence of asthma, sickle cell disease and acute pain. [33]	Hong Kong Observatory released advice to "avoid prolonged exposure to wintry winds." [34] No literature was found to evaluate the local population's wind-related behaviour.

Table 1. Cont.

Protective Measure	Linkage with Human Health	Related Health Benefits from Literature	Personal Characteristics Associated with the Behaviour from Literature
Use of Heaters	Maintaining adequate indoor temperature. [35]	Increase resistance to respiratory and vascular complications, such as myocardial infractions. Improvement in symptoms of asthma in children and reduced time off school. [8,36]. Ensure thermoregulatory function in elderly people, as the minimum indoor temperature for them should be a few degrees higher than average. [35]	Availability of heating system(s) such as heaters, fireplace, central heating, etc. [30]
Ensure Indoor Ventilation	Intended to remove pollutants emitted from indoor sources, e.g., building materials, furnishings, unvented combustions, etc.	Associated with reduced prevalence of sick building syndrome and allergic manifestation in children. Literature suggests low ventilation rates are associated with inflammation and respiratory infections [37].	A few elders in the UK opened windows for air circulation, mostly for a short while. Most considered it potentially wasteful of heat. [30] Some elders opened windows at night to sleep and turned off the heater [35].

Remark: Protective measures included were references from the Hong Kong Observatory.

Measurement of Risk Perception Accuracy

To assess the risk perception accuracy of subjects, the objective risk of subjects was compared with their self-risk perception. Subjects fulfilling at least one of these four factors in 2017, old age (≥60 years), history of chronic diseases, living alone and receiving comprehensive social security assistance (CSSA), were considered to be at high health risk during low temperatures. This assumes that old age and a history of chronic diseases increase vulnerability physiologically, while living alone and receiving CSSA are related to less resources and support. Underestimation of risk was defined as subjects who fulfilled one or more of these risk factors (the high-risk group) but did not consider themselves high risk. Considering that there might be other risk factors of cold related health problems not included in this study, people who appeared to be overestimating their risk (reported themselves as high risk but fulfilled none of the four pre-set criteria) were grouped as "potentially overestimated". Subjects from the high-risk group who considered themselves high risk, and those who did not have any of the pre-set criteria and considered themselves low risk were defined as having correct perception.

2.3. Statistical Method

Chi-square test was used to compare the uptake rate of the PCPB between the two cold waves. Associated factors for the uptake of protective behaviours in 2017 cold wave were identified using multiple logistic regression models. A two-stage model selection approach, univariate analyses (chi-square test) followed by multiple logistic regression, was adopted. Factors with $p < 0.2$ in univariate analyses were entered a logistic regression for examining the independent associations in the second stage. Chi-square test was performed to examine the characteristics of the lost-to-follow-up group. All analyses were performed using IBM SPSS 21(IBM, Armonk, NY, USA).

2.4. Model Selections in Identifying Associated Factors of PCPB

Socio-demographic factors such as age, sex and income have been reported to be associated factors of heat protective behaviours [17,18]. Age-group, gender, household income and residential district were therefore included in all regression models as the core model. Other independent variables considered in the model selection process included education level, CSSA status, occupation, marital status, history of chronic diseases, risk perception, risk perception accuracy, feeling cold at home during the 2017 cold period and experience of adverse health effect during the 2016 cold waves that needed medical treatment or medicine. Dependent variables, the uptake of the four PCPBs during the 2017 cold wave (Yes/ No), were examined separately.

3. Results

3.1. Descriptive Results

A total of 1017 subjects were recruited for the 2016 baseline survey and 429 of these subjects have completed the follow-up survey in 2017 (follow-up rate 42.2 %). A diagram demonstrating the subject recruitment process is shown in Supplementary Figure S1.

Descriptive statistics of the personal characteristics of the 2016–2017 cohort are shown in Table 2 with the comparison to the characteristics of the Census. Although the baseline sample was comparable to the 2011 census characteristics, it should be noted that the proportion of the elderly ≥65 years old in the follow-up sample in 2017 was higher than that in the baseline, due to the lower follow-up rate among the working population (25–44 years) (lost-to-follow-up analysis available in Supplementary Table S2).

Table 2. Descriptive statistics of socio-demographic variables, history of chronic diseases and health perception of subjects in 2017 follow-up survey, with comparison to the major socio-demographic characteristics in Hong Kong Census 2016 and 2016 baseline sample.

Demographics	HK 2016 Population By-Census Data ($n = 6,506,130$)		Sampled Participants in 2016 ($n = 1017$)		Follow-Up Participants in 2017 ($n = 429$)		2017 Sample vs. Census p-Value [a]
	n	%	n	%	n	%	
Gender							1 [b]
Male	2,947,073	45.3%	437	43.0%	194	45.20%	
Female	3,559,057	54.7%	580	57.0%	235	54.80%	
Age							<0.001
15–24	785,981	12.1%	126	12.4%	49	11.40%	
25–44	2,228,566	34.3%	315	31.0%	109	25.40%	
45–64	2,328,430	35.8%	384	37.8%	165	38.50%	
≥65	1,163,153	17.9%	192	18.9%	106	24.70%	
Geographical distribution *							0.43
Hong Kong Island	1,120,143	17.2%	182	17.9%	83	19.30%	
Kowloon	1,987,380	30.6%	315	31.0%	133	31.00%	
New Territories	3,397,499	52.2%	518	51.0%	213	49.70%	
Education attainment							<0.01
Primary and below	1,673,431	25.7%	137	13.5%	59	13.80%	
Secondary	2,841,510	43.7%	501	49.4%	215	50.10%	
Post-secondary	1,991,189	30.6%	377	37.1%	154	35.90%	
Marital status							0.34 [b]
Single	2,708,709	41.6%	410	40.5%	188	43.80%	
Married	3,797,421	58.4%	602	59.5%	239	55.70%	
Monthly household income (HKD)							
<10,000					67	15.60%	
10,000–19,999					72	16.80%	
20,000–29,999					72	16.80%	
30,000–39,999					60	14.00%	
40,000 or above					128	29.80%	

Table 2. Cont.

Demographics	HK 2016 Population By-Census Data (n = 6,506,130)		Sampled Participants in 2016 (n = 1017)		Follow-Up Participants in 2017 (n = 429)		2017 Sample vs. Census p-Value [a]
	n	%	n	%	n	%	
Comprehensive social security assistant (CSSA)							
Yes					17	4.00%	
No					412	96.00%	
Occupation							
Clerical					66	15.40%	
Non clerical					108	25.20%	
Housewife					88	20.50%	
Student					37	8.60%	
Retired/ unemployed					123	28.70%	
History of chronic diseases							
Yes					113	26.30%	
No					316	73.70%	
Living alone							
Yes					38	8.90%	
No					388	91.40%	
Own heating equipment at home							
Yes					252	58.70%	
No					175	40.80%	
Felt cold at home during the study cold period in 2017							
Very cold					24	5.60%	
Cold					253	59.00%	
Not cold					149	34.70%	
Reporting any adverse health effects during the 2016 cold waves (needed medical treatment or medicine)							
Yes					49	11.40%	
No					380	88.60%	
Self- risk perception in low temperature							
High					100	23.30%	
Low					324	75.50%	
Risk at low temperature based on pre-defined factors							
High					193	45.00%	
Low					234	54.50%	
Health perception accuracy [c]							
Correct					267	62.2%	
Underestimated					123	28.7%	
Potentially overestimated					32	7.5%	

[a] χ^2 test was used to measure the overall difference in proportions between this survey and the 2016 Hong Kong Population Census data. p-value < 0.05 indicates significant difference. [b] χ^2 test with continuity correction was used. [c] Underestimated: People fulfilled at least one of the four preset criteria (old age, history of chronic diseases, living alone and receiving CSSA) but did not consider themselves high risk. Correct: People fulfilled at least one of the four preset criteria and considered themselves high risk AND People did not have any of the preset criteria and considered themselves low risk. Overestimated: People did not have any of the preset criteria but considered themselves high risk. * Marine population are excluded. Remarks: Percentage may not add up to 100% due to missing data.

3.1.1. Risk Perception and Risk Perception Accuracy

In the 2017 survey, 45.0% of the subjects fulfilled at least one of the pre-defined risk factors and were considered as high risk in low temperatures. Overall, 23.3% of subjects considered themselves having higher health risk during low temperature (Table 2). Regarding risk perception accuracy,

62.2% had correct risk perception, 28.7% had underestimated their risk and 7.5% had potentially overestimated the risk. Among the high-risk group, 63.7% (123/193) had underestimated their risk.

3.1.2. PCPB Patterns

In general, warm-keeping PCPB uptake rate was statistically significantly higher during the colder cold wave in 2016 ($p < 0.0005$ in chi-square test) (Figure 1). During the colder cold wave in 2016, 95.3% had reported putting on more clothes, 83.4% had avoid staying in windy area and 55.0% has used heating equipment during the cold wave (80.2 % among those owning heating equipment). In the milder cold wave in 2017, 81.4% had reported putting on more clothes, 59.2% had avoided staying in windy area and 28.7% had used heating equipment (41.0 % among those owning heating equipment). In contrast, the proportion of subjects that had ensured indoor ventilation increased from 79.0% in 2016 to 89.5% in 2017.

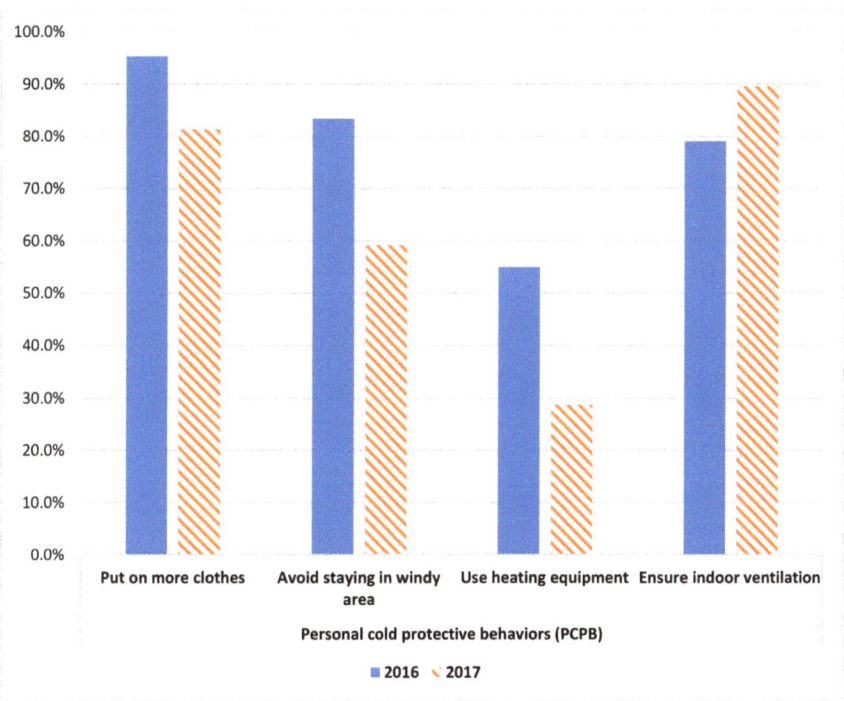

Figure 1. Uptake rate of personal cold protection behaviour among the same group of subjects in 2016 and 2017 cold wave ($n = 429$). Remarks: p-values of Chi-square test comparing the four personal cold protective behaviours between 2016 (the colder cold wave) and 2017 (a warmer cold wave) are all <0.0005.

3.2. Associated Factors of PCPB

The selected distribution of PCPB across levels of covariates and the respective chi-square test results are presented in Table 3. A full table of results of all variables considered can be found in Supplementary Table S1. Subjects with previous experience of adverse health effect in the 2016 cold wave were more likely to consider themselves as high risk at low temperature (p-value for chi-square test = 0.003). To avoid multicollinearity, self-risk perception was excluded from multiple logistic regression models whenever previous experience of adverse health effect was included in the model, and vice versa.

Table 3. Association between personal characteristics and uptake of personal cold protection behaviour in 2017 cold wave using Chi-square test.

Personal Characteristics		Put on More Cloths			Avoid Staying at Windy Area			Use Heating Equipment			Keep Indoor Ventilation		
		No	Yes	* p-Value	No	Yes	* p-Value	No	Yes	* p-Value	No	Yes	* p-Value
Gender													
Male		39	155	0.37	89	104	0.03	155	39	<0.0005	21	173	0.84
		50.0%	44.4%		51.4%	40.9%		50.7%	31.7%		46.7%	45.1%	
Female		39	194		84	150		151	84		24	211	
		50.0%	55.6%		48.6%	59.1%		49.3%	68.3%		53.3%	54.9%	
Age													
15–24		10	39	0.64	21	28	0.09	42	7	0.08	13	36	<0.0005
		12.8%	11.2%		12.1%	11.0%		13.7%	5.7%		28.9%	9.4%	
24–39		18	65		36	47		58	25		11	72	
		23.1%	18.6%		20.8%	18.5%		19.0%	20.3%		24.4%	18.8%	
40–59		22	117		45	94		98	41		18	121	
		28.2%	33.5%		26.0%	37.0%		32.0%	33.3%		40.0%	31.5%	
60–69		18	68		35	52		64	23		2	85	
		23.1%	19.5%		20.2%	20.5%		20.9%	18.7%		4.4%	22.1%	
≥70		10	60		36	33		44	27		1	70	
		12.8%	17.2%		20.8%	13.0%		14.4%	22.0%		2.2%	18.2%	
Education													
Primary or below		8	51	0.46	28	30	0.29	41	18	0.78	3	56	0.06
		10.3%	14.6%		16.2%	11.9%		13.4%	14.8%		6.7%	14.6%	
Secondary		38	176		80	134		157	58		19	196	
		48.7%	50.4%		46.2%	53.0%		51.3%	47.5%		42.2%	51.2%	
Post-secondary or above		32	122		65	89		108	46		23	131	
		41.0%	35.0%		37.6%	35.2%		35.3%	37.7%		51.1%	34.2%	

Table 3. *Cont.*

Personal Characteristics	Put on More Cloths			Avoid Staying at Windy Area			Use Heating Equipment			Keep Indoor Ventilation		
	No	Yes	*p-Value	No	Yes	*p-Value	No	Yes	*p-Value	No	Yes	*p-Value
Residential districts												
Hong Kong Island	17	65	0.05	48	35	0.001	64	19	0.15	12	71	0.41
	21.8%	18.6%		27.7%	13.8%		20.9%	15.4%		26.7%	18.5%	
Kowloon	15	117		53	80		87	46		12	121	
	19.2%	33.5%		30.6%	31.5%		28.4%	37.4%		26.7%	31.5%	
New Territories	46	167		72	139		155	58		21	192	
	59.0%	47.9%		41.6%	54.7%		50.7%	47.2%		46.7%	50.0%	
Self-risk perception at low temperature												
Low risk	64	259	0.03	137	185	0.18	249	75	<0.0005	34	290	0.89
	86.5%	74.4%		79.7%	74.0%		81.9%	65.5%		75.6%	76.5%	
High risk	10	89		35	65		55	45		11	89	
	13.5%	25.6%		20.3%	26.0%		18.1%	37.5%		24.4%	23.5%	
Risk-perception accuracy												
Correct	50	207	0.12	102	156	0.34	188	70	0.26	28	230	0.05
	68.5%	59.7%		59.6%	62.7%		62.0%	58.8%		63.6%	60.8%	
Under-estimate	22	115		61	75		100	38		10	128	
	30.1%	33.1%		35.7%	30.1%		33.0%	31.9%		22.7%	33.9%	
Potentially over-estimate	1	25		8	18		15	11		6	20	
	1.4%	7.2%		4.7%	7.2%		5.0%	9.2%		13.6%	5.3%	
Experience of adverse health effect in 2016 cold wave and needed medical consultation/ any form of treatment												
No	75	303	0.02	157	221	0.23	278	102	0.02	37	343	0.16
	96.2%	86.8%		90.8%	87.0%		90.8%	82.9%		82.2%	89.3%	
Yes	3	46		16	33		28	21		8	41	
	3.8%	13.2%		9.2%	13.0%		9.2%	17.1%		17.8%	10.7%	

* *p*-value for Chi-square test.

Table 4. Adjusted Odds-ratio (OR) of associated factors of personal cold protective behaviours in 2017 cold wave using multiple logistic regression.

Associated Factor	Personal Cold Protective Measures											
	Put on More Cloths (n = 398)			Avoid Staying at Windy Area (n = 398)			Use Heating Equipment (n = 399)			Keep Indoor Ventilation (n = 398)		
	OR	95%CI		OR	95%CI		OR	95%CI		OR	95%CI	
		Lower	Upper		Lower	Upper		Lower	Upper		Lower	Upper
^ Gender												
Male	1.00	-	-	1.00	-	-	1.00	-	-	1.00	-	-
Female	1.08	0.62	1.85	1.34	0.88	2.04	1.85	1.14	3.00	0.92	0.46	1.85
^ Age												
15–24	1.00	-	-	1.00	-	-	1.00	-	-	1.00	-	-
25–39	0.86	0.33	2.23	1.22	0.57	2.62	3.31	1.12	9.77	1.74	0.64	4.73
40–59	1.70	0.66	4.35	2.15	1.03	4.50	3.34	1.18	9.50	1.12	0.38	3.36
60–69	0.74	0.27	2.06	1.52	0.68	3.41	2.52	0.82	7.74	7.22	1.13	46.02
≥70	1.02	0.32	3.26	0.95	0.39	2.30	4.00	1.210	13.19	14.57	1.33	159.55
^ Residential districts												
Hong Kong Island	1.00	-	-	1.00	-	-	1.00	-	-	1.00	-	-
Kowloon	2.64	1.15	6.04	2.18	1.20	3.97	1.94	0.97	3.91	3.07	1.16	8.16
New Territories	1.15	0.57	2.29	2.65	1.50	4.67	1.44	0.73	2.84	2.10	0.88	5.02
^ Income												
<10000	1.00	-	-	1.00	-	-	1.00	-	-	1.00	-	-
10000–19999	0.70	0.24	2.03	1.50	0.69	3.26	0.51	0.221	1.18	2.02	0.36	11.34
20000–29999	0.66	0.22	1.99	1.14	0.53	2.45	0.73	0.32	1.68	0.77	0.15	3.85
30000–39999	0.42	0.14	1.29	1.20	0.52	2.74	0.63	0.25	1.56	1.22	0.22	6.73
≥40000	0.42	0.15	1.18	1.00	0.47	2.11	0.70	0.31	1.56	1.49	0.29	7.74
^ Marital status												
Currently not married	-	-	-	-	-	-	-	-	-	1.00	-	-
Currently married	-	-	-	-	-	-	-	-	-	3.33	1.34	8.28
^ Felt cold at home during the cold period in 2017												
No	-	-	-	-	-	-	1.00	-	-	-	-	-
Cold	-	-	-	-	-	-	1.24	0.77	2.08	-	-	-
Very cold	-	-	-	-	-	-	3.72	1.29	10.72	-	-	-

Table 4. Cont.

	Personal Cold Protective Measures											
	Put on More Cloths (n = 398)			Avoid Staying at Windy Area (n = 398)			Use Heating Equipment (n = 399)			Keep Indoor Ventilation (n = 398)		
Associated Factor	OR	95%CI		OR	95%CI		OR	95%CI		OR	95%CI	
		Lower	Upper		Lower	Upper		Lower	Upper		Lower	Upper
^ Experience of adverse health effect in 2016 cold wave and needed medical consultation/ any form of treatment												
No	1.00	-	-	-	-	-	1.00	-	-	-	-	-
Yes	5.48	1.26	23.83	-	-	-	1.89	0.97	3.71	-	-	-
# Health risk perception at low temperatures												
Low	1.00	-	-	-	-	-	1.00	-	-	-	-	-
High	2.30	1.03	5.16	-	-	-	2.57	1.48	4.44	-	-	-

ORs were estimated from Logistic Regression models. **Bold:** p-value < 0.05 in Logistic Regression. ^ Not adjusted for "Health risk perception at low temperatures". # Not adjusted for "Experience of adverse health effect in 2016 cold wave and needed medical consultation/any form of treatment".

3.2.1. Put on More Clothes

Those who lived in Kowloon (compared to those who lived on Hong Kong Island) (Odds Ratios (OR) (95% confidence interval) 2.64 (1.15 to 6.04)), those who had experienced adverse health effects during the 2016 cold wave (5.48 (1.26 to 23.83)) and those who perceived high health risk at low temperatures (2.30 (1.03 to 5.16)) were more likely to put on more clothes (Table 4).

3.2.2. Avoid Staying in Windy Area

Compared to residents from the Hong Kong Island, those living in Kowloon (2.18 (1.20 to 3.97)) and the New Territories (2.65 (1.50 to 4.67)) were more likely to avoid staying in a windy area. Age group 40–59 (2.15 (1.03 to 4.50)) were also more likely to stay away from the wind compared to the youngest age-group 15–24.

3.2.3. Use Heating Equipment

Females (1.85 (1.14 to 3.00)), those who felt very cold at home (3.72 (1.29 to 10.72)), the older age-groups (vs. 15–24) and those who had high health risk perception (2.57 (1.48 to 4.44)) were more likely to use heating equipment during the cold wave. The ORs of using heating equipment for the older age-groups (vs. 15–24) ranged from 3.31 to 4.00 (Table 4). In subgroup analysis among those who owned any heating equipment at home by age, feeling cold at home remained statistically significant.

3.2.4. Ensure Indoor Ventilation

The elderly aged above 60 years (ORs range from 7.22 to 14.57), those who lived in Kowloon (3.07 (1.16 to 8.16)) and were married (3.33 (1.34 to 8.28)) were more likely to ensure indoor ventilation.

4. Discussion

In summary, 45.0% of the subjects were considered under high health risk during cold weather but more than 60% (28.7% of all subjects) of this vulnerable group had underestimated their health risk. The uptake rates of cold protective measures were generally higher in a stronger cold wave except for ensuring indoor ventilation. Regarding associated factors of PCPB, those who had experienced adverse health effects during the 2016 cold wave, who perceived high health risk in low temperatures, females and the older groups (≥60) were more likely to apply PCPB in the cold waves studie.

Risk perception was associated with warm-keeping, cold protective behaviours in this study (wearing more clothes and using heating equipment). This was consistent with the results from previous hot effect studies from the UK [19], China [20] and Pakistan [21]. However, a significant proportion of subjects did not consider themselves more vulnerable in extremely low temperatures regardless of their age and history of chronic diseases and similar results have been reported in UK [38] and North American based cities (proportions not reported) [39]. The findings did highlight the gap in health literacy and self-risk perception and reconfirmed the need for targeted health education and services for the vulnerable groups, such as people with chronic disease and the elderly, to reduce exposures, and also highlighted the corresponding health outcomes and the related health burden. The two-year survey-based study has also suggested the adaptation ability of the population to low temperature by implementing personal protective measures based on personal experiences.

Our study found that females were more likely to uptake cold protective behaviours which agreed with the findings from previous studies [17,18]. Previous studies suggested this may be associated with less willingness to seek care or help among men than women, as reported previously [40]. Targeted health promotion can be considered for the male group. Older age was another demographic factor associated with higher adoption of PCPB, which was contradictory to the previous hot effect studies in the UK [18] and New York City [22]. Although the effect of age on uptake of health protection behaviours is unclear, the differences in physiological conditions that affect homeostatic process between age groups may explain our result. Older people generally have lower metabolic rate and compromised thermoregulation [41,42], which may make the elderly more sensitive to cold than heat [43]. Income or CSSA status, which was associated with hot protective behaviour in the UK [18], and education level, which was associated with cold protective behaviour in Europe, were not found to be associated in this study. One possibility is that most of the PCPBs in this study are straight forward, well-promoted by the Hong Kong Observatory and financially affordable (e.g., avoid staying in windy area), which made them less likely to affected by income and education level.

Special attention should be paid to results for ensuring indoor ventilation. While the population were more likely to adopt warm-keeping measures in the colder winter (2016), they were less likely to manage indoor ventilation. Hong Kong is a subtropical city in which central heating and housing design for cold insulation are not common. On cold days, people tend to shut doors and windows to reduce the drop in indoor temperature. Unlike regions with colder climates, facilities enhancing ventilation, such as trickle vent on window frames, are rarely found in Hong Kong. Shutting doors and windows leads to poor indoor ventilation. Poor ventilation is associated with higher risk of infectious diseases [4]. Indoor air quality and heating have been raised as an important element in building a sustainable living environment [44]. More investigation is needed to seek practical solutions in balancing indoor warming and ventilation during cold days in different settings to reduce relevant health risks.

To the authors' knowledge, this is the first study examining personal cold protective behaviours in a setting without central heating systems and cold-insulation housing design. This study covered PCPB on the coldest day in the region in the past six decades which allowed us to capture PCPB in response to an unusual cold wave and compare it to a that in a normal cold wave. The sample was representative in terms of gender and residential districts. The immediate outreach to subjects after the cold waves also helped reduce recall bias. This study has several limitations. Although the land-based telephone list covered 94% of fix line telephones in Hong Kong, the households that were not in the list of land-based telephone service were not included [28]. The follow-up rate was low due to the length of the survey (about 30 minutes). Thus, the age distribution of the 2017 follow-up sample might not be comparable to that of the general population. We adjusted age-group in statistical models for identifying associated factors of PCPB to reduce the bias. Due to the relatively small sample size, all chronic diseases were grouped and assessed as a single variable which might also introduce bias as behaviour may vary by disease. Effects of microclimate that might affect personal protective behaviours were not included in this study. The prompt interviews conducted, starting one week after the cold waves, might not be able to capture all adverse health effects, as cold-related health effects tended to have long lags [45–47]. The proportion of reporting unwell might be underestimated.

5. Conclusions

Our results showed that PCPB changed according to the intensity of cold waves, age, gender, past experiences and risk perception. Study findings agree with previous studies that vulnerable groups commonly underestimated their health-risk which might deter PCPB and increase risk of adverse health effects. Targeted health promotion should be provided to vulnerable groups, such as those with chronic diseases, old aged and living alone, to increase risk perception, and to males to raise their awareness of health protection against cold to reduce avoidable cold-related health risks. This study also raised the concern in balancing indoor warming and ventilation in warmer regions that are less prepared for low temperature. Studies investigating warm-keeping solutions without compromising ventilation should inform cold-related health protection strategies.

Supplementary Materials: The following are available online at http://www.mdpi.com/1660-4601/17/5/1672/s1, Table S1: Association between personal characteristics and uptake of personal cold protection behaviour in 2017 cold wave using Chi-square test; Table S2: Table showing age distribution in participants in the lost-to-follow-up group and 2016-17 cohort group; Figure S1: Diagram showing subject recruitment process.

Author Contributions: Conceptualization, E.Y.Y.C.; methodology, E.Y.Y.C., Z.H., S.L. and C.G.; data curation, Z.H., S.L., and C.G.; formal analysis, Z.H. and H.C.Y.L.; investigation, Z.H. and H.C.Y.L.; writing—original draft:

H.C.Y.L.; writing—review & editing and approval of the final version, E.Y.Y.C., Z.H., S.L., C.G., W.B.G., Z.H. and H.C.Y.L. All authors have read and agreed to the published version of the manuscript.

Funding: This work was supported by the Chinese University of Hong Kong (CUHK) Focused Innovations Scheme – Scheme A: Biomedical Sciences (Phase 2); the CUHK Climate Change and Health research project fund.

Acknowledgments: The authors would like to thank Hong Kong Observatory and all the participants for their support.

Conflicts of Interest: The authors declare no conflict of interest.

References

1. Gasparrini, A.; Guo, Y.; Hashizume, M.; Lavigne, E.; Zanobetti, A.; Schwartz, J.; Tobias, A.; Tong, S.; Rocklöv, J.; Forsberg, B.; et al. Mortality risk attributable to high and low ambient temperature: A multicountry observational study. *Lancet* **2015**, *386*, 369–375. [CrossRef]
2. Bunker, A.; Wildenhain, J.; Vandenbergh, A.; Henschke, N.; Rocklöv, J.; Hajat, S.; Sauerborn, R. Effects of air temperature on climate-sensitive mortality and morbidity outcomes in the elderly; A systematic review and meta-analysis of epidemiological evidence. *EBioMedicine* **2016**, *6*, 258–268. [CrossRef] [PubMed]
3. Handmer, J.; Honda, Y.; Arnell, N.; Benito, G.; Hatfield, J.; Fadl Mohamed, I.; Peduzzi, P.; Wu, S.; Sherstyukov, B.; Takahashi, K.; et al. Changes in impacts of climate extremes: Human systems and ecosystems. In *Managing the Risks of Extreme Events and Disasters to Advance Climate Change Adaptation*; Field, C.B., Barros, V., Stocker, T.F., Eds.; Cambridge University Press: Cambridge, UK; New York, NY, USA, 2012; pp. 231–290.
4. Seltenrich, N. Between extremes: Health effects of heat and cold. *Environ. Health Perspect.* **2015**, *123*, A275–A280. [CrossRef] [PubMed]
5. Curriero, F.C.; Heiner, K.S.; Samet, J.M.; Zeger, S.L.; Strug, L.; Patz, J.A. Temperature and mortality in 11 cities of the Eastern United States. *Am. J. Epidemiol.* **2002**, *155*, 80–87. [CrossRef] [PubMed]
6. Xu, Z.; Huang, C.; Hu, W.; Turner, L.R.; Su, H.; Tong, S. Extreme temperatures and emergency department admissions for childhood asthma in Brisbane, Australia. *Occup. Environ. Med.* **2013**, *70*, 730–735. [CrossRef]
7. Yu, W.; Guo, Y.; Ye, X.; Wang, X.; Huang, C.; Pan, X.; Tong, S. Science of the total environment the effect of various temperature indicators on different mortality categories in a subtropical city of Brisbane, Australia. *Sci. Total Environ.* **2011**, *409*, 3431–3437. [CrossRef]
8. Lin, Y.; Wang, Y.; Lin, P.; Li, M.; Ho, T. Science of the total environment relationships between cold-temperature indices and all causes and cardiopulmonary morbidity and mortality in a subtropical island. *Sci. Total Environ.* **2013**, *461–462*, 627–635. [CrossRef]
9. Chan, E.Y.Y.; Goggins, W.B.; Kim, J.J.; Griffiths, S.M. A study of intracity variation of temperature-related mortality and socioeconomic status among the Chinese population in Hong Kong. *J. Epidemiol. Community Health* **2012**, *66*, 322–327. [CrossRef]
10. Zhou, M.G.; Wang, L.J.; Liu, T.; Zhang, Y.H.; Lin, H.L.; Luo, Y.; Xiao, J.P.; Zeng, W.L.; Zhang, Y.W.; Wang, X.F.; et al. Health impact of the 2008 cold spell on mortality in subtropical China: The climate and health impact national assessment study (CHINAs). *Environ. Health* **2014**, *13*, 60. [CrossRef]
11. Goggins, W.B.; Chan, E.Y.Y.; Yang, C.; Chong, M. Associations between mortality and meteorological and pollutant variables during the cool season in two Asian cities with sub-tropical climates: Hong Kong and Taipei. *Environ. Health* **2013**, *12*, 59. [CrossRef]
12. Chau, P.H.; Wong, M.; Woo, J. Ischemic heart disease hospitalization among older people in a subtropical city — Hong Kong: Does winter have a greater impact than summer? *Int. J. Environ. Res. Public Health* **2014**, *11*, 3845–3858. [CrossRef] [PubMed]
13. Qiu, H.; Sun, S.; Tang, R.; Chan, K.-P.; Tian, L. Pneumonia hospitalization risk in the elderly attributable to cold and hot temperatures in Hong Kong, China. *Am. J. Epidemiol.* **2016**, *184*, 555–569. [CrossRef] [PubMed]
14. *United Nations Sendai Framework for Disaster Risk Reduction 2015–2030*; UNISDR: Geneva, Switzerland, 2015.
15. Ryti, N.R.I.; Guo, Y.; Jaakkola, J.J.K. Global association of cold spells and adverse health effects: A systematic review and meta-analysis. *Environ. Health Perspect.* **2016**, *124*, 12–22. [CrossRef] [PubMed]
16. Turner, L.R.; Barnett, A.G.; Connell, D.; Tong, S. Ambient temperature and cardiorespiratory morbidity: A systematic review and meta-analysis. *Epidemiology* **2012**, *23*, 594–606. [CrossRef]

17. Donaldson, G.; Rintamäki, H.; Näyhä, S. Outdoor clothing: Its relationship to geography, climate, behaviour and cold-related mortality in Europe. *Int. J. Biometeorol.* **2001**, *45*, 45–51. [CrossRef]
18. Khare, S.; Hajat, S.; Kovats, S.; Lefevre, C.E.; De Bruin, W.B.; Dessai, S.; Bone, A. Heat protection behaviour in the UK: Results of an online survey after the 2013 heatwave. *BMC Public Health* **2015**, *15*, 1–12. [CrossRef]
19. Lefevre, C.E.; Bruine de Bruin, W.; Taylor, A.L.; Dessai, S.; Kovats, S.; Fischhoff, B. Heat protection behaviors and positive affect about heat during the 2013 heat wave in the United Kingdom. *Soc. Sci. Med.* **2015**, *128*, 282–289. [CrossRef]
20. Ban, J.; Shi, W.; Cui, L.; Liu, X.; Jiang, C.; Han, L.; Wang, R.; Li, T. Health-risk perception and its mediating effect on protective behavioral adaptation to heat waves. *Environ. Res.* **2019**, *172*, 27–33. [CrossRef]
21. Rauf, S.; Bakhsh, K.; Abbas, A.; Hassan, S.; Ali, A.; Kächele, H. How hard they hit? Perception, adaptation and public health implications of heat waves in urban and peri-urban Pakistan. *Environ. Sci. Pollut. Res.* **2017**, *24*, 10630–10639. [CrossRef]
22. Lane, K.; Wheeler, K.; Charles-Guzman, K.; Ahmed, M.; Blum, M.; Gregory, K.; Graber, N.; Clark, N.; Matte, T. Extreme heat awareness and protective behaviors in New York City. *J. Urban Health* **2014**, *91*, 403–414. [CrossRef]
23. Burns, W.J.; Slovic, P. Risk perception and behaviors: Anticipating and responding to crises. *Risk Anal.* **2012**, *32*, 579–582. [CrossRef]
24. Ferrer, R.; Klein, W.M. Risk perceptions and health behavior. *Curr. Opin. Psychol.* **2015**, *5*, 85–89. [CrossRef] [PubMed]
25. Sund, B.; Svensson, M.; Andersson, H. Demographic determinants of incident experience and risk perception: Do high-risk groups accurately perceive themselves as high-risk? 2017, 20, 99–117. *J. Risk Res.* **2017**, *20*, 99–117. [CrossRef]
26. IPCC Summary for policymakers. In *Climate Change 2014: Impacts, Adaptation, and Vulnerability. Part A: Global and Sectoral Aspects. Contribution of Working Group II to the Fifth Assessment Report of the Intergovernmental Panel on Climate Change*; Field, C.B.; Barros, V.R.; Dokken, D.J. (Eds.) Cambridge University Press: Cambridge, UK; New York, NY, USA, 2014; pp. 1–32.
27. Hong Kong Observatory Cold and Very Hot Weather Warnings. Available online: http://www.hko.gov.hk/wservice/warning/coldhot.htm. (accessed on 2 March 2020).
28. Ying, E.; Chan, Y.; Huang, Z.; Ka, C.; Mark, M. Weather information acquisition and health significance during extreme cold weather in a subtropical city: A cross-sectional survey in Hong Kong. *Int. J. Disaster Risk Sci.* **2017**, *8*, 134–144.
29. Færevik, H. Clothing and protection in arctic environments. *J. Amb. Intel. Smart En.* **2015**, *14*, 7–9.
30. Day, R.; Hitchings, R. *Older People and Their Winter Warmth Behaviours: Understanding the Contextual Dynamics*; University of Birmingham: Birmingham, UK, 2009.
31. Tanner, L.M.; Moffatt, S.; Milne, E.M.G.; Mills, S.D.H.; White, M. Socioeconomic and behavioural risk factors for adverse winter health and social outcomes in economically developed countries: A systematic review of quantitative observational studies. *J. Epidemiol. Community Health* **2013**, *67*, 1061–1067. [CrossRef]
32. Budd, G.M. Ergonomic aspects of cold stress and cold adaptation. *Scand. J. Work Environ. Health* **2017**, *1*, 15–26.
33. Jones, S.; Duncan, E.R.; Thomas, N.; Walters, J.; Dick, M.C.; Height, S.E.; Stephens, A.D.; Thein, S.L.; Rees, D.C. Windy weather and low humidity are associated with an increased number of hospital admissions for acute pain and sickle cell disease in an urban environment with a maritime temperate climate. *Br. J. Haematol.* **2005**, *131*, 530–533. [CrossRef]
34. Li, P.; Chan, S. Application of a weather stress index for alerting the public to stressful weather in Hong Kong. *Meteorol. Appl.* **2000**, *7*, 369–375. [CrossRef]
35. McKee, C.M. Deaths in winter: Can Britain learn from Europe? *Eur. J. Epidemiol.* **1989**, *5*, 178–182. [CrossRef]
36. Olsen, N.D. Prescribing warmer, healthier homes. *Br. Med. J.* **2001**, *322*, 748–749. [CrossRef]
37. Sundell, J.; Levin, H.; Nazaroff, W.W.; Cain, W.S.; Fisk, W.J.; Grimsrud, D.T.; Gyntelberg, F.; Li, Y.; Persily, A.K.; Pickering, A.C.; et al. Ventilation rates and health: Multidisciplinary review of the scientific literature. *Indoor Air* **2011**, *21*, 191–204. [CrossRef]
38. Abrahamson, V.; Wolf, J.; Lorenzoni, I.; Fenn, B.; Kovats, S.; Wilkinson, P.; Adger, W.N.; Raine, R. Perceptions of heatwave risks to health: Interview-based study of older people in London and Norwich, UK. *J. Public Health (Bangkok)* **2008**, *31*, 119–126. [CrossRef]

39. Sheridan, S.C. A survey of public perception and response to heat warnings across four North American cities: An evaluation of municipal effectiveness. *Int. J. Biometeorol.* **2007**, *52*, 3–15. [CrossRef]
40. Doward, J. Men Risk Health by Failing to Seek NHS Help, Survey Finds. Available online: https://www.theguardian.com/society/2012/nov/04/men-failing-seek-nhs-help (accessed on 11 August 2017).
41. Frisard, M.I.; Broussard, A.; Davies, S.S.; Roberts, L.J.; Rood, J.; Jonge, L.D.; Fang, X.; Jazwinski, S.M.; Deutsch, W.A.; Ravussin, E. Aging, resting metabolic rate, and oxidative damage results from the Louisiana healthy aging study. *J. Gerontol. A Biol. Sci. Med. Sci.* **2007**, *62*, 752–759. [CrossRef]
42. Barzilai, N.; Huffman, D.M.; Muzumdar, R.H.; Bartke, A. The critical role of metabolic pathways in aging. *Diabetes* **2012**, *61*, 1315–1322. [CrossRef]
43. Guergova, S.; Dufour, A. Thermal sensitivity in the elderly: A review. *Ageing Res. Rev.* **2011**, *10*, 80–92. [CrossRef]
44. Sharpe, R.A.; Machray, K.E.; Fleming, L.E.; Taylor, T.; Henley, W.; Chenore, T.; Hutchcroft, I.; Taylor, J.; Heaviside, C.; Wheeler, B.W. Household energy efficiency and health: Area-level analysis of hospital admissions in England. *Environ. Int.* **2019**, *133*. [CrossRef]
45. Liu, J.; Ma, Y.; Wang, Y.; Li, S.; Liu, S.; He, X.; Li, L.; Guo, L.; Niu, J.; Luo, B.; et al. The impact of cold and heat on years of life lost in a Northwestern Chinese city with temperate continental climate. *Int. J. Environ. Res. Public Health* **2019**, *16*, 3529. [CrossRef]
46. Chai, G.; He, H.; Su, Y.; Sha, Y.; Zong, S. Lag effect of air temperature on the incidence of respiratory diseases in Lanzhou, China. *Int. J. Biometeorol.* **2020**, *64*, 83–93. [CrossRef]
47. Yi, W.; Chan, A.P.C. Effects of temperature on mortality in Hong Kong: A time series analysis. *Int. J. Biometeorol.* **2015**, *59*, 927–936. [CrossRef]

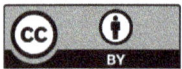

© 2020 by the authors. Licensee MDPI, Basel, Switzerland. This article is an open access article distributed under the terms and conditions of the Creative Commons Attribution (CC BY) license (http://creativecommons.org/licenses/by/4.0/).

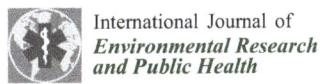

Review

A Literature Review on Psychosocial Support for Disaster Responders: Qualitative Synthesis with Recommended Actions for Protecting and Promoting the Mental Health of Responders

Maki Umeda [1,*], Rie Chiba [2], Mie Sasaki [1], Eni Nuraini Agustini [3,4] and Sonoe Mashino [1]

[1] Research Institute of Nursing Care for People and Community, University of Hyogo, 13-71 Kitaoji-cho, Akashi, Hyogo 673-8588, Japan; mie_sasaki@cnas.u-hyogo.ac.jp (M.S.); sonoe_mashino@cnas.u-hyogo.ac.jp (S.M.)
[2] Graduate School of Health Sciences, Kobe University, 7-10-2 Tomogaoka, Suma-ku, Kobe, Hyogo 654-0142, Japan; crie-tky@umin.ac.jp
[3] Graduate School of Nursing Art and Science, University of Hyogo, 13-71 Kitaoji-cho, Akashi, Hyogo 673-8588, Japan; eni.nuraini@uinjkt.ac.id
[4] School of Nursing, Faculty of Health Sciences, Syarif Hidayatullah State Islamic University, Jl. Kertamukti No.5 Cireundeu CiputatTangerang Selatan, Banten 15419, Indonesia
* Correspondence: maki_umeda@cnas.u-hyogo.ac.jp; Tel.: +81-78-925-9652

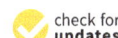

Received: 3 February 2020; Accepted: 16 March 2020; Published: 18 March 2020

Abstract: Little scientific evidence exists on ways to decrease the psychological stress experienced by disaster responders, or how to maintain and improve their mental health. In an effort to grasp the current state of research, we examined research papers, agency reports, the manuals of aid organisations, and educational materials, in both English and Japanese. Using MEDLINE, Ichushi-Web (Japanese search engine), Google Scholar, websites of the United Nations agencies, and the database of the Grants System for Japan's Ministry of Health, Labour, and Welfare, 71 pertinent materials were identified, 49 of which were analysed. As a result, 55 actions were extracted that could potentially protect and improve the mental health of disaster responders, leading to specific recommendations. These include (1) during the pre-activity phase, enabling responders to anticipate stressful situations at a disaster site and preparing them to monitor their stress level; (2) during the activity phase, engaging in preventive measures against on-site stress; (3) using external professional support when the level of stress is excessive; and (4) after the disaster response, getting back to routines, sharing of experiences, and long-term follow-up. Our results highlighted the need to offer psychological support to disaster responders throughout the various phases of their duties.

Keywords: disaster responders; support; psychosocial; risk management

1. Introduction

Natural disasters threaten every aspect of people's lives and are a significant burden on the health of those affected [1,2]. The alleviation of the health impacts resulting from disasters is of great concern to all countries, as the number and scope of disasters have been increasing worldwide due to global trends in urbanisation, environmental degradation, and climate change [3].

In the acute phase of a disaster response, treating physical health problems has often been prioritised. However, over the past two decades, the psychological impact of disasters has come to be a major focus of disaster health management [4–6]. The morbidity of psychiatric disorders after disasters has been reported to be as high as 60% [7], with an increased risk for anxiety, depression, stress-related disorders, and alcohol and substance abuse [8]. Deteriorating psychological health substantially decreases quality of life, and negatively affects physical and social functioning [9]. These facts highlight the importance of enhancing psychological health as critical to alleviating the health impact of disasters [10,11].

Disaster responders, such as health professionals, relief workers, public-service providers, and volunteer workers in disaster-affected areas, are at high risk for extreme stress, as are disaster survivors. Being a disaster responder involves exposure to traumatic events, a high level of work demands with limited resources, working with highly stressed populations in critical moments, and separation from home and family [4]. In addition, earlier studies have demonstrated that disaster responders generally felt unprepared and were not confident they would be able to effectively support others [12,13], which can result in psychological exhaustion and burn out.

In spite of the high likelihood of disaster responders experiencing mental health problems, little research has been conducted on ways to decrease their psychological stress and maintain or improve their mental health [14]. Existing studies suggest that programs providing knowledge about stress and stress management could improve the self-esteem of disaster responders, facilitate their self-care, and motivate them to engage in self-directive learning regarding their duties [15–18]. Programs aiming to alleviate existing psychological symptoms have also been found to be useful by some researchers [19]. On the other hand, a few studies did not find such programs effective [20,21]. Still other programs targeting disaster responders' mental health lack empirical evidence to support their effectiveness [22,23].

The present review was part of a project that aimed to develop a psychosocial support guide for disaster responders that could be used in a global setting. The purpose of this review was to identify the types of psychosocial support considered appropriate for disaster responders as a preliminary item pool for guide development. To achieve this aim we reviewed the non-academic literature, such as guides, manuals, and educational materials, to identify field-based knowledge and practices. Although the information in this review may not necessarily be tested scientifically, it does provide a comprehensive picture of field experiences that could be further scrutinised by scientific measures. Academic articles examining the effectiveness of psychosocial support specific to disaster responders were also reviewed as a primary source of evidence. Materials in English and Japanese do not cover all the generated information in other parts of the world, but it is anticipated that reports from Japan, which is one of the most disaster-prone countries and thus has a rich experience in disaster responses [24], could provide a solid knowledge base for exploring this issue.

In the following sections, we describe the procedure of our review and our analytical framework. Accordingly, our findings are presented using an analytical framework that groups the identified actions by their goals. To enhance their applicability to the field, the identified actions were further grouped by disaster response phase and actors. Lastly, we discuss the characteristics of these actions, and challenges in their implementation.

2. Material and Methods

2.1. Review Authors

All five authors conducted the literature search, and four of them analysed the data. All authors were from a nursing research institute specializing in disaster health management. Two of the authors are specialised in psychiatric nursing; one in nursing management and disaster nursing, one in acute care management, and the other in public health and epidemiology. All authors were project members for the development of a guide on psychosocial support for disaster responders, and all have field or research experience in disaster-affected areas.

2.2. Search Strategy

The search was conducted by all authors on MEDLINE (OVID), Ichushi-Web (Japanese search engine), Google Scholar, websites of United Nations (UN) agencies, and the database of the Grants System for Japan's Ministry of Health, Labour, and Welfare. The employed key search terms were "disaster"; "providers or responder"; "mental or psychological or psychosocial"; "support, education, or intervention"; and "critical incidence stress". The reference lists of relevant studies and reviews were also checked, and as a result, individual book chapters and educational brochures were included in our examination. Language was limited to English and Japanese. Below is a flow chart showing the study selection process (Figure 1).

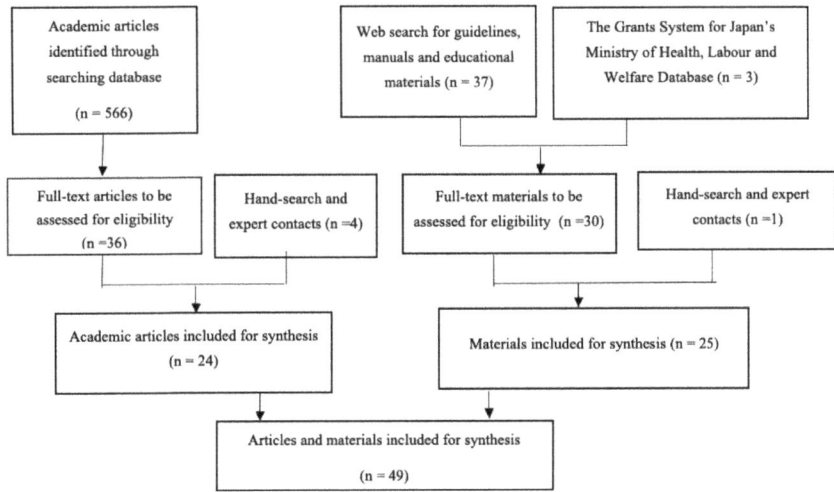

Figure 1. Selection of sources of evidence: academic articles and guidelines, manuals, and educational materials included for synthesis.

2.3. Inclusion Criteria

All types of materials, such as guidelines, manuals, educational materials, and research reports, were reviewed if they provided detailed information about actual or recommended psychosocial support for disaster responders. The initial focus of this review was psychosocial support for disaster responders who had not received formal training to respond to a natural disaster. Materials developed for firefighters and army personnel were not included because the support needs of these professionals would most likely differ from our target responders, owing to the difference in preparedness for critical-disaster-related incidents. On the other hand, we did not exclude materials with a broader scope than natural disasters when they provided applicable information to disaster responders.

2.4. Term Definitions

Psychological support is a composite term that was defined as any type of internal and external support that aims to protect or promote psychosocial well-being, prevent mental disorders, and facilitate treatment if needed [25].

2.5. Analysis

The analysis procedure was conducted by four review authors. At the beginning of the analysis, the authors discussed the analytical framework. With the aim of developing a guide applicable to broad societal contexts, goals were developed which were focused on enhancing field applicability by allowing variations in local contexts. Before setting the goals, we derived some actions from identified materials, and sorted these by disaster-response phase. Next, we categorised the actions into a group that aimed at the same goal (these were labelled "Goals"). Here, we explain in greater detail the procedures in each step by asking research questions.

The first question was "What should be done to protect or improve the mental health of responders?" To answer this question, the recommended actions for protecting and improving the mental health of disaster responders were extracted from the materials, and each action was separately recorded on a Post-It note. Upon reviewing these notes, it became apparent that there were two groups initiating these actions. The first was organisations that dispatch responders to disaster-affected areas or co-ordinate responders on site. The second was made up of disaster responders themselves, who were expected to maintain and enhance their own mental health.

The second question was "When should these actions be taken?" To answer this question, the various Post-It notes were grouped together on the basis of which activity phase the action was part of: the pre, during, or after phase of the disaster response. At this stage, similar types of data were gathered as a set of cards, and examined on the basis of whether they should be grouped as a single unit or independent sets. Then, a label was selected for a set of cards on the basis of reviewer consensus.

Once all information was classified by phase and actor, the final question was "For what reason should these actions be taken?" In exploring the goals of these actions, we focused on the stress and coping theory of Lazarus that conceptualises coping as a process of interpreting the cause of psychological stress (stressors), evaluating coping options, taking actions to reduce stress, and reappraising the coping process [26]. The three identified goals were (1) understanding stressors and making them manageable, (2) reducing stressors and preventing chronically stressful situations, and (3) responding to crises for those whose level of stress was overwhelming and something that could not be handled with normal coping strategies. Each action on the cards was classified under one of these goals to demonstrate the expected achievement of these actions.

3. Results

The search identified 71 materials and, eventually, 49 were used for analysis (Tables 1–3). Fifty-five actions that potentially protect and improve the mental health of disaster responders were extracted. Each action is explained below on the basis of its goal.

3.1. Goal 1: Understanding Stressors and Making them Manageable

Seventeen actions were identified under this goal (Table 1). Responders were encouraged to gather information on their duties and the area of operation, and then assess their readiness to join the disaster response team before enrolment [27–35]. Organisations were recommended to train responders to monitor their own stress levels for better stress self-management during a disaster response [17,21,27,28,31,32,35–47]. Making a thoughtful decision on who should be a member of the response team was also considered part of the role of the organisation before enrolment [28,36,37,42,43,47].

During the activity phase, monitoring stressors and their impact was considered a significant action for protecting responders' mental health at both the individual and the organisational level [25,27,29,30,37,38,41,45,48,49]. The re-conceptualisation of experience and feelings was specifically suggested for individuals as a way of taking an objective view of stressors and enhancing their coping ability [29,30,41,50].

After the activity, a reappraisal of experience and feelings during the activities was also recommended. In this post-phase, organisations were expected to provide opportunities for this reappraisal in the form of workshops, seminars, and the like [25,35,39,44,45,50–55]. Furthermore, organisations were encouraged to recognise the responders' work as an essential contribution to the organisational goals, and to demonstrate their appreciation to members of the organisation [30,35,41,50,56]. Continuous monitoring of responders' mental health was another action to be taken by both individuals and organisations [30,41,57–60].

Table 1. Actions for Goal 1: Understanding stressors and making them manageable.

Disaster Time	Actors	Actions	References
Before	Individual Actions	1. Gather information on one's duties and area of operation. 2. Identify possible challenges on site. 3. Assess the readiness of one's health, work, and family for enrolment. 4. Make an honest decision on whether they could join a disaster-response team.	[27–35]
	Organisational Actions	1. Train responders in monitoring their stress levels. 2. Address potential work-related stressors. 3. Consider thoroughly who should or should not be dispatched to disaster-affected areas.	[23,24,27,28,31,32,35–47]
During	Individual Actions	1. Use a stress checklist to assess the impact of stressors. 2. Accept one's own emotional reactions and tensions. 3. Re-conceptualise one's experience during duties, and feelings about them, from different angles.	[29,30,41,48,50]
	Organisational Actions	1. Enable responders to monitor their level of stress. 2. Monitor the physical and mental health of responders.	[25,27,37,38,41,43,45,49,50]
After	Individual Actions	1. Look back on what they experienced and take an objective view of those experiences. 2. Monitor one's mental health over the long term.	[29,30,35,41,59]
	Organisational Actions	1. Recognise disaster-response activities as a contribution to the missions of organisation. 2. Provide responders with opportunities for frankly talking about their experience and feelings. 3. Monitor responder's mental health over the long term.	[25,28,35,38,41,43,50–58,60]

3.2. Goal 2: Reducing Stressors and Preventing Chronically Stressful Situations

Twenty-five actions were found under this goal (Table 2). In addition to maintaining physical and mental wellbeing, solving concerns at home and work before enrolment were considered necessary preparation for lightening possible stressors that might add to the burden during disaster-response activities [25,28,35]. It was also recommended that responders learn stress-management skills and make their own self-care plan so that they can effectively respond to on-site stress [28,32,40,41,50], while organisations were expected to provide the relevant training opportunities [23,25,27–29,35,37–39,43,47,48,50,60–62]. In addition, improving teamwork, ensuring responders have clear ideas about their duties, and making an efficient operational system prior to deployment were considered effective ways of preventing stressful situations [28,41,44,48,50].

During the activities, responders were encouraged to take care of their physical and mental health. Maintaining their routines, refraining from use of stimulants or addictive substances such as caffeine, tobacco, and alcohol, and carrying out their own self-care plans were highly recommended [24,27–32,38,41,42,45,48,53,59,63]. On the organisational side, several actions were recommended, such as managing the responders' workload and duties, providing them with opportunities for informal communication and peer support, and holding defusing sessions [25,27–30,37,38,43–46,48,50,54,64–66].

After completing on-site duties, responders were encouraged to take time off from work in order to promote recovery from physical and psychological fatigue [27,29,40,59,67–69]. Making sure that responders can take this rest before coming back to routine work was recommended for organisations [24,25,39,41,50,57,70]. Changing from "disaster-response mode" to "routine mode" was seen as another effective means for maintaining the mental health of responders [30]. Offering a clear declaration of mission accomplishment and keeping responders informed about self-care were effective actions that could be taken by organisations [24,28,37,39,48,57,70].

Table 2. Actions for Goal 2: Reducing stressors and preventing chronically stressful situations.

Disaster Time	Actors	Actions	References
Before	Individual Actions	1. Promote and maintain one's physical and mental states. 2. Develop one's own self-care plan. 3. Explain to family members about the duties, and set up support and communication. 4. Disentangle one's concerns at home and at work.	[28,32,40,41,50]
	Organisational Actions	1. Improve responders' basic knowledge and skills of stress management. 2. Improve responders' teamwork skills. 3. Give responders a concrete idea of what their duties will be. 4. Develop means of communication with responders' family. 5. Develop an efficient operational system with a clear command chain. 6. Have a written and active policy for preventing and managing the stress of responders.	[23,25,27–29,32, 35,37–39,41,44,47, 48,50,60,61,70]
During	Individual Actions	1. Maintain routines for one's health. 2. Get enough rest and refresh oneself using the self-care plan. 3. Refrain from too much alcohol, tobacco, and caffeine. 4. Create mutually supportive teams with co-workers. 5. Keep connected with family and friends. 6. Keep a positive attitude in one's role.	[24,27–32,38,41, 42,45,48,50,53,59, 63,67,68]
	Organisational Actions	1. Control the volume and content of work given to responders. 2. Hold a defusing meeting to normalise responders' reactions to stressors. 3. Support responders' informal communication with their peers. 4. Develop a peer support system within the team (buddy system).	[25,27–30,37,38, 43–46,48,50,54,60, 64–66]
After	Individual Actions	1. Switch from a disaster-response to routine mode. 2. Take time off from work to recover from physical and psychological fatigue. 3. Spend time with family and friends.	[27,29,30,59,67–69]
	Organisational Actions	1. Clearly announce the end of disaster-response activities. 2. Ensure that responders can take time off work before returning to their routine there. 3. Provide responders with information on self-care.	[24,25,27,28,35,37, 39,41,48,50,57,70, 72]

Table 3. Actions for Goal 3: Responding to crises and alleviating stress.

Disaster Time	Actors	Actions	References
Before	Individual Actions	Develop personal indicators for extreme fatigue or crisis.	[32]
	Organisational Actions	1. Provide training of psychological first aid to make it immediately available to all responders in times of crisis. 2. Develop a system that responds to the traumatic experiences of responders.	[28,36,37,43,45,47, 50,56]
During	Individual Actions	1. Ask for help from mental health professionals. 2. Make a decision as to whether to continue with or resign one's duties.	[28,30,37,50,55]
	Organisational Actions	1. Give the responder time off, or lighten the volume and content of work. 2. Provide support that is specific to the crisis of that responder. 3. Ensure access to professional support from external organisations. 4. Make a decision as to whether the stressed-out responder should remain at the site or be replaced.	[24,25,28,31,37,42, 46,48,56,66]
After	Individual Actions	1. Ask for help from professionals. 2. Take rest until recovery from the mental health crisis.	[37,48,53,56,57,61, 71]
	Organisational Actions	Link responders and their families to social resources, including mental health professionals, to provide the responder with mental health care.	[24,25,27,28,30,36, 41,48,49,57,59,72]

Family was considered as a significant source of informal support for responders. Communication between responders and family members about their duties prior to deployment could be key to ensuring their families are supportive during and after deployment [28,32]. Organisations were also encouraged, prior to deployment, to develop a means of communicating with the responders' family during the deployment [43,50]. Staying connected to their family during deployment was also recognised as an effective way for responders to cope with their stress [25,28].

3.3. Goal 3: Alleviating Stressful Situations and Managing Crises

Thirteen actions were identified under this goal (Table 3). Becoming aware of one's own indicators of extreme fatigue and crisis before enrolment could be helpful to capture signs of crisis on site in a timely manner [32]. On the part of organisations [28,36,37,43,45,48,50,56], providing responders with psychological first-aid training was highly recommended in order to enable responders to be effective supporters to their peers. Building a system that effectively responds to the traumatic experience of responders prior to deployment was also considered an organisational responsibility.

Once stress becomes unavoidable, responders' workload and duties should be adjusted in order to ease their physical and psychological burden [25,28,37,42,46,48,56]. If the level of stress seems overwhelming, the use of mental-health professionals was suggested, and a decision as to whether an individual responder should continue with or resign their duties should be made [24,25,28,31,37,42,46,48,56,66].

After the completion of activities, responders who suffered from stress need rest for a considerable amount of time [37,56,57,71]. The use of resources, including mental health professionals, was also suggested in this phase [24,48,49,53,57–59]. In addition, adjusting the responder's routine work if the level of stress continued was considered part of the organisation's role [24,25,27,28,30,36,41,48,49,59,72].

4. Discussion

The identified actions in this study were implemented throughout all phases of disaster-response activities. Fifty-five actions to protect and promote the mental health of disaster responders were identified from the reviewed materials, and the three following goals were derived from these actions: "understanding stressors and making them manageable" (Goal 1), "reducing stressors and preventing chronically stressful situations" (Goal 2), and "alleviating stressful situations and managing crises" (Goal 3). These three goals can be summarised as the following three steps: "be aware", "prevent", and "respond".

Among the 55 actions, 17 fell under Goal 1, 25 under Goal 2, and 13 under Goal 3. Therefore, about 70% of the actions were preventive measures ("be aware" and "prevent"). Although responding to a stressor once it occurs is still an important countermeasure against negative impacts on metal health among disaster responders [9], understanding and reducing the occurrence of stressors and enhancing resilience can also be a major part of psychosocial support for disaster responders.

In regards to the timing of actions, most actions were to be performed before and during a disaster response, with 20 actions during the pre-period, 21 during an activity, and 14 during the post-period. Specifically, the largest number of actions for Goal 1 ("be aware") were found in the pre-period, for Goal 3 ("respond") in the activity period, and for Goal 2 ("prevent") in both the pre- and during periods. These results indicate that many types of psychosocial support were expected to be performed at the earlier stages of a disaster response. This notion echoes the view that pre- and peri-disaster preparation aimed at reducing stressors and responding to stress reactions can help prevent post-disaster mental-health problems [5].

Our findings also suggest that individual actions are as important as organisational support for the mental health of disaster responders, as almost the same number of actions were identified for individuals as for organisations. Individual actions, such as monitoring one's own stress level, managing stressors, and performing self-care, were considered to be essential, especially in disaster-affected areas, where each responder is perceived as a caregiver and works under very high-stress conditions with limited human and social resources [4]. Many organisational actions, such as "train responders to monitor their stress" (Goal 1), "improve the responders' basic knowledge and stress-management skills" (Goal 2), and "provide information on self-care" (Goal 2), were undertaken to support such individual actions.

Another important role of organisations was to develop a system to monitor, reduce, and respond to responders' stressors and stress reactions, including "develop an efficient operational system with a clear command chain", "have a written and active policy for preventing and managing stress among responders", "control the volume and content of work", and "develop a system that responds to the traumatic experiences of responders". Furthermore, recommendations such as "create mutually supportive teams with co-workers", "support responders' informal communications with their peers", and "develop a peer support system within the team" suggest that the use of a peer support system may be a promising psychosocial approach to building a resilient response team.

On the basis of these results, the following types of psychosocial support were considered to be helpful. The first focuses on preparing disaster responders for stressor management. Psychosocial support of this kind can be offered through training and knowledge dissemination on stress management, disaster-response duties, and team-building skills [4]. The second is to build the operational system, specifically in terms of reducing stressors from daily activities. Ongoing support, both informal and formal, needs to be established on a daily basis and over the long term [37]. Such support is crucial to maximising the productivity of the response team and achieving organisational goals, as well as protecting workers from stress-related mental disorders [37,50]. The third type is crisis support and management. When there is the need for timely support, external professional support can be helpful [37]. Clear written policies and manuals for its administration are needed to make it effective [37,41,48,49].

However, recommending these actions does not necessarily mean that they were implemented in the field. For example, a study conducted in the area affected by the Great East Japan Earthquake [50] found that a significant proportion of firefighters (42%) reported that long-term leave was the most prioritised measure for treating critical stress-related incidents caused by the disaster response. On the other hand, only 2% reported that their affiliated department offered them leave after completion of their response duties. Considering that human-resource management for firefighters is often better prepared for disaster situations, the unmet needs of other types of disaster responders, especially volunteer responders, may be even larger.

One of the possible barriers causing the gap between recommendations and implementation may be conflicts between routine work and disaster response. In the case that disaster response is not part of a routine, organisations may not be prepared when their staff leave work behind to respond to a disaster. A lack of supplementary staff to make up for their work would heavily burden their colleagues and the management department. Under such conditions, psychosocial support, such as training, monitoring, and offering long-term leave, may not be readily available for responders. In addition, personal characteristics, such as "calm and emotionally collected, acts on logic over emotion, exercises emotional control and self-control", are highly valued among disaster responders [73]. Therefore, seeking support for one's mental health conditions can be stigmatised in the culture of responders [50]. Individual counselling for all involved workers may be an effective way of reaching out to such responders [50]. This approach could eventually promote awareness that psychological reactions caused by a disaster response can affect anyone.

This study has the following limitations. First, the reviewed materials were all written in either Japanese or English. Although the derived information from the Japanese materials grew out of extensive experience in disaster response, the contexts of the disasters and the roles of the disaster responders may differ on the basis of geographical areas and cultural regions. In addition, our review covered recommended actions written in reports, guides, manuals, and research articles. Therefore, how many of these actions were performed in the field, and whether they were effective for protecting and improving the mental health of responders, remain unclear. For example, a systematic review conducted by Guilaran et al. [74] reported that the positive impact of interpersonal support was limited in the prevention of mental health problems among disaster responders. Thus, to develop an evidence-based package of psychosocial support for disaster responders, further studies examining the feasibility and effectiveness of these actions are needed.

5. Conclusions

Our results highlighted the need to offer psychological support to disaster responders throughout different activity phases. Support during the pre- and during activity periods may be crucial to preventing and minimising the negative impact of stressors associated with disaster response. Promoting self-care in accordance with stress monitoring can play a central role in psychosocial support. Therefore, organisational efforts in routinising self-care by controlling the workload and ensuring self-care opportunities are recommended. Disaster responders often work in an environment where team members and resources from different departments, organisations, and countries are assembled in an ad hoc manner. This condition makes it very difficult to build and operationalise a consistent support system. Co-ordinating disaster-response activities, including workload management and health monitoring of responders, cannot be viewed as dispensable, and the use of external resources may be one of the solutions. Barriers against these recommendations need to be identified in future research to bridge the gap between recommendations and implementation.

Author Contributions: All authors made substantial contributions, from the design stages of this study through to the final draft of the manuscript. All authors conducted the search and reviewed the articles. M.U., R.C., M.S., and S.M. conducted analysis for qualitative synthesis. M.U. wrote the first draft of the manuscript, and all the authors reviewed and made important, substantial input to the manuscript. The final draft was reviewed and approved by all authors. All authors have read and agreed to the published version of the manuscript.

Funding: This research received no external funding.

Conflicts of Interest: The authors declare no conflict of interest.

References

1. Brooks, S.K.; Dunn, R.; Amlôt, R.; Greenberg, N.; Rubin, G.J. Training and post-disaster interventions for the psychological impacts on disaster-exposed employees: A systematic review. *J. Ment. Health* **2018**. [CrossRef] [PubMed]
2. Dückers, M.L.A.; Thormar, S.B.; Juen, B.; Ajdukovic, D.; Newlove-Eriksson, L.; Olff, M. Measuring and modelling the quality of 40 post-disaster mental health and psychosocial support programmes. *PLoS ONE* **2018**, *13*, e0193285. [CrossRef] [PubMed]
3. Leaning, J.; Guha-Sapir, D. Natural disasters, armed conflict, and public health. *N. Engl. J. Med.* **2013**, *369*, 1836–1842. [CrossRef] [PubMed]
4. Benedek, D.M.; Fullerton, C.; Ursano, R.J. First responders: Mental health consequences of natural and human-made disasters for public health and public safety workers. *Annu. Rev. Public Health* **2007**, *28*, 55–68. [CrossRef] [PubMed]
5. Goldmann, E.; Galea, S. Mental health consequences of disasters. *Annu. Rev. Public Health* **2014**, *35*, 169–183. [CrossRef] [PubMed]
6. Shinfuku, N. Disaster mental health: Lessons learned from the Hanshin Awaji earthquake. *World Psychiatry* **2002**, *1*, 158–159.
7. Beaglehole, B.; Mulder, R.T.; Frampton, C.M.; Boden, J.M.; Newton-Howes, G.; Bell, C.J. Psychological distress and psychiatric disorder after natural disasters: Systematic review and meta-analysis. *Br. J. Psychiatry* **2018**, *213*, 716–722. [CrossRef]
8. Cox, R.S.; Danford, T. The need for a systematic approach to disaster psychosocial response: A suggested competency framework. *Prehosp. Disaster Med.* **2014**, *29*, 183–189. [CrossRef]
9. Foa, E.B.; Stein, D.J.; McFarlane, A.C. Symptomatology and psychopathology of mental health problems after disaster. *J. Clin. Psychiatry* **2006**, *67* (Suppl. 2), 15–25.
10. Lee, J.S.; You, S.; Choi, Y.K.; Youn, H.; Shin, H.S. A preliminary evaluation of the training effects of a didactic and simulation-based psychological first aid program in students and school counselors in South Korea. *PLoS ONE* **2017**, *12*, e0181271. [CrossRef]

11. Thorpe, L.E.; Assari, S.; Deppen, S.; Glied, S.; Lurie, N.; Mauer, M.P.; Mays, V.M.; Trapido, E. The role of epidemiology in disaster response policy development. *Ann. Epidemiol.* **2015**, *25*, 377–386. [CrossRef] [PubMed]
12. Fahim, C.; O'Sullivan, T.L.; Lane, D. Support needs for canadian health providers responding to disaster: New insights from a grounded theory approach. *PLoS Curr.* **2015**, *7*. [CrossRef] [PubMed]
13. O'Sullivan, T.L.; Dow, D.; Turner, M.C.; Lemyre, L.; Corneil, W.; Krewski, D.; Phillips, K.P.; Amaratunga, C.A. Disaster and emergency management: Canadian nurses' perceptions of preparedness on hospital front lines. *Prehosp. Disaster Med.* **2008**, *23*, s11–s18. [CrossRef] [PubMed]
14. Haugen, P.T.; Evces, M.; Weiss, D.S. Treating posttraumatic stress disorder in first responders: A systematic review. *Clin. Psychol. Rev.* **2012**, *32*, 370–380. [CrossRef]
15. Matsui, Y.; Tatewaki, Y. Countermeasures for thecritical incident stress from occupational mental health perspective: The care for the critical incidentstress of firefighters, the critical incident stress careand crisis intervention system. *Occup. Ment. Health* **2013**, *21*, 24–30.
16. Kobayashi, T.; Eguchi, M.; Imaki, H.; Saito, J.; Yoshinaga, Y.; Ishikawa, R.; Nakagaki, M.; Tuchiya, H. Effect of multidisciplinary training workshop related to mental health care after a disaster. *Bull. Cent. Educ. Res. Tech. Dev. Shizuoka Univ.* **2015**, *24*, 103–107.
17. Reid, W.M.; Ruzycki, S.; Haney, M.L.; Brown, L.M.; Baggerly, J.; Mescia, N.; Hyer, K. Disaster mental health training in florida and the response to the 2004 hurricanes. *J. Public Health Manag. Pract.* **2005**, *11*, S57–S62. [CrossRef]
18. Kuhls, D.A.; Chestovich, P.J.; Coule, P.; Carrison, D.M.; Chua, C.M.; Wora-Urai, N.; Kanchanarin, T. Basic Disaster Life Support (BDLS) training improves first responder confidence to face mass-casualty incidents in Thailand. *Prehosp. Disaster Med.* **2017**, *32*, 492–500. [CrossRef]
19. Kamena, M.; Galvez, H. Intensive residential treatment program: Efficacy for emergency responders' critical incident stress. *J. Police Crim. Psych.* **2019**. [CrossRef]
20. Miyamichi, R.; Ishikawa, S.; Omi, S. Efficacy of significant event analysis for stress management among disaster relief operation doctors: A non-blinded randomized control study. *Nihon Kyukyu Igakukai Zasshi* **2013**, *24*, 321–328. [CrossRef]
21. Salita, C.; Liwanag, R.; Tiongco, R.E.; Kawano, R. Development, implementation, and evaluation of a lay responder disaster training package among school teachers in Angeles City, Philippines: Using Witte's behavioral model. *Public Health* **2019**, *170*, 23–31. [CrossRef] [PubMed]
22. Hammond, J.; Brooks, J. The world trade center attack. Helping the helpers: The role of critical incident stress management. *Crit. Care Lond. Engl.* **2001**, *5*, 315–317. [CrossRef]
23. Yajima, J. The role of clinical psychologist in the support for disaster workers after disaster. *Jpn. J. Stress Sci.* **2019**, *33*, 330–332.
24. Yamamoto, T.; Tsunoda, T.; Yamashita, R. Operational stress management for members of Japan self-defense forces on the disaster relief mission of great east Japan earthquake. *Trauma. Stress Stud.* **2013**, *11*, 125–132.
25. Inter-Agency Standing Committee. *Guidelines on Mental Health and Psychosocial Support in Emergency Settings*; Inter-Agency Standing Committee: Geneva, Switzerland, 2007; Available online: https://www.who.int/mental_health/emergencies/guidelines_iasc_mental_health_psychosocial_june_2007.pdf (accessed on 2 September 2019).
26. Lazarus, R.S. *Emotion and Adaptation*; Oxford University Press: New York, NY, USA, 1991.
27. Asada, T. Psychological Care on Disaster. Psychological Support, Medical and Welfare, Life Support. Procedure Manual Version 1.0. 2015. Available online: http://www.jrc.or.jp/vcms_lf/care2.pdf (accessed on 2 September 2019).
28. Young, B.H.; Ford, J.D.; Ruzek, J.I.; Friedman, M.J.; Gusman, F.D. *Disaster Mental Health Handbook: Disaster Services: A Guidebook for Clinician and Administrators*; Department of Veterans Affairs, the National Center for Post-Traumatic Stress Disorder: California, USA, 2006; Available online: https://www.hsdl.org/?view&did=441325 (accessed on 18 March 2020).
29. Japanese Red Cross Society. *Mental Health Care in Disaster*; Japanese Red Cross Society: Tokyo, Japan, 2004; Available online: http://www.jrc.or.jp/vcms_lf/care2.pdf (accessed on 2 September 2019).
30. Japanese Red Cross Society. *Training Manual of Mental Health Care in Disaster for Trainers of Relief Workers*; Japanese Red Cross Society: Tokyo, Japan, 2012. Available online: http://ndrc.jrc.or.jp/infolib/cont/01/G0000001nrcarchive/000/070/000070821.pdf (accessed on 2 September 2019).

31. Takahashi, Y. Principles of mental health among care providers. *Hum. Mind* **2016**, *190*, 92–96.
32. United Nations High Commissioner for Refugees. *Emergency Handbook: Staff Wellbeing Version 2.9*; United Nations High Commissioner for Refugees: Geneva, Swizterland; Available online: https://emergency.unhcr.org/ (accessed on 2 September 2019).
33. World Health Organisation. *War Trauma Foundation and World Vision International: Psychological First Aid: Facilitator's Guide for Field Workers*; WHO: Geneva, Switzerland, 2011; Available online: https://apps.who.int/iris/bitstream/handle/10665/44615/9789241548205_eng.pdf;jsessionid=0AB6486F31E96F87EBAEE6F4772388FE?sequence=1 (accessed on 2 September 2019).
34. World Health Organization. *War Trauma Foundation and World Vision International: Psychological First Aid: Facilitator's Guide for Field Workers*; WHO: Geneva, Switzerland, 2013; Available online: https://apps.who.int/iris/bitstream/handle/10665/102380/9789241548618_eng.pdf?sequence=1&isAllowed=y (accessed on 2 September 2019).
35. Yamada, H.; Kujyu, M.; Yoshida, H. The research on the mental health and body health condition toward public health nurses working for the victims of East Japan Great Earthquake. *Jpn. Soc. Health Sci. Mind Body* **2013**, *9*, 26–36.
36. Office of Disaster Psychiatric Assistance Team. Activity Manual on Disaster Psychiatric Assistance Team: DPAT Version 2.0. Available online: http://www.dpat.jp/images/dpat_documents/3.pdf (accessed on 2 September 2019).
37. Antares Foundation. *Managing Stress in Humanitarian Workers: Guidelines for Good Practice*; Published 2012; Antares Foundation: Amsterdam, Netherlands, 2012; Available online: http://www.socialserviceworkforce.org/resources/managing-stress-humanitarian-workers-guidelines-good-practice (accessed on 2 September 2019).
38. Cabinet Office. *Psychological Care for Disaster Survivors: Management Guidelines for Prefectural Governments*; Cabinet Office: Tokyo, Japan, 2012.
39. Fukaya, H.; Yamamoto, K. A study of care for the nonprofessional supporters during large regional disaster. *Ritsumeikan Ningenkagaku Kenkyu* **2013**, *26*, 77–83.
40. Kim, Y.; Shimazu, K.; Kobayashi, M. Disaster Mental Health Activity Guidelines 2016: Review of domestic and international literature for developing a new comprehensive guidelines. In *Report for Health Labour Sciences Research Grant*; National Center of Neurology and Psychiatry: Tokyo, Japan, 2017.
41. Local Government Officials Association for the Promotion of Safety and Health. *Mental Health Promotion against Critical Incidence Stress in Disaster—Self-care and Organizational Measures*; Health Promotion Series of Workplace 61; Local Government Officials Association for the Promotion of Safety and Health: Tokyo, Japan, 2011.
42. Nagamine, M. Care for care providers during relief activities. *Hum. Mind* **2017**, *194*, 117–121.
43. Nagano Mental Health and Welfare Center. *Mental Health Care during Disasters—Manual for Disaster Responders*, 3rd ed.; Nagano Mental Health and Welfare Center: Nagano, Japan, 2015.
44. Narisawa, T.; Suzuki, Y.; Fukasawa, M. Toward development of a guideline for work-related stress management of care-providers in natural disasters; Consensus building through the Delphi process. *Jpn. J. Trauma. Stress* **2013**, *10*, 59–69.
45. Ohtsuka, E.; Matsumoto, J. Secondary traumatization of rescue workers and the mental health care system. *Bull. Nagano Coll. Nurs.* **2007**, *9*, 19–27.
46. Osawa, T. Critical Incident stress measures led by the fire and disaster management agency-from the Great Hanshin-Awaji Earthquake to the great east Japan earthquake, and future prospects. *Jpn. J. Trauma. Stress* **2013**, *11*, 17–24.
47. Shimizu, K. Preparation ahead of the relief activities: Education and training. *Hum. Mind* **2017**, *193*, 124–129.
48. International Recovery Platform Secretariat & United Nations Development Program. *Guidance Note on Recovery: Psychosocial*; International Recovery Platform Secretariat & United Nations Development Program: Hyogo, Japan, 2010; Available online: https://www.unisdr.org/files/18781_irppsychosocial.pdf (accessed on 2 September 2019).
49. Sawaguchi, R.; Misao, H. Support activities for care providers: Lessons learned from the Great East Japan Earthquake. *Nursing (London)* **2014**, *34*, 108–115.

50. Suzuki, Y.; Fukasawa, M.; Nakajima, S.; Narasawa, T.; Kono, K.; Kim, Y. *Manual for Disaster Mental Health*; National Institute of Mental Health, National Center of Neurology and Psychiatry: Tokyo, Japan, 2011; Available online: https://www.ncnp.go.jp/nimh/seijin/H22DisaManu110311.pdf (accessed on 2 September 2019).
51. Abe, Y. Yuragi of volunteer operating in distressed areas and her/his need of care: In terms of volunteer as learner. *Waseda Educ. Res.* **2012**, *3*, 27–41.
52. Fujishiro, T. Critical incident stress management in Japanese police. *Jpn. J. Trauma. Stress* **2013**, *11*, 41–49.
53. Nakanobu, R. How to support nurses who provided disaster nursing care in affected area. *Kochi Women Univ. J. Nurs. Acad.* **2012**, *37*, 7–11.
54. Setou, N. Challenges in supporting the aid workers at the areas afflicted by the Great East Japan earthquake and tsunami -findings through support activities for the bereaved in the disaster areas. *Konan Womens Coll. Res.* **2013**, *7*, 49–55.
55. Yamazaki, T. Support for nurses who experienced critical incident stress in the line of duty. *Occup. Ment. Health* **2013**, *21*, 4–8.
56. Ministry of Health, Labor and Welfare. *About the Disaster Health Emergency Assistance Team*; Ministry of Health, Labor and Welfare: Tokyo Japan. Available online: http://www.mhlw.go.jp/file/05-Shingikai-10901000-Kenkoukyoku-Soumuka/0000131931.pdf (accessed on 2 September 2019).
57. Kato, H. Helper's help following major disaster. *J. Clin. Psychiatry* **2013**, *55*, 1011–1016.
58. Takahashi, S. Follow up for care providers. *Hum. Mind* **2017**, *196*, 113–119.
59. Mental Health Working Group of Osaka Center for Disabled. Osaka Disabled Liaison Conference for Countermeasure for Emergencies in Great East Japan Earthquake. Available online: http://www.ritsumei.ac.jp/~{}kohei-y/lab/staff.pdf (accessed on 2 September 2019).
60. Ministry of Health, Labor and Welfare. *Guidelines for Activities of Child Guidance Center at the Time of Disaster*; Ministry of Health, Labor and Welfare: Tokyo, Japan, 2013. Available online: https://www.mhlw.go.jp/bunya/kodomo/pdf/dv130424_1.pdf (accessed on 2 September 2019).
61. Ito, T.; Tsukada, Y.; Suzuki, S. Briefing to the nursing staff to be dispatched for the disaster assistance—Attempt of the briefing in Graduate School of Nursing, Chiba University at the 2016 Kumamoto Earthquake. *J. Grad. Sch. Nurs. Chiba Univ.* **2017**, *39*, 59–63.
62. Occupational Safety and Health Administration (OSHA): Outreach Training Program, Disaster Site Worker Procedures. Available online: https://www.osha.gov/dte/outreach/disaster/disaster_procedures.pdf (accessed on 2 September 2019).
63. Sato, D.; Shimoyama, M.; Yoshida, T. Evaluation of fatigue among staff in areas stricken by the Great East Japan Earthquake for disaster-related condition nursing. *J. Jpn. Soc. Disaster Nurs.* **2017**, *18*, 24–35.
64. Fuji, N. Group-based support for care providers. *Hum. Mind* **2017**, *192*, 68–72.
65. Osawa, T.; Kato, H. *Disaster Stress and Mental Health Countermeasures in Disaster Relief Organization Past and Future*; Hyogo Institute for Traumatic Stress: Hyogo, Japan, 2016; Available online: http://www.j-hits.org/function/research/pdf/28_4chouki.pdf (accessed on 2 September 2019).
66. UNICEF: Staff Well-Being Guidelines and Good Practice. Available online: http://unicefinemergencies.com/downloads/eresource/docs/3.3%20Human%20Resources/Staff%20Well-Being%20Guidelines%20and%20Good%20Practices%20-%207%20December%202009.pdf (accessed on 2 September 2019).
67. Hyogo Nursing Association. *Disaster Support Nurse: Manual for Nursing Practice*; Hyogo Nursing Association, 2012. Available online: https://www.hna.or.jp/archives/001/201512/saigai_manual.pdf (accessed on 2 September 2019).
68. Study Group of Press Workers' Stress. *Manual for Responding Critical Incidence Stress*; Study Group of Press Workers' Stress: Ibaraki, Japan, 2016; Available online: http://www.human.tsukuba.ac.jp/~{}ymatsui/disaster_manual3.html (accessed on 2 September 2019).
69. Suzuki, Y.; Fukasawa, M.; Nakajima, S.; Narisawa, T.; Kim, Y. Development of disaster mental health guidelines through the Delphi process in Japan. *Int. J. Ment. Health Syst.* **2012**, *6*, 7. [CrossRef] [PubMed]
70. Fujiwara, T. Care for care providers after relief activities. *Hum. Mind* **2017**, *195*, 92–96.
71. Ozaki, A.; Osaka, T.; Ikeda, M.A. Systematic review of psychosocial support by clinical psychologists in disaster. *Obirin Psychol. Res.* **2016**, *7*, 33–41.
72. Japan Psychiatric Hospitals Association. In *Guide for Manual Preparation of Disaster Countermeasures at Psychiatric Hospital*; Japan Psychiatric Hospitals Association: Tokyo, Japan, 2015.

73. King, R.V.; North, C.S.; Larkin, G.L.; Downs, D.L.; Klein, K.R.; Fowler, R.L.; Swienton, R.E.; Pepe, P.E. Attributes of effective disaster responders: Focus group discussions with key emergency response leaders. *Disaster Med. Public Health Prep.* **2010**, *4*, 332–338. [CrossRef]
74. Guilaran, J.; de Terte, I.; Kaniasty, K.; Stephens, C. Psychological outcomes in disaster responders: A systematic review and meta-analysis on the effect of social support. *Int. J. Disaster Risk Sci.* **2018**, *9*, 344–358. [CrossRef]

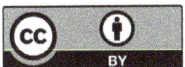

© 2020 by the authors. Licensee MDPI, Basel, Switzerland. This article is an open access article distributed under the terms and conditions of the Creative Commons Attribution (CC BY) license (http://creativecommons.org/licenses/by/4.0/).

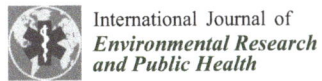

Article

Sociodemographic Predictors of Health Risk Perception, Attitude and Behavior Practices Associated with Health-Emergency Disaster Risk Management for Biological Hazards: The Case of COVID-19 Pandemic in Hong Kong, SAR China

Emily Ying Yang Chan [1,2,3,*], Zhe Huang [1], Eugene Siu Kai Lo [1], Kevin Kei Ching Hung [1,4], Eliza Lai Yi Wong [3] and Samuel Yeung Shan Wong [3]

1. Collaborating Centre for Oxford University and CUHK for Disaster and Medical Humanitarian Response (CCOUC), The Chinese University of Hong Kong, Hong Kong, China; huangzhe@cuhk.edu.hk (Z.H.); euglsk@cuhk.edu.hk (E.S.K.L.); kevin.hung@cuhk.edu.hk (K.K.C.H.)
2. Nuffield Department of Medicine, University of Oxford, Oxford OX37BN, UK
3. JC School of Public Health and Primary Care, The Chinese University of Hong Kong, Hong Kong, China; lywong@cuhk.edu.hk (E.L.Y.W.); yeungshanwong@cuhk.edu.hk (S.Y.S.W.)
4. Accident & Emergency Medicine Academic Unit, The Chinese University of Hong Kong, Prince of Wales Hospital, Hong Kong, China
* Correspondence: emily.chan@cuhk.edu.hk; Tel.: +852-2252-8411

Received: 28 April 2020; Accepted: 28 May 2020; Published: 29 May 2020

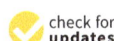

Abstract: In addition to top-down Health-Emergency and Disaster Risk Management (Health-EDRM) efforts, bottom-up individual and household measures are crucial for prevention and emergency response of the COVID-19 pandemic, a Public Health Emergency of International Concern (PHEIC). There is limited scientific evidence of the knowledge, perception, attitude and behavior patterns of the urban population. A computerized randomized digital dialing, cross-sectional, population landline-based telephone survey was conducted from 22 March to 1 April 2020 in Hong Kong Special Administrative Region, China. Data were collected for socio-demographic characteristics, knowledge, attitude and risk perception, and various self-reported Health-EDRM behavior patterns associated with COVID-19. The final study sample was 765. Although the respondents thought that individuals (68.6%) had similar responsibilities as government (67.5%) in infection control, less than 50% had sufficient health risk management knowledge to safeguard health and well-being. Among the examined Health-EDRM measures, significant differences were found between attitude and practice in regards to washing hands with soap, ordering takeaways, wearing masks, avoidance of visiting public places or using public transport, and travel avoidance to COVID-19-confirmed regions. Logistic regression indicated that the elderly were less likely to worry about infection with COVID-19. Compared to personal and household hygiene practices, lower compliance was found for public social distancing.

Keywords: COVID-19; urban; health risks; Health-Emergency and Disaster Risk Management; biological hazard; pandemic; PHEIC; Hong Kong

1. Introduction

The COVID-19 pandemic was considered a Public Health Emergency of International Concern (PHEIC) by the World Health Organization (WHO) on 30 January 2020 [1]. The SARS-CoV2 belongs to the coronavirus family, which is the same family as the severe acute respiratory syndrome (SARS) and middle east respiratory syndrome (MERS) viruses [2]. It was first reported as a cluster of respiratory illnesses in Wuhan, China, on 30 December 2019. As of 12 April 2020, there were 1,844,863 confirmed cases and 117,021 deaths according to the World Health Organization report [3]. The case-fatality rate resulting from SARS-CoV2 is believed to be around 1%–2% for symptomatic cases [4,5], and the proportion of asymptomatic cases of COVID-19 is much higher [6]. With a higher basic reproductive number than SARS and MERS, and the finding of viral shedding in asymptomatic patients [7], the total number of people infected and killed by COVID-19 exceeds SARS and MERS combined, even though it is less deadly than them [8]. As of April 2020, although more than 200 countries have reported confirmed cases and have implemented travel restrictions [9], social distancing [10] and other response measures to this PHEIC, the global COVID-19 epidemic is yet to end.

The Situation in Hong Kong and Past Experiences of Similar Pandemics

Figure 1 shows that on 23 January 2020, Hong Kong reported its first imported case of COVID-19 [11] and the first local transmission emerged on 31 January 2020 [12]. As of 14 April, there were 1013 confirmed cases [13]. As soon as cases were confirmed in Hong Kong, the Hong Kong government implemented various infection control measures (Figure 1a), including declaring emergency response levels in relation to COVID-19 infection [14], suspending class resumption for all schools and community services [15,16], and prohibiting citizen outdoor activities and gatherings [17–20]. At that time, there were a substantial number of confirmed cases of the epidemic (Figure 1b).

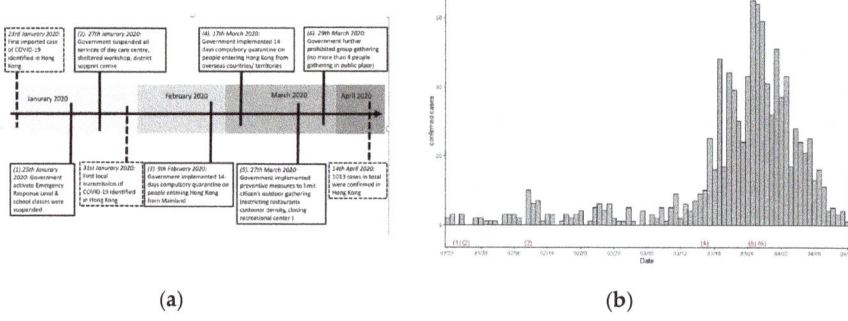

Figure 1. (a) Timeline of the COVID-19 outbreak in Hong Kong and the preventive measures implemented by the Hong Kong government. (b) The confirmed cases in Hong Kong from 23 January 2020 to 16 April 2020. Note: (1) to (6) in Figure 1b correspond to (1) to (6) in Figure 1a.

The Health-Emergency and Disaster Risk Management (Health-EDRM) Framework provides a common language and a comprehensive approach for all actors in health and other sectors, to reduce health risks and consequences of emergencies and disasters [21]. Biological hazards, such as infectious disease outbreaks, are considered one of the major health risks for the human population. Besides top-down government efforts in infection control and management, efforts at the individual and household level also have crucial roles in bottom-up resilience of Health-EDRM for biological hazards. Currently, limited scientific evidence is available to understand patterns of knowledge, perception, attitude and behavior undertaken by urban populations for relevant disaster risk reduction programs and policy planning. Hong Kong, as an Asian metropolis in Southern China, has encountered various infectious disease outbreaks, like SARS [22] and avian influenza (e.g., H5N1 and H7N9) [23,24]. Its healthcare system has pre-existing policies and practices against emerging infectious diseases [25]. For example, wearing face masks, washing hands, and disinfecting living quarters for SARS [26], and avoiding contact with birds for the avian influenza [27], are examples of community bottom-up Health-EDRM practices for self-help and contribution to infection control. This study, using a population-based, computerized randomized digital dialing landline telephone survey, intends to examine and explore various primary Health-EDRM prevention efforts in the community through self-reported knowledge, perception and behaviors related to COVID-19 and various droplet borne-transmission control-related Health-EDRM preventive measures among the Hong Kong population [28,29].

2. Materials and Methods

2.1. Study Design and Study Population

A computerized randomized digital dialing (RDD), cross-sectional, population landline-based telephone survey was conducted from 22 March to 1 April 2020. The study population consisted of Hong Kong residents aged 18 years or above, including those holding valid work or study visas. Sample exclusion criteria included (i) non-Cantonese-speaking respondents; (ii) overseas visitors holding tourist visas to Hong Kong or two-way permit holders from mainland China; (iii) those unable to be interviewed due to medical reasons; and iv) non-institutional residents. For the sample size estimation, an assumption was made that 50% of the Hong Kong population were concerned about contracting COVID-19. A sample size of 750 participants was calculated with a 3.6% margin of error and 95% confidence interval.

2.2. Data Collection

The computerized random digit dialing (RDD) method was used for each of Hong Kong's 18 districts to randomly select a representative sample. Stratified random sampling was used to ensure the demographic representation of the general population in Hong Kong in terms of age, gender, and district of residence. This data collection method has been used for other similar local studies on infectious diseases [30,31]. Most of the calls were made during evenings (6:30 pm to 10:00 pm) to avoid an under-representation of the working population. An eligible family member whose birthday was closest to the survey date was invited to participate in the study. If the selected participant was busy at the time, up to four follow-up calls would be made before that number was considered unanswered. All telephone interviews were conducted by trained interviewers in Cantonese. Figure 2 shows that 765 eligible participants were recruited to account for missing values and increase the modelling flexibility.

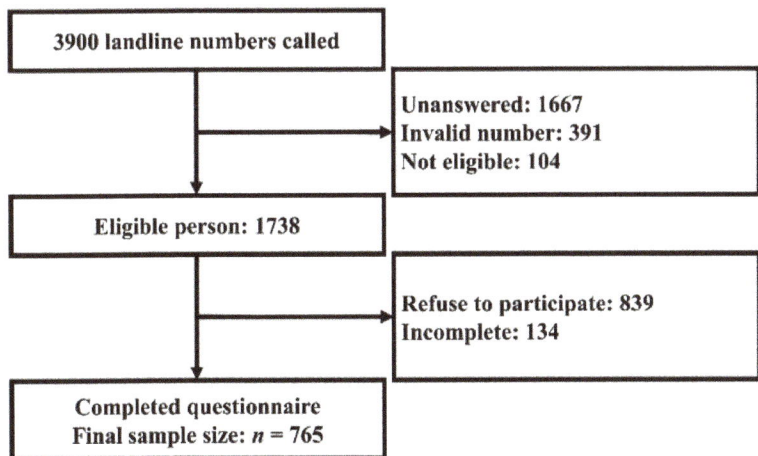

Figure 2. The algorithm of the final data collection.

2.3. Study Instrument

A self-reported structured Chinese questionnaire with 141 questions was designed on the basis of a literature review and previous research experience [27,30–34] on data collection. Information was collected on socio-demographic characteristics, knowledge, attitude and risk perception, and various behavior patterns associated with COVID-19. Sociodemographic information, current and preferred channels of information acquisitions were similar to a number of published study tools of human behavior in extreme events in the same context [30,35,36]. Questions related to "knowledge about COVID-19", "risk perception", "self-reported perception and Health-EDRM practices" and "caregiving", were adopted from previous studies [27,30,31]. A summary of the survey questions can be grouped into six major subgroups as follows.

1. Sociodemographic information was collected for age, gender, district of residence, household income, household size, marital status, education, size of housing, occupation and employment status.
2. Knowledge about COVID-19, including the transmission route, and the comparison between COVID-19 and other respiratory diseases.
3. Risk perception of Health-EDRM behavior associated with COVID-19, including the perceived impacts (e.g., physical, mental, social, financial and the whole impact), perceived sufficient knowledge to manage COVID-19, perceived severity and infectivity. Five-point Likert scales were used to measure the level of agreement or disagreement for the questions (from 1 to 5, 1 = strongly disagree, 2 = disagree, 3 = neutral, 4 = agree, 5 = strongly agree). The 6-item short form of the State-Trait Anxiety Inventory (STAI) was used for measuring their current anxiety level concerning the outbreak [32]. A binary question of whether the respondent was worried about getting infected with COVID-19 was asked.
4. Self-reported perceived usefulness and actual Health-EDRM behavioral practice of nine personal or household health emergency disaster risks management related behaviors and practices of COVID-19 prevention behavior. These include: (1) washing hands before meals and after toileting, (2) washing hands with soaps, (3) avoiding dining or gathering together, (4) using serving utensils, (5) ordering takeaways more often, (6) bringing one's own utensil when dining out, (7) wearing a mask when going out, (8) avoiding going to public places or using public transport, and (9) avoiding going to COVID-19-confirmed regions outside Hong Kong. The four-point Likert scale was used to ascertain the level of the practices (from 1 to 4, 1 = always, 2 = usually, 3 = sometimes, 4 = never).
5. Current and preferred channels of information acquisition, the information they were interested in and the awareness of COVID-19.
6. Questions about home quarantine and caregiving to non-suspected family members during the COVID-19 outbreak were also asked.

We focused on the general patterns of health risk perception, attitude and behavior practices associated with Health-Emergency Disaster Risk Management. Each interview took about 20–40 min. A pilot survey study ($n = 28$) was conducted in March 2020 to ensure interpretability and feasibility of the questions. Verbal consent was obtained from the participants and ethics approval and the consent procedure of the study were reviewed and obtained from the Survey and Behavioral Research Ethics Committee at The Chinese University of Hong Kong (SBRE-19-498).

2.4. Statistical Analysis

Descriptive statistics were reported for the study sample socio-demographic characteristics, awareness, perception and knowledge of COVID-19. Statistical association tests (Pearson's χ^2 test, Fisher's exact test, or McNemar's test) were conducted where appropriate. A binary variable of whether the respondent was worried about getting infected with COVID-19 was used as the dependent variable in logistic regression. Explanatory variables entered into multivariable logistic regression if the *p*-value < 0.10 in bivariate analysis. Apart from the worry, various community patterns and individual uptake of Health-EDRM behavior associated with COVID-19 as dependent variables were dichotomized for logistic regression ("always" or "usually" versus "sometimes" or "never"). The level of significance of the statistical test was 0.05. All statistical analyses were conducted by using IBM SPSS 21 (IBM Corp., Armonk, NY, USA) for Windows.

3. Results

The final study sample consisted of 765 respondents and a response rate of 44.0% (765/1738) (Table 1). The final study sample was comparable and representative of the population data in the Hong Kong Census 2016 [37] with respect to their age, gender, marital status and residential districts. However, the level of education and household income in our sample were higher than the population census.

Table 1. The respondent's socioeconomic characteristics and comparison with Census population data.

Demographics	2016 Population Census		Study Sample		*p*-Value [d]
Age	*n*	%	*n*	%	0.332
18–24	600,726	9.50%	71	9.30%	
25–44	2,228,566	35.26%	248	32.40%	
45–64	2,328,430	36.84%	303	39.60%	
65 or older	1,163,153	18.40%	143	18.70%	
Gender					0.425 [e]
Male	2,850,731	45.10%	356	46.50%	
Female	3,470,144	54.90%	409	53.50%	
Marital status					0.962 [e]
Non-married	2,523,742	39.93%	304	39.80%	
Married	3,797,133	60.07%	459	60.20%	
Residential district [a,b]					0.334
Hong Kong Island	1,120,143	17.2%	147	19.20	
Kowloon	1,987,380	30.6%	231	30.20	
New Territory	3,397,499	52.2%	387	50.60	
Education [a]					<0.001
Primary level or below	1,673,431	25.7%	61	8.00%	
Secondary	2,841,510	43.7%	330	43.30%	
Tertiary level	1,991,189	30.6%	371	48.70%	
Household Income [c]					<0.001
<2000–7999	378,451	15.1	66	9.3	
8000–19999	649,450	25.9	101	14.1	
20000–39999	699,450	27.8	191	26.6	
40000 or more	782,383	31.2	360	50.2	

[a] The Hong Kong population Census data additionally included age 15 to 17 years old. [b] Marine population was excluded. [c] The analysis was conducted with household data; only 718 households were available in our sample. [d] The χ^2 test was used to measure the overall difference between this survey and the 2016 Hong Kong Population Census data. A *p*-value < 0.05 indicates a significant difference. [e] The χ^2 test with continuity correction was used.

3.1. Perception of Various Health and Economic Impacts of COVID-19

Figure 3 describes the respondents' perception of various health impacts brought on by COVID-19. Although 94.4% (722/765) of the study respondents believed that COVID-19 had a large impact on their community, social health was reported as the most affected (72.0%). In addition, participants reported the role of government policy (68.6%) would be similar to the effort put in at the household or individual level (67.5%). However, although 63.9% (489/765) believed they had enough knowledge for regular communicable diseases (e.g., influenza), less than half of the participants (47.8%) reported that they had sufficient knowledge to manage the health risk and safety during the outbreak of COVID-19. After adjusting for age, gender, education, household income, and occupation, multiple logistic regression suggested that people aged 65 or above were less likely to be impacted by COVID-19 in terms of their mental, social and financial status, while people with less household income were more likely to be affected financially. In addition, females were more likely to report a large impact on their mental health, but none of the above sociodemographic variables were associated with the reported physical health (Appendix A Table A1).

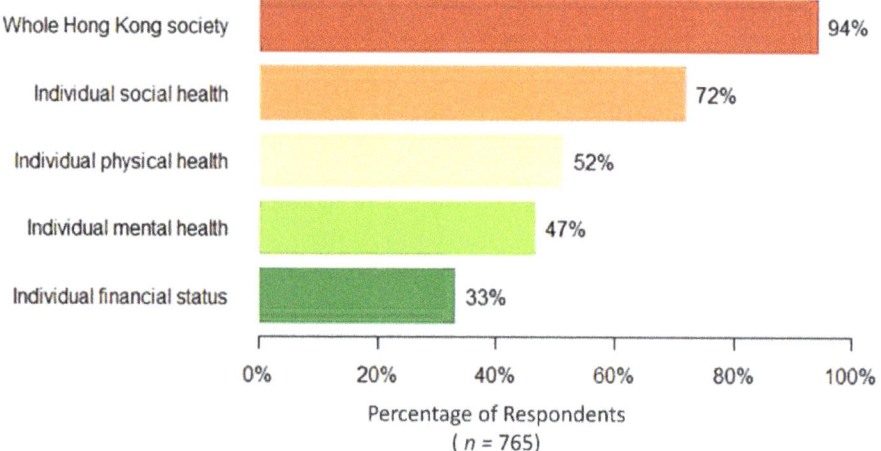

Figure 3. Self-reported large or very large impacts of COVID-19 on various dimensions.

3.2. Knowledge and Risk Perception of COVID-19

Regarding the overall knowledge and understanding of COVID-19, results indicated that most respondents could identify that the disease could be transmitted through droplets, direct or indirect hand contact, fecal contamination, and contact with asymptomatic patients (Figure 4). Yet, confusion was found with some reporting of unconfirmed transmission routes (e.g., insects as vectors) and about 24% (181/764) of the respondents did not believe that asymptomatic patients could transmit the disease, which might affect adoption of appropriate practices. Respondents with a higher level of education were more likely to correctly identify whether insects and asymptomatic patients can transmit the virus (Appendix A Table A1).

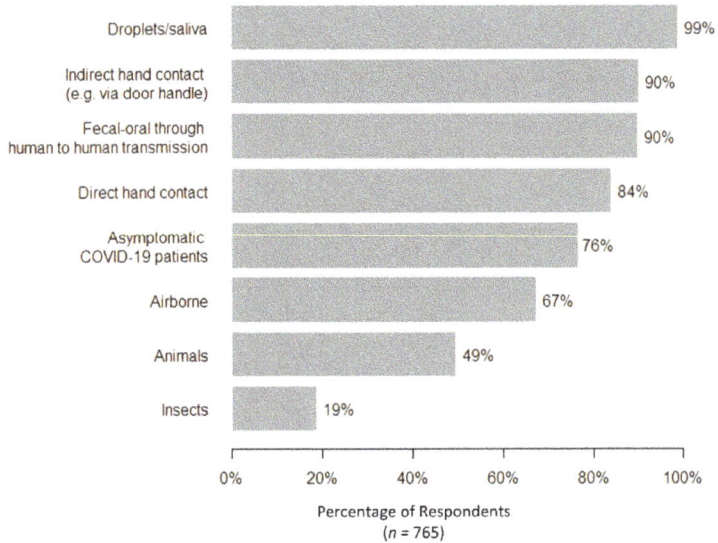

Figure 4. Reported believed transmission mode for COVID-19.

For the perceived infectivity of COVID-19, about 96% (34/765) believed the infectivity was high or very high and that it was much higher than SARS (78.0%) and seasonal influenza (52.5%). For the perceived severity, about 80% (156/765) believed it had a severe or very severe harm to health, which was less than SARS (90.5%) but higher than seasonal influenza (21.6%).

3.3. Attitude and Uptake of Health-EDRM Behavior Practice towards COVID-19

Although the uptake of Health-EDRM practice varied, most respondents agreed that personal or household preventive measures could reduce the transmission of COVID-19 (Table 2). Significant statistical differences were found between attitude and practice in regards to washing hands with soap, ordering takeaways more often, wearing masks when going out, avoidance of visiting public places or using public transport, and avoidance of travelling beyond COVID-19-confirmed regions outside Hong Kong. Furthermore, a comparison of the behavior of wearing masks before and after the epidemic found that when going outdoors, mask wearing had increased from 11.3% (86/764) before the epidemic to 97.4% after the disease outbreak (McNemar's test, p-value < 0.001). Compared to personal and household hygiene, compliance of social distancing in public was lower. After adjusting for age, gender, education, household income, and occupation, multiple regression revealed that male gender was significantly negatively associated with the behavior of washing hands with soap and the avoidance of dining and gathering together. Compared to white collar workers, housewives and the unemployed or retired were more likely to avoid going to public places or using public transport (Appendix A Table A2).

Table 2. Perceived usefulness and practice of preventive measures against COVID-19.

Control Measures that Can Protect from COVID-19 Infections	Thought It Was Useful for Prevention		Always or Usually Practicing Currently		Attitude vs. Practice [a]
	n	%	n	%	p-Value
Wash hands before meals and after toilet	749	97.9	749	97.9	0.555 [b]
Wash hands with soaps	740	96.7	706	92.3	<0.001
Wear mask when going out	753	98.4	745	97.4	<0.001 [b]
Use serving utensil	708	92.5	568	74.2	0.174
Bring own utensils when dining out [†]	542	81.9	52	7.9	0.199
Order takeaway more often	474	62.0	262	34.4	<0.001
Avoid dining or gathering together	742	97.0	616	85.0	0.178
Avoid going to public place or using public transport	713	93.4	408	53.5	0.002
Avoid going to COVID-19 confirmed regions outside Hong Kong	714	93.3	628	88.0	<0.001

[a] Chi-square or Fisher's exact test was used to test whether the perceived usefulness and practice are dependent. [b] Fisher's exact test was used. [†] This analysis only included people who will go outdoors for a meal during the epidemic (n = 662).

Around 32.7% (n = 249) of respondents believed in religion. Among them, analysis of mass gathering activity showed that 68.7% (171/249) reported that they reduced their religious gathering behavior during this pandemic. In addition, about a quarter of the study population (n = 181) reported that they had traveled abroad since January 2020. Mainland China (30.6%) and Japan (25.0%) were the most popular travelling areas.

3.4. Sociodemographic Factors Affecting Anxiety around Getting COVID-19

Among all the respondents, 66.7% (252/757) worried that they would become infected with COVID-19 with a mean STAI score of 2.57. Bivariate analyses of different socio-demographics, perception of the effect of COVID-19, and perceived infectivity and severity towards the worry about getting COVID-19 were conducted (Table 3). A multivariable logistic regression (Omnibus tests of model coefficients chi-square: 86.9, df = 10) revealed that young age, respondents who perceived significant COVID-19 impact on their physical, mental health, and/or social life were more likely to express anxiety of being infected. In addition, as the first global metropolis to report house pet SARS-CoV2 infection, our study showed that among the 124 respondents who are house pet owners, 18.5% (23/124) worried that their pets will also be infected with COVID-19.

The multivariable regression revealed that except for age, sociodemographic factors including gender, chronic disease status, education, marital status, household income, household floor area and district of residence were not significantly associated with the concern of becoming infected, which suggested that the worry of COVID-19 was indiscriminate across different sociodemographic factors in Hong Kong. Meanwhile, believing COVID-19 had a large effect on their physical, mental or social health was more likely to cause worry that they will be infected.

Table 3. Factors affecting concern of getting COVID-19.

Characteristics		Not Worry or Don't Know † (n = 252)	Worry (n = 505)	p-Value	AOR (95% CI)	p-Value
Age	18–24	15 (6.0%)	55 (10.9%)	0.037	1	
	25–44	77 (30.6%)	169 (33.5%)		0.567 (0.294–1.095)	0.091
	45–64	103 (40.9%)	198 (39.2%)		0.606 (0.318–1.153)	0.127
	65 or more	57 (22.6%)	83 (16.4%)		0.493 (0.244–0.995)	0.048
Gender	Male	132 (52.4%)	220 (43.6%)	0.022	1	
	Female	120 (47.6%)	285 (56.4%)		1.323 (0.956–1.831)	0.092
Chronic disease	No	206 (81.7%)	412 (81.6%)	0.957		
	Yes	46 (18.3%)	93 (18.3%)			
Education level	Primary level or below	25 (10.0%)	33 (6.6%)	0.249		
	Secondary level	108 (43.0%)	220 (43.7%)			
	Tertiary level	118 (47.0%)	250 (49.7%)			
Marital status	Non-married	99 (39.4%)	201 (39.9%)	0.908		
	Married	152 (60.2%)	303 (60.1%)			
Residential district	Hong Kong Island	52 (21.0%)	93 (18.4%)	0.207		
	Kowloon	83 (32.9%)	145 (28.7%)			
	New Territories	116 (46.0%)	267 (52.9%)			
Families members with chronic disease	No or don't know	209 (82.9%)	393 (77.8%)	0.100		
	Yes	43 (17.1%)	112 (22.2%)			
Household floor area	350 ft or below	53 (21.6%)	100 (21.1%)	0.964		
	351 ft to 800 ft	157 (64.1%)	304 (64.0%)			
	801 ft or above	35 (14.3%)	71 (14.9%)			

Table 3. *Cont.*

Characteristics		Not Worry or Don't Know [†] (n = 252)	Worry (n = 505)	p-Value	AOR (95% CI)	p-Value
Household income	<2000–7999	29 (12.1%)	36 (7.6%)	0.147		
	8000–19,999	36 (15.0%)	65 (13.8%)			
	20,000–39,999	66 (27.5%)	123 (26.1%)			
	40,000 or more	109 (45.4%)	248 (52.5%)			
Believing COVID-19 had large effect on their physical health	No	158 (62.9%)	206 (40.9%)	<0.001	1	
	Yes	93 (37.1%)	298 (59.1%)		1.583 (1.111–2.256)	0.011
Believing COVID-19 had large effect on their mental health	No	183 (72.6%)	219 (43.4%)	<0.001	1	
	Yes	69 (27.4%)	286 (56.6%)		2.490 (1.719–3.608)	<0.001
Believing COVID-19 had large effect on their financial status	No	181 (71.8%)	324 (64.2%)	0.035	1	
	Yes	71 (28.2%)	181 (35.8%)		0.927 (0.644–1.336)	0.685
Believing COVID-19 had large effect on their social life	No	104 (41.3%)	108 (21.4%)	<0.001	1	
	Yes	148 (58.7%)	397 (78.6%)		1.657 (1.138–2.413)	0.008
Believing COVID-19 had large effect on whole Hong Kong society	No	22 (8.7%)	20 (4.0%)	0.007	1	
	Yes	230 (91.3%)	485 (96.0%)		1.205 (0.608–2.385)	0.593
Perceived sufficient knowledge to manage COVID-19	No	127 (50.4%)	269 (53.3%)	0.456		
	Yes	125 (49.6%)	236 (43.7%)			
Perceived COVID-19 infectivity	Very low to medium or don't know	16 (6.3%)	17 (3.4%)	0.058	1	
	High or very high	236 (93.7%)	488 (96.6%)		1.290 (0.610–2.728)	0.505
Perceived COVID-19 severity	Very low to medium or don't know	58 (23.0%)	63 (19.0%)	0.197		
	High or very high	194 (77.0%)	409 (81.0%)			

[†] 248 participants reported "not worried" and 4 reported "don't know".

3.5. Other Related Behavioral Experiences: Home Quarantine and Caregiving to Non-Infected Family Members during COVID-19

Of the study respondents, 4.2% (32/765) reported that they practiced home-quarantine for COVID-19, where 71.9% (23/32) were volunteers and 28.1% (9/32) were compulsory quarantined. Most cited reasons for home-quarantine was history of recent travel abroad (13/32 = 40.6%) and close contact with confirmed patients (6/32 = 18.8%). About 83.8% subjects believed that quarantine was effective in infection control. During the COVID-19 epidemic, 25.1% of respondents (n = 192) reported that they engage in regular home and social care responsibilities. Among all the care providers, around 20% reported that they previously used community services and centers (e.g., school and day care centers) before COVID-19. Meanwhile, among these community service users, about 40% had stopped or decreased the use of those services due to closure during the epidemic. Respondents reported the need to take care of one (45.8%) or two family members (35.4%). About 28% and 7.4% of these respondents had been caring for frail older adults and those with disabilities, respectively. More details on caregiving to non-infected family members will be reported separately.

3.6. Information Channel and Type of Information of Health Information Seeking for COVID-19

More than 95% of the respondents reported that they were continuously concerned about the development of the COVID-19 epidemic. The main reported information seeking channels were television (36.1%), internet (28.8%) and smartphone apps (27.6%). When asked what kind of information they wanted to know, 88.3% and 87.7% of respondents wanted to know information about a vaccine and the situation of the epidemic, respectively.

4. Discussion

Using the standard computerized RDD method, this population landline-based study showed the self-reported perceived health impact, and the health emergency and disaster risk management (Health-EDRM) related preventive measures uptake (both individual or household level, and government level) against COVID-19 among the Hong Kong population. Consistent with other telephone survey results at early stages of the pandemic reported in Hong Kong, most respondents continued to report high perceived severity of COVID-19 [38]. In addition, a higher anxiety level during COVID-19 (STAI of 2.57) was seen in this study when compared with previous studies using the comparable scales conducted during SARS (2.24) in 2003 [39], and the H7N9 epidemic (1.85) in 2014 [27].

For various health impacts on demographic subgroups, people aged 65 or above reported that they were less affected by COVID-19 in terms of mental and social health, and these factors were also found to be significantly associated with concern of COVID-19. Findings were consistent with the online survey study results in mainland China [40] that also reported a higher anxiety level among younger respondents. The previous published online survey held in Hong Kong in February 2020 [41] had reported a higher proportion of respondents in distress from COVID-19, which might be explained by the differences in sampling of that study, which had recruited a lower proportion of the elderly. In contrast, the health severity perception of COVID-19 in this telephone survey was lower. This could be due to feeling fatigue with the epidemic news [42] or due to receiving more information about the situation and the virus, as the epidemic had evolved when compared with previous reported findings. Study findings indicated that respondents with chronic disease did not have higher levels of worry of getting COVID-19 when compared with those without chronic disease, even though the literature suggested that having chronic disease was considered as a risk factor for disease severity (complications and mortality) in COVID-19 [43–46]. Strengthening of information about those at higher risk in the community should be provided to raise the awareness of people at risk. Of note, the local population reported their belief that individuals (68.6%) bore comparable responsibility compared to the government (67.5%) to engage in infection control. Less than half of the respondents reported to have sufficient knowledge and accurate concepts to manage the health risk and safety during the outbreak [47]. For example, a quarter of the respondents did not perceive asymptomatic patients as infectious, which was similar to published findings in Egypt [48]. This misconception may affect the effectiveness of COVID-19 prevention efforts because the literature indicates that infected people can transmit the virus regardless of symptoms [7] and a high asymptomatic proportion of all infected patients was reported in Japan and Italy [6,49]. Furthermore, respondents with a misconception of the transmission route were found to be more likely to use television or radio as their main information source. As this misconception may likely be due to the lack of emphasis on asymptomatic patients as a transmission route, additional information related to the transmission route should be tailored to those with a lower education level.

Health-EDRM encompasses a wide range of components, where the component "Community Capacities for Health-EDRM" highlights the importance of the participation of the local population for managing the health risks in an emergency. Among the Health-EDRM behavioral practices [28], which are related to primary disease prevention practices [29], significant differences were found between attitude and practice in regards to washing hands with soap, ordering takeaways more often, wearing masks when going out, and avoiding going to COVID-19-confirmed regions outside Hong Kong. People who regarded these behaviors as useful tended to have a higher uptake rate. Consistent with Kwok et al. and Cowling et al. [38,41], the Hong Kong population showed a high compliance of wearing masks (94.2%), and there was a significant difference before and after the outbreak, which might be due to the high awareness of the outbreak, mass public health information announced through different channels, and the previous experience of SARS. However, more than half of respondents still reported traveling to COVID-19-confirmed regions before and during the study period. In addition, moderate and low uptake rates were found in using serving utensils (74.2%) and bringing their own utensils to meals (7.9%). Uptake patterns were found to be higher when compared with a previous study conducted during the H7N9 pandemic [27], where rates of 45.9% and 1.6%, respectively, were reported.

Meanwhile, no significant differences were found between perceived usefulness and practice of avoidance of dining or gathering together. This might suggest that even though people thought social avoidance might be useful to prevent COVID-19, they were unwilling to practice this socially limiting preventive behavior. As our study findings showed, males were less likely to avoid dining or gathering together, this might also provide the hypothesis that gender behavior might at least be associated with the gender imbalance in confirmed cases (with male predominance) at the beginning of the local outbreak [50]. In addition, "ordering takeaway food" was found to have increased by respondents during the epidemic. This increase may due to the social distancing promotion and regulations by the government (e.g., encouraging restaurants to provide takeaways as an option and avoiding table sharing) [51,52]. To promote better self-protection against infectious diseases, targeted interventions may focus on increasing the awareness towards the outbreak for the behaviors with a significant attitude–practice gap, while for the behaviors without an attitude–practice gap, additional measures to reinforce the practice were suggested. Further studies focusing on the barriers and self-efficacy might also be needed. Appropriate Health-EDRM health education and risk communication might wish to target subgroups who revealed suboptimal behavioral practices to further improve bottom-up response efforts.

Television, internet and smartphone apps were the top three channels for obtaining infectious disease information, covering more than 90% of the population. In Hong Kong, habits of television consumption have developed among the middle-aged and elderly, while the use of internet or smartphone apps were more popular in the younger age group. Consistent with the survey previously held in Hong Kong in February [41], almost all of the respondents would like to know more about the current situation of the outbreak, and how the government and themselves should respond. The availability and safety of COVID-19 vaccine were also of interest to general population.

Study limitations included the methodological limitations of telephone surveys. Firstly, households with no land-based telephone service may be missed. Nonetheless, the penetration rate of residential fixed line services in Hong Kong was 85.5% in December 2019 [53]. In addition, our study was conducted during the peak period of confirmed cases of COVID-19 in Hong Kong. During the data collection period, Hong Kong had 492 confirmed cases, accounting for almost half of the cases as of 14 April. Furthermore, the data collection occurred during the lockdown period in Hong Kong when people were advised to stay at home, and the government prohibited group gatherings of more than four people in public places under the Prohibition on Group Gathering Regulation. In addition, a landline telephone survey allows for more accurate geographic and demographic targeting when compared with mobile and online surveys. In general, specific subgroups, such as the elderly and the poor are more likely to be reached via landline than young adults [54]. Moreover, the landline telephone study methodology might capture populations that might be less technological or digital literate and it also offers the opportunity for researchers to compare with previous study findings with similar study methodology of other extreme events and disaster context. Finally, our sample was collected over a short period and comparable with the population census data in terms of age, gender, district of residence and marital status, which was generalizable to the Hong Kong population.

Secondly, the cross-sectional study design can only demonstrate associations between patterns and social-demographic predictors and causation cannot be attributed to the findings. A further cohort-based study design should be considered to monitor and assess changes in knowledge, attitude and practice patterns. Thirdly, this study might be subject to reporting bias since the information collected was self-reported, and data from non-respondents could not be obtained. In addition, the enquired personal or household health emergency disaster risks management (Health-EDRM) related behaviors and practices of COVID-19 prevention behavior were developed based on previous health and hygiene behavioral practices that might be relevant to contact transmission of the disease [33]. Yet, there are other relevant Health-EDRM behavioral practices in other cultural (non-Asia) and living contexts (e.g., rural community's settings) that are worth exploring to generate evidence and develop health-risk education.

Last but not least, as the survey study was conducted after the implementation of the government preventive social distancing measures (e.g., restricting restaurant's customer density, prohibition of group gathering), behavioral patterns might be subject to further changes if authorities have regulation and policy changes.

5. Conclusions

The Health-EDRM Framework is an integrated approach to manage health risks and build resilience. The COVID-19 pandemic offers an opportunity for the global community to understand how community and individuals might engage in disease prevention and health protection Health-EDRM behaviors that address a major biological hazard. The study findings indicated elderly and people with low education attainment had relatively poor knowledge and were less likely to adopt preventive Health-EDRM practices toward COVID-19. Tailored information with relevant information channels should be considered to reach these at-risk groups. Better understanding of uptake of knowledge, perception, attitude and behavior patterns by urban populations might facilitate better program and policy planning for Health-EDRM.

Author Contributions: Conceptualization, E.Y.Y.C.; methodology, E.Y.Y.C. and E.S.K.L.; validation, Z.H.; formal analysis, E.S.K.L.; investigation, E.S.K.L., E.Y.Y.C., Z.H., E.L.Y.W., S.Y.S.W. and K.K.C.H.; data curation, E.S.K.L. and Z.H.; writing—original draft preparation, E.S.K.L., E.Y.Y.C. and Z.H.; writing—review and editing, E.S.K.L. E.Y.Y.C., Z.H., E.L.Y.W., S.Y.S.W. and K.K.C.H.; visualization, E.S.K.L.; supervision, E.Y.Y.C.; project administration, Z.H. All authors have read and agreed to the published version of the manuscript.

Funding: This research received no external funding.

Conflicts of Interest: The authors declare no conflict of interest.

Appendix A

Table A1. Association between demographic variables and risk perception and knowledge about COVID-19.

Demographics	Large Impact on Mental Health	Large Impact on Social Health	Large Impact on Financial Status	Large Impact on Hong Kong	Can be Prevented at Government Level	Can Be Spread by Insect	Can Be Spread by Asymptomatic Patient
Education							
Primary			1.10 (0.51–2.38)	0.15 (0.04–0.51) *		2.89 (1.35–6.18) *	0.45 (0.21–0.96) *
Secondary			1.81 (1.22–2.69) *	0.51 (0.21–1.23)		1.40 (0.87–2.26)	0.50 (0.32–0.78) *
Post-secondary			1	1		1	1
Gender							
Male	1	1					
Female	1.41 (1.02–1.95) *	1.60 (1.10–2.33) *					
Age							
18–24	2.00 (0.77–5.18)	6.12 (1.78–21.54) *	7.93 (2.76–22.76) *		3.06 (0.88–10.61)		
25–44	2.21 (1.19–4.12) *	4.03 (1.99–8.15) *	7.05 (3.35–14.81) *		2.12 (1.10–40.9) *		
45–64	1.26 (0.73–2.19)	2.98 (1.60–5.55) *	4.32 (2.22–8.42) *		0.96 (0.55–1.69)		
65+	1	1	1		1		
Household income							
<2000–7999			1				
8000–19,999			0.43 (0.20–0.92) *				
20,000–39,999			0.33 (0.16–0.72) *				
40,000 or more			0.25 (0.12–0.54) *				
Occupation							
White collar		1					
Blue collar		1.70 (0.99–2.93)					
Housewife		1.95 (0.98–3.90)					
Student		1.35 (0.36–5.05)					
Unemployment or retired		3.41 (1.72–6.76) *					

Note: Multivariable regression was not performed on outcome variables with a small number of cases (probability of that happening <0.05 or >0.95). Only variables with significant odds ratios in the multivariable logistic regression are shown in the table. None of these five demographic variables were significantly associated with believing COVID-19 had a large impact on their physical health, perceived sufficient knowledge of COVID-19, believing COVID-19 can be prevented at the household or individual level, perceived high infectivity and perceived severity of COVID-19. * indicates $p < 0.05$.

Table A2. Association between demographic variables and the practices (always or usually) of preventive measures against COVID-19.

Demographics	Wash Hands with Soaps	Avoid Dining or Gathering Together	Use Serving Utensil	Avoid Going to Public Place or Using Public Transport
Education				
Primary	0.31 (0.12–0.84) *		0.15 (0.04–0.51) *	
Secondary	0.68 (0.33–1.42)		0.51 (0.21–1.23)	
Post-secondary	1		1	
Gender				
Male	1	1		
Female	2.27 (1.17–4.43) *	1.82 (1.21–2.74) *		
Age				
18–24	2.15 (0.39–11.97)			2.48 (0.93–6.65)
25–44	4.62 (1.47–14.52) *			2.08 (1.09–3.98) *
45–64	2.83 (1.15–6.95) *			1.37 (0.77–2.44)
65+	1			1
Household income				
<2000–7999				
8000–19,999				
20,000–39,999				
40,000 or more				
Occupation				
White collar				1
Blue collar				0.70 (0.44–1.23)
Housewife				3.47 (1.87–6.42) *
Student				0.99 (0.37–2.65)
Unemployment or retired				2.29 (1.28–4.07) *

Note: Multivariable regression was not performed on outcome variables with a small number of cases (probability of that happening <0.05 or >0.95). Only variables with significant odds ratio in the multivariable logistic regression are shown in the table. None of these five demographic variables were significantly associated with bringing one's own utensils when dining out, ordering takeaway food more often, and avoiding going to COVID-19-confirmed regions outside Hong Kong. * indicates $p < 0.05$.

References

1. Rolling Updates on Coronavirus Disease (COVID-19). Available online: https://www.who.int/emergencies/diseases/novel-coronavirus-2019/events-as-they-happen (accessed on 23 April 2020).
2. Ye, Z.W.; Yuan, S.; Yuen, K.S.; Fung, S.Y.; Chan, C.P.; Jin, D.Y. Zoonotic origins of human coronaviruses. *Int. J. Biol. Sci.* **2020**, *16*, 1686. [CrossRef]
3. Coronavirus Disease 2019 (COVID-19) Situation Report–85. Available online: https://www.who.int/docs/default-source/coronaviruse/situation-reports/20200414-sitrep-85-covid-19.pdf?sfvrsn=7b8629bb_2 (accessed on 23 April 2020).
4. Rajgor, D.D.; Lee, M.H.; Archuleta, S.; Bagdasarian, N.; Quek, S.C. The many estimates of the COVID-19 case fatality rate. *Lancet Infect. Dis.* **2020**. [CrossRef]
5. Kim, D.D.; Goel, A. Estimating case fatality rates of COVID-19. *Lancet Infect. Dis.* **2020**. [CrossRef]
6. Day, M. Covid-19: Identifying and isolating asymptomatic people helped eliminate virus in Italian village. *BMJ* **2020**, *368*, m1165. [CrossRef] [PubMed]
7. Kimball, A. Asymptomatic and presymptomatic SARS-CoV-2 infections in residents of a long-term care skilled nursing facility—King County, Washington, March 2020. *Morb. Mortal. Wkly. Rep.* **2020**, *69*, 377–381. [CrossRef]
8. Mahase, E. Coronavirus: COVID-19 has killed more people than SARS and MERS combined, despite lower case fatality rate. *BMJ* **2020**, m641. [CrossRef]
9. Wells, C.R.; Sah, P.; Moghadas, S.M.; Pandey, A.; Shoukat, A.; Wang, Y.; Galvani, A.P. Impact of international travel and border control measures on the global spread of the novel 2019 coronavirus outbreak. *Proc. Natl. Acad. Sci. USA* **2020**, *117*, 7504–7509. [CrossRef]
10. Lewnard, J.A.; Lo, N.C. Scientific and ethical basis for social-distancing interventions against COVID-19. *Lancet Infect. Dis.* **2020**. [CrossRef]

11. Novel Coronavirus (2019-nCoV) SITUATION REPORT-3 23 JANUARY 2020. Available online: https://www.who.int/docs/default-source/coronaviruse/situation-reports/20200123-sitrep-3-2019-ncov.pdf?sfvrsn=d6d23643_8 (accessed on 23 April 2020).
12. CHP Investigates Two Additional Cases of Novel Coronavirus Infection. Available online: https://www.info.gov.hk/gia/general/202001/31/P2020013100015.htm?fontSize=1 (accessed on 23 April 2020).
13. Latest Situation of Cases of COVID-19 (as of 14 April, 2020). Available online: https://www.chp.gov.hk/files/pdf/local_situation_covid19_en.pdf (accessed on 15 April 2020).
14. CE Announces Activation of Emergency Response Level in Relation to Novel Coronavirus Infection (with Photo). Available online: https://www.info.gov.hk/gia/general/202001/26/P2020012600087.htm (accessed on 23 April 2020).
15. LNY Welfare Services Set. Available online: https://www.news.gov.hk/eng/2020/01/20200127/20200127_233955_845.html (accessed on 23 April 2020).
16. Deferral of Class Resumption for All Schools Together, We Fight the Virus. Available online: https://www.edb.gov.hk/attachment/en/sch-admin/admin/about-sch/diseases-prevention/edb_20200331_eng.pdf (accessed on 23 April 2020).
17. Compulsory Quarantine Implemented Smoothly. Available online: https://www.info.gov.hk/gia/general/202002/09/P2020020900715.htm?fontSize=1 (accessed on 23 April 2020).
18. Quarantine Measures Enhanced. Available online: https://www.news.gov.hk/eng/2020/03/20200317/20200317_202509_713.html (accessed on 23 April 2020).
19. Prevention and Control of Disease (Requirement and Directions) (Business and Premises) Regulation Gazette. Available online: https://www.info.gov.hk/gia/general/202003/27/P2020032700878.htm?fontSize=1 (accessed on 23 April 2020).
20. Prevention and Control of Disease (Prohibition on Group Gathering) Regulation. Available online: https://www.info.gov.hk/gia/general/202003/28/P2020032800720.htm?fontSize=1 (accessed on 23 April 2020).
21. Health Emergency and Disaster Risk Management Framework. Available online: https://www.who.int/hac/techguidance/preparedness/health-emergency-and-disaster-risk-management-framework-eng.pdf?ua=1 (accessed on 23 April 2020).
22. Wan, Y.K.P. A comparison of the governance of tourism planning in the two Special Administrative Regions (SARs) of China–Hong Kong and Macao. *Tour. Manag.* **2013**, *36*, 164–177.
23. Kung, N.Y.; Morris, R.S.; Perkins, N.R.; Sims, L.D.; Ellis, T.M.; Bissett, L.; Peiris, M.J. Risk for infection with highly pathogenic influenza A virus (H5N1) in chickens, Hong Kong, 2002. *Emerg. Infect. Dis.* **2007**, *13*, 412. [CrossRef]
24. Cheng, V.C.C.; Lee, W.M.; Sridhar, S.; Ho, P.L.; Yuen, K.Y. Prevention of nosocomial transmission of influenza A (H7N9) in Hong Kong. *J. Hosp. Infect.* **2015**, *90*, 355–356. [CrossRef] [PubMed]
25. Wong, A.T.; Chen, H.; Liu, S.H.; Hsu, E.K.; Luk, K.S.; Lai, C.K.; Tong, A.Y. From SARS to avian influenza preparedness in Hong Kong. *Clin. Infect. Dis.* **2017**, *64* (Suppl. S2), S98–S104. [CrossRef] [PubMed]
26. Lau, J.T.; Tsui, H.; Lau, M.; Yang, X. SARS transmission, risk factors, and prevention in Hong Kong. *Emerg. Infect. Dis.* **2004**, *10*, 587. [CrossRef] [PubMed]
27. Chan, E.Y.Y.; Cheng, C.K.; Tam, G.; Huang, Z.; Lee, P. Knowledge, attitudes, and practices of Hong Kong population towards human A/H7N9 influenza pandemic preparedness, China, 2014. *BMC Public Health* **2015**, *15*, 943. [CrossRef] [PubMed]
28. West, R.; Michie, S.; Rubin, G.J.; Amlôt, R. Applying principles of behaviour change to reduce SARS-CoV-2 transmission. *Nat. Hum. Behav.* **2020**, *4*, 1–9. [CrossRef] [PubMed]
29. Chan, E.Y.Y.; Shahzada, T.S.; Sham, T.; Dubois, C.; Huang, Z.; Liu, S.; Shaw, R. Non-Pharmaceutical Behavioural Measures for Droplet-Borne Biological Hazards Prevention: Health-EDRM for COVID-19 (SARS-CoV-2) Pandemic. 2020; Manuscript Submitted for Publication.
30. Chan, E.Y.Y.; Cheng, C.K.Y.; Tam, G.; Huang, Z.; Lee, P. Willingness of future A/H7N9 influenza vaccine uptake: A cross-sectional study of Hong Kong community. *Vaccine* **2015**, *33*, 4737–4740. [CrossRef] [PubMed]
31. Tam, G.; Huang, Z.; Chan, E.Y.Y. Household preparedness and preferred communication channels in public health emergencies: A cross-sectional survey of residents in an Asian developed urban city. *Int. J. Environ. Res. Public Health* **2018**, *15*, 1598. [CrossRef]
32. Marteau, T.M.; Bekker, H. The development of a six-item short-form of the state scale of the Spielberger State-Trait Anxiety Inventory (STAI). *Br. J. Clin. Psychol.* **1992**, *31 Pt 3*, 301–306. [CrossRef]

33. Chan, E.Y.Y.; Wong, C.S. Public health prevention hierarchy in disaster context. In *Public Health and Disasters-Health Emergency and Disaster Risk Management in Asia*; Chan, E.Y.Y., Shaw, R., Eds.; Springer: Tokyo, Japan, 2020; pp. 7–17.
34. Chan, E.Y.Y. *Building Bottom-up Health and Disaster Risk Reduction Programmes*; Oxford University Press: Oxford, UK, 2018.
35. Chan, E.Y.Y.; Huang, Z.; Mark, C.K.M.; Guo, C. Weather information acquisition and health significance during extreme cold weather in a subtropical city: A cross-sectional survey in Hong Kong. *Int. J. Disaster Risk Sci.* **2017**, *8*, 134–144. [CrossRef]
36. Chan, E.Y.Y.; Huang, Z.; Hung, K.K.C.; Chan, G.K.W.; Lam, H.C.Y.; Lo, E.S.K.; Yeung, M.P.S. Health emergency disaster risk management of public transport systems: A population-based study after the 2017 subway fire in Hong Kong, China. *Int. J. Environ. Res. Public Health* **2019**, *16*, 228. [CrossRef]
37. Hong Kong SAR Census and Statistics Department. Available online: https://www.bycensus2016.gov.hk/en/bc-dp.html (accessed on 23 April 2020).
38. Cowling, B.J.; Ali, S.T.; Ng, T.W.; Tsang, T.K.; Li, J.C.; Fong, M.W.; Wu, J.T. Impact assessment of non-pharmaceutical interventions against coronavirus disease 2019 and influenza in Hong Kong: An observational study. *Lancet Public Health* **2020**, *5*, e279–e288. [CrossRef]
39. Leung, G.M.; Lam, T.H.; Ho, L.M.; Ho, S.Y.; Chan, B.H.Y.; Wong, I.O.L.; Hedley, A.J. The impact of community psychological responses on outbreak control for severe acute respiratory syndrome in Hong Kong. *J. Epidemiol. Community Health* **2003**, *57*, 857–863. [CrossRef] [PubMed]
40. Huang, Y.; Zhao, N. Generalized anxiety disorder, depressive symptoms and sleep quality during COVID-19 epidemic in China: A web-based cross-sectional survey. *MedRxiv* **2020**, *288*, 112954.
41. Kwok, K.O.; Li, K.K.; Chan, H.H.; Yi, Y.Y.; Tang, A.; Wei, W.I.; Wong, S.Y. Community Responses during Early Phase of COVID-19 Epidemic, Hong Kong. *Emerg. Infect. Dis.* **2020**, *26*. [CrossRef]
42. Collinson, S.; Khan, K.; Heffernan, J.M. The effects of media reports on disease spread and important public health measurements. *PLoS ONE* **2015**, *10*, e0141423. [CrossRef]
43. Shahid, Z.; Kalayanamitra, R.; McClafferty, B.; Kepko, D.; Ramgobin, D.; Patel, R.; Jain, R. COVID-19 and older adults: What we know. *J. Am. Geriatr. Soc.* **2020**, *68*, 926–929. [CrossRef]
44. Kalligeros, M.; Shehadeh, F.; Mylona, E.K.; Benitez, G.; Beckwith, C.G.; Chan, P.A.; Mylonakis, E. Association of Obesity with Disease Severity among Patients with COVID-19. *Obesity* **2020**. [CrossRef]
45. Hussain, A.; Bhowmik, B.; do Vale Moreira, N.C. COVID-19 and diabetes: Knowledge in progress. *Diabetes Res. Clin. Pract.* **2020**, *162*, 108142. [CrossRef]
46. Cook, T.M. The importance of hypertension as a risk factor for severe illness and mortality in COVID-19. *Anaesthesia* **2020**. [CrossRef]
47. World Health Organization. Modes of Transmission of Virus Causing COVID-19: Implications for IPC Precaution Recommendations: Scientific Brief, 27 March 2020 (No. WHO/2019-nCoV/Sci_Brief/Transmission_modes/2020.1). Available online: https://apps.who.int/iris/bitstream/handle/10665/331601/WHO-2019-nCoV-Sci_Brief-Transmission_modes-2020.1-eng.pdf (accessed on 23 April 2020).
48. Abdelhafiz, A.S.; Mohammed, Z.; Ibrahim, M.E.; Ziady, H.H.; Alorabi, M.; Ayyad, M.; Sultan, E.A. Knowledge, Perceptions, and Attitude of Egyptians Towards the Novel Coronavirus Disease (COVID-19). *J. Community Health* **2020**, 1–10. [CrossRef]
49. Mizumoto, K.; Kagaya, K.; Zarebski, A.; Chowell, G. Estimating the asymptomatic proportion of coronavirus disease 2019 (COVID-19) cases on board the Diamond Princess cruise ship, Yokohama, Japan, 2020. *Eurosurveillance* **2020**, *25*, 2000180. [CrossRef] [PubMed]
50. Coronavirus Disease (COVID-19) in HK. Available online: https://chp-dashboard.geodata.gov.hk/covid-19/en.html (accessed on 23 April 2020).
51. Let's Beat COVID-19 Together. Available online: https://www.cfs.gov.hk/english/whatsnew/whatsnew_fstr/whatsnew_fstr_Beat_COVID-19.html (accessed on 18 May 2020).
52. New Regulations to Fight COVID-19. Available online: https://www.news.gov.hk/eng/2020/03/20200327/20200327_202339_445.html (accessed on 18 May 2020).

53. Office of the Communications Authority Key Communications Statistics. Available online: https://www.ofca.gov.hk/en/data_statistics/data_statistics/key_stat/ (accessed on 23 April 2020).
54. Petrovčič, A.; Vehovar, V.; Dolničar, V. Landline and mobile phone communication in social companionship networks of older adults: An empirical investigation in Slovenia. *Technol. Soc.* **2016**, *45*, 91–102. [CrossRef]

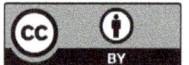

© 2020 by the authors. Licensee MDPI, Basel, Switzerland. This article is an open access article distributed under the terms and conditions of the Creative Commons Attribution (CC BY) license (http://creativecommons.org/licenses/by/4.0/).

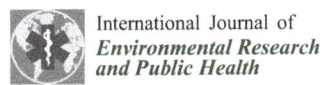

International Journal of
Environmental Research and Public Health

Article

The Association between Utilization of Media Information and Current Health Anxiety Among the Fukushima Daiichi Nuclear Disaster Evacuees

Masatsugu Orui [1,2,*], Chihiro Nakayama [1], Yujiro Kuroda [3], Nobuaki Moriyama [1], Hajime Iwasa [1,4], Teruko Horiuchi [1], Takeo Nakayama [5], Minoru Sugita [6] and Seiji Yasumura [1]

1. Department of Public Health, Fukushima Medical University School of Medicine, Fukushima 960-1295, Japan; nakac@fmu.ac.jp (C.N.); moriyama@fmu.ac.jp (N.M.); hajimei@fmu.ac.jp (H.I.); t-hori@fmu.ac.jp (T.H.); yasumura@fmu.ac.jp (S.Y.)
2. Sendai City Mental Health and Welfare Center, Sendai 980-0845, Japan
3. Center for Integrated Science and Humanities, Fukushima Medical University, Fukushima 960-1295, Japan; kuroday@fmu.ac.jp
4. Tokyo Metropolitan Institute of Gerontology, Tokyo 173-0015, Japan
5. Department of Health Informatics, School of Public Health, Kyoto University, Kyoto 606-8501, Japan; nakayama.takeo.4a@kyoto-u.ac.jp
6. Toho University, Tokyo 143-8540, Japan; sugitamnr@a05.itscom.net
* Correspondence: oruima@fmu.ac.jp; Tel.: +81-24-547-1180

Received: 19 May 2020; Accepted: 29 May 2020; Published: 1 June 2020

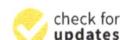

Abstract: The 2011 nuclear disaster in Fukushima was not only a health disaster, but also an information disaster. Although media can promote health communication following disasters, studies have revealed associations between media information and negative psychological reactions. To clarify the relationship between media utilization and current health anxiety due to radiation exposure, a cross-sectional questionnaire survey was conducted in Fukushima. We selected 2000 subjects from evacuation (i.e., 500) and non-evacuation (i.e., 1500) areas by two-stage stratified random sampling. As the independent variable, participants were asked about current health anxiety due to radiation exposure at the time of answering the questionnaire. For utilization of media about radiation exposure, local media, national media, Internet media, public broadcasts, and public relations information from local government were set as the dependent variables. Questionnaire data were analyzed by evacuation type (i.e., forced/voluntary). In a multivariate logistic regression analysis, the use of public relations information was significantly associated with lower anxiety for the forced evacuees (odds ratio: 0.72; 95% confidence interval: 0.56–0.93). Our findings highlight the importance of public relations information from local government in terms of it being associated with lower current health anxiety, and this could potentially aid in preparing for future disasters.

Keywords: Fukushima nuclear accident; mass media; Internet; public health practice; community mental health services

1. Introduction

The Great East Japan Earthquake, which occurred on 11 March 2011, was the largest earthquake ever recorded in Japan's history. The earthquake (magnitude 9.0) generated a massive tsunami that caused enormous damage to the Pacific Coast. This was followed by a separate tsunami, which hit the Fukushima Daiichi Nuclear Power Plant operated by the Tokyo Electric Power Company, causing radiation disasters in Fukushima Prefecture and requiring the long-term evacuation of residents from many surrounding municipalities. Due to this triple disaster, more than 92,000 residents who lived in an area designated by the national government as an evacuation area were forced to leave their homes (as of May 2016) [1]. Moreover, some residents decided to evacuate voluntarily to avoid the effects of the nuclear disaster, even residents who lived in non-evacuation areas.

The nuclear accident at the Fukushima Daiichi Nuclear Power Station caused multiple public health problems, including increased anxiety and mental health issues due to perceived risk among the evacuees and residents of Fukushima. In addition, Yamashita, who supported the nuclear accident response on-site as a radiation specialist, have argued that the Fukushima event was not only a health disaster, but also an information disaster [2], because the accident was an unprecedented experience for evacuees, and their perceived radiation exposure risk may have been related to the mass media. Consequently, their disaster-related stress and/or psychological distress levels may have been affected [3]. Indeed, newspaper coverage of the accident focused mainly on the crisis response relating to immediate issues, actions, and decisions in the aftermath of the accident (e.g., information of on-site actions undertaken, communications about the INES (International Nuclear Event Scale), food restrictions, cost, and number of people affected and being evacuated) [4].

One of the recommendations of the Chernobyl Forum report was to address the lack of accurate information available to local populations on the health risks as a result of the disaster itself, as well as wider health risks such as non-communicable diseases [5]. Moreover, the United Nations Sendai Framework for Disaster Risk Reduction aims to understand disaster risk while sharing non-sensitive information and appropriate communications, and to strengthen the utilization of media, including social media and traditional media [5]. In fact, the media functioned as a form of interpersonal communication with others, or as a channel for local government and other organizations during the immediate aftermath of the Great East Japan Earthquake [6]. However, the media are not always helpful. Several studies have examined disaster-related television viewing in the context of terrorism and have explored a range of outcomes, including post-traumatic stress disorder (PTSD), depression, anxiety, stress reactions, and substance use [7]. One study reported a significant association between the consumption of television and Internet coverage of the 2011 Great East Japan Earthquake and Tsunami, and post-traumatic reactions [8]. This suggests that the media (including Internet and television) can trigger negative psychological responses in evacuees and residents who use it.

Against this backdrop, the present study aims to clarify the association between media utilization (e.g., Internet media, public relations information from local government, and other traditional media) and current strong health anxiety at the time of the survey in the context of the Fukushima nuclear disaster, in order to consider effective modes of disaster communication among evacuees. These findings will likely be useful for future disaster risk reduction and management.

2. Materials and Methods

2.1. Participants

This cross-sectional questionnaire survey targeted 2000 residents of Fukushima Prefecture aged 20–79 years. Participant selection was based on two-stage stratified random sampling (stage one, survey of the region; stage two, survey of individuals). A random selection occurred of 33–34 individuals per point from municipal resident registration files to obtain 2000 representative participants. Of the 2000 subjects, 500 were from the three types of evacuation area that the Japanese government designated according to spatial radiation dose rates, as follows: (1) difficult-to-return areas, with a radiation dose rate ≥50 millisieverts (mSv) per year; (2) residence restriction areas, with a radiation dose rate ≥20 and <50 mSv per year; and (3) areas where evacuation orders were ready to be lifted as of 22 April 2011. The remaining 1500 people lived in the non-evacuation areas of Fukushima Prefecture (500 people were selected from each of the three areas of Hama-Dori, Naka-Dori, and Aizu) (Figure 1). We sent an anonymous, self-reporting postal questionnaire to participants between August and October 2016. The survey was approved by the ethics review committee of Fukushima Medical University on 12 April 2016 (approval number: 2699).

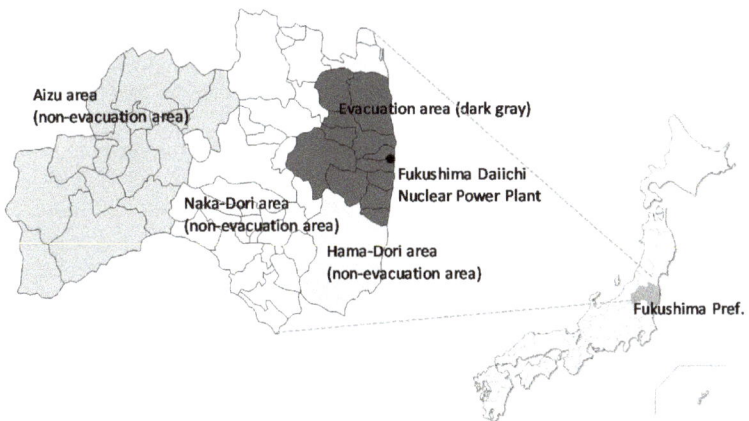

Figure 1. Evacuation and non-evacuation areas in Fukushima. Regions colored in dark gray correspond to the municipalities where evacuation orders were issued. Hama-Dori, Naka-Dori, and Aizu were the non-evacuation areas.

2.2. Survey Variables

For the independent variable, i.e., current anxiety regarding perceived radiation health risks, participants were asked to subjectively rate at the time of answering the questionnaire "Your current level of anxiety about the effects of radiation on your health due to the nuclear disaster" on a five-point scale: "Not at all," "Only a little," "Somewhat," "Very," and "Extremely." "Very" and "Extremely" were categorized as the "current strong anxiety group," with the other levels of anxiety as the "no or weak anxiety group." This questionnaire was investigator-designed.

For utilization of media about radiation, respondents selected up to three items from the following 13 options: local newspapers, national newspapers, NHK (Nippon Hoso Kyokai) television (public broadcast television, both national and local), private local broadcast television, private national broadcast television, radio, Internet news, Internet sites/blogs, social network services (SNS), magazines/books, public relations information from local government, word of mouth, and none of the above. To assess the association between media utilization and current strong health anxiety, we categorized "any local media (local newspapers and broadcasting)," "any national media (national newspapers and broadcasting)," "public broadcasting (NHK)," "any Internet media (Internet news, Internet sites/blogs, SNS)," and "public relations information from local government" as dependent variables, since these types of media were utilized by a relatively large number of respondents.

Regarding current health anxiety due to radiation exposure, participants were asked about: (1) anxiety related to delayed effects (e.g., severe diseases) with the statement "I am worried I might suffer from serious diseases due to the influence of radiation in the future"; (2) anxiety related to unhealthy status with the statement "Every time my condition gets worse, I become anxious about radiation exposure"; (3) anxiety related to genetic effects with the statement "I am worried that the influence of radiation will be inherited by the next generation, such as my children and grandchildren"; and (4) anxiety relating to broadcasting about nuclear issues with the statement "Looking at reports on nuclear power plant accidents, I become very anxious." These four single-item questions were part of a reliable questionnaire regarding radiation anxiety (i.e., the 7-item Radiation Anxiety Scale developed by Umeda et al. [9] and presented by Fukasawa et al. [10]). The Cronbach's alpha coefficient of the scale has been reported as 0.81, and in the present study sample, it was 0.84.

The other questionnaire than the 7-item Radiation Anxiety Scale was investigator-designed. All questionnaire items were shown in a previous report presented by Nakayama et al. [11].

2.3. Statistical Analysis

Data were also analyzed by evacuation type: (1) forced evacuation (or forced evacuees), which refers to evacuation due to living in an area designated by the national government as an evacuation area, as of 11 March 2011; and (2) voluntary evacuation (or voluntary evacuees), which refers to voluntary evacuation to avoid the effects of the nuclear disaster, even among residents living in non-evacuation areas, as of 11 March 2011. The chi-square test and multivariate logistic regression analysis were used to examine the association between media utilization and current strong health anxiety due to the nuclear disaster, as well as the characteristics of current strong health anxiety among evacuees by evacuation type. Statistical significance was evaluated using two-sided, design-based tests with a 5% level of significance. All statistical analyses were performed using SPSS 23.0 (IBM Corp., Armonk, NY, USA).

3. Results

3.1. Participants

We sent out 1985 questionnaires (excluding those returned to the sender due to no one residing at the address) and received 916 responses from August to December 2016 (response rate, 46.1%). After excluding 55 respondents who failed to provide information regarding sex or age, as well as 636 respondents who were not evacuees or did not answer a question about relocation due to nuclear disaster, the final study population consisted of 225 respondents who were either forced ($n = 156$) or voluntary ($n = 69$) evacuees (Figure 2).

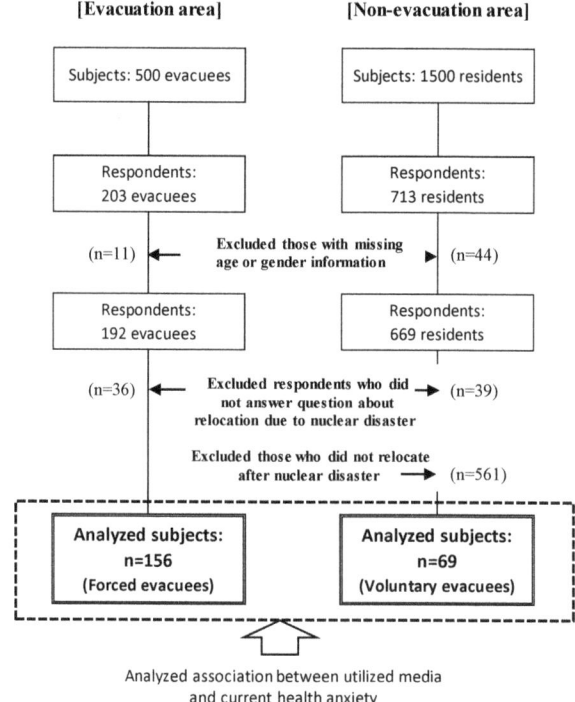

Figure 2. Sample selection in the evacuation and non-evacuation areas. The analyzed subjects included 156 forced evacuees and 69 voluntary evacuees.

3.2. Respondent Characteristics

The proportions of respondents aged 65 years and older, of respondents with a junior/senior high school education, and of respondents who were unemployed were higher among forced evacuees compared to voluntary evacuees (Table 1).

Table 1. Basic characteristics of the participants (forced/voluntary evacuees).

	Total		Forced Evacuees		Voluntary Evacuees		p-Value (χ^2)
	($n = 225$)		($n = 156$)		($n = 69$)		
	n	(%)	n	(%)	n	(%)	
Age (as of August 2016)							
<40 years	32	(14.2)	16	(10.3)	16	(23.2)	
40–64 years	110	(48.9)	76	(48.7)	34	(49.3)	0.02
≥65 years	83	(36.9)	64	(41.0)	19	(27.5)	($\chi^2 = 7.99$)
Gender							
Male	89	(39.6)	61	(39.1)	28	(40.6)	0.83
Female	136	(60.4)	95	(60.9)	41	(59.4)	($\chi^2 = 0.04$)
Education							
Junior/senior high school	145	(65.6)	110	(71.9)	35	(51.5)	<0.01
Vocational college, university, or graduate school	76	(34.4)	43	(28.1)	33	(48.5)	($\chi^2 = 8.70$)
Occupational category							
Employed or owner	105	(47.5)	58	(37.9)	47	(69.1)	
Suspended from job	7	(3.2)	7	(4.6)	0	(0.0)	<0.01
Unemployed	109	(49.3)	88	(57.5)	21	(30.9)	($\chi^2 = 19.5$)
Living area as of March 11, 2011							
Evacuation areas	156	(69.3)	156	(100.0)	0	(0.0)	<0.01
Non-evacuation areas	69	(30.7)	0	(0.0)	69	(100.0)	($\chi^2 = 220.3$)
(Hama-Dori area)	50	(22.2)	-	-	50	(72.5)	
(Naka-Dori area)	15	(6.7)	-	-	15	(21.7)	
(Aizu area)	4	(1.8)	-	-	4	(5.8)	

3.3. Utilization of Media Relating to Nuclear Exposure

The type of media with the highest utilization rate was any local media (69.8%), followed by public broadcasting (NHK) (45.3%), and then public relations information from local government (44.0%). There was no significant difference in the utilization of local, national, or public broadcasting (NHK) between forced and voluntary evacuees. In contrast, the utilization rate of Internet media and public relations information from local governments differed significantly between forced and voluntary evacuees (Table 2). Moreover, the characteristics of the users of media relating to nuclear exposure are shown in Supplementary Tables S1 and S2. The Internet media users in this study tended to be of a younger generation and of a higher educational level than users of the other types of media. Furthermore, the proportion of those who utilized any Internet media among voluntary evacuees was higher in comparison to forced evacuees.

Table 2. Utilization of media relating to nuclear exposure among evacuees (forced/voluntary).

	Total (n = 225) n (%)	Forced Evacuees (n = 156) n (%)	Voluntary Evacuees (n = 69) n (%)	p-Value (χ^2)
Local media				
Local newspapers	140 (62.2)	102 (65.4)	38 (55.1)	0.14 ($\chi^2 = 2.16$)
Local broadcasting	71 (31.6)	42 (26.9)	29 (42.0)	0.03 ($\chi^2 = 5.05$)
Any local media	157 (69.8)	112 (71.8)	45 (65.2)	0.32 ($\chi^2 = 9.81$)
National media				
National newspapers	29 (12.9)	23 (14.7)	6 (8.7)	0.21 ($\chi^2 = 1.56$)
National broadcasting	39 (17.3)	26 (16.7)	13 (18.8)	0.69 ($\chi^2 = 0.16$)
Any nationwide media	63 (28.0)	46 (29.5)	17 (24.6)	0.46 ($\chi^2 = 0.56$)
Public broadcasting (NHK)	102 (45.3)	76 (48.7)	26 (37.7)	0.13 ($\chi^2 = 2.35$)
Internet media				
Internet news	33 (14.7)	16 (10.3)	17 (24.6)	0.01 ($\chi^2 = 7.91$)
Other information on Internet	21 (9.3)	8 (5.1)	13 (18.8)	<0.01 ($\chi^2 = 10.6$)
Social networking sites (SNS)	12 (5.3)	5 (3.2)	7 (10.1)	0.03 ($\chi^2 = 4.56$)
Any Internet media	54 (24.0)	24 (15.4)	30 (43.5)	<0.01 ($\chi^2 = 20.7$)
Public relations from local government	99 (44.0)	79 (50.6)	20 (29.0)	<0.01 ($\chi^2 = 9.11$)

3.4. Specifics of Current Strong Anxiety

The proportion of respondents with current strong health anxiety due to radiation exposure at the time of answering the questionnaire was 20.3% (43/223). Among evacuees who expressed current health anxiety at the time of answering the questionnaire, most were concerned about the delayed effects (92.9%), the genetic effects (92.9%), and the broadcasting about nuclear issues (95.3%). Only anxiety about unhealthy status was of relatively low concern among evacuees (63.4%). The proportion of evacuees with these concerns was significantly higher among those who expressed current strong health anxiety compared to those who did not. There was no significant difference between forced and voluntary evacuees (Table 3).

Table 3. Characteristics of current anxiety (forced/voluntary evacuees).

	Total			Forced Evacuees			Voluntary Evacuees		
	Current Strong Anxiety about Health due to Nuclear Disaster			Current Strong Anxiety about Health due to Nuclear Disaster			Current Strong Anxiety about Health due to Nuclear Disaster		
	(+) (n = 43) n (%)	(−) (n = 178) n (%)	p-Value (χ^2)	(+) (n = 29) n (%)	(−) (n = 124) n (%)	p-Value (χ^2)	(+) (n = 14) n (%)	(−) (n = 54) n (%)	p-Value (χ^2)
Anxiety about delayed effects	39 (92.9)	81 (45.5)	<0.01 ($\chi^2 = 30.7$)	25 (89.3)	54 (43.5)	<0.01 ($\chi^2 = 19.1$)	14 (100.0)	27 (50.0)	<0.01 ($\chi^2 = 11.6$)
Anxiety about unhealthy status	26 (63.4)	34 (19.2)	<0.01 ($\chi^2 = 32.6$)	17 (60.7)	26 (21.0)	<0.01 ($\chi^2 = 17.8$)	9 (69.2)	8 (15.1)	<0.01 ($\chi^2 = 16.0$)
Anxiety about genetic effects	39 (92.9)	84 (47.2)	<0.01 ($\chi^2 = 28.7$)	26 (92.9)	57 (46.0)	<0.01 ($\chi^2 = 20.3$)	13 (92.9)	27 (50.0)	<0.01 ($\chi^2 = 8.43$)
Anxiety from broadcasting about a nuclear event	41 (95.3)	129 (73.3)	<0.01 ($\chi^2 = 9.68$)	27 (93.1)	85 (69.7)	0.01 ($\chi^2 = 6.72$)	14 (100.0)	44 (81.5)	0.08 ($\chi^2 = 3.04$)

3.5. Association between Current Strong Health Anxiety and Utilization of Media Information

Among all evacuees, a significant negative association was observed between utilization of public relations information from local government and current strong health anxiety at the time of answering the questionnaire. Among the voluntary evacuees, there was a non-significant trend between utilization of Internet media and current strong health anxiety (Table 4).

Table 4. Association between current strong anxiety and media utilization (forced/voluntary evacuees).

	Total					Forced Evacuees					Voluntary Evacuees				
	Current Strong Anxiety about Health due to Nuclear Disaster					Current Strong Anxiety about Health due to Nuclear Disaster					Current Strong Anxiety about Health due to Nuclear Disaster				
	(+)		(−)		p-Value (χ^2)	(+)		(−)		p-Value (χ^2)	(+)		(−)		p-Value (χ^2)
	(n = 43)		(n = 180)			(n = 29)		(n = 126)			(n = 14)		(n = 54)		
	n	(%)	n	(%)		n	(%)	n	(%)		n	(%)	n	(%)	
Any local media	31	(72.1)	124	(68.9)	0.68 ($\chi^2 = 0.17$)	22	(75.9)	89	(70.6)	0.57 ($\chi^2 = 0.32$)	9	(64.3)	35	(64.8)	0.97 ($\chi^2 = 0.01$)
Any national media	14	(32.6)	49	(27.2)	0.49 ($\chi^2 = 0.49$)	11	(37.9)	35	(27.8)	0.28 ($\chi^2 = 1.16$)	3	(21.4)	14	(25.9)	0.73 ($\chi^2 = 0.12$)
Public broadcasting (NHK)	15	(34.9)	85	(47.2)	0.14 ($\chi^2 = 2.13$)	11	(37.9)	64	(50.8)	0.21 ($\chi^2 = 1.56$)	4	(28.6)	21	(38.9)	0.48 ($\chi^2 = 0.51$)
Any Internet media	13	(30.2)	40	(22.2)	0.27 ($\chi^2 = 1.23$)	4	(13.8)	20	(15.9)	0.78 ($\chi^2 = 0.08$)	9	(64.3)	20	(37.0)	0.07 ($\chi^2 = 3.38$)
Public relations from local government	12	(27.9)	87	(48.3)	0.02 ($\chi^2 = 5.87$)	9	(31.0)	70	(55.6)	0.17 ($\chi^2 = 5.67$)	3	(21.4)	17	(31.5)	0.46 ($\chi^2 = 0.54$)

In the multivariate logistic regression analysis, utilization of public relations information from local government was significantly associated with lower current strong health anxiety at the time of answering the questionnaire among all evacuees (odds ratio (OR): 0.76; 95% confidence interval (CI): 0.61–0.94) and among forced evacuees (OR: 0.72; 95% CI: 0.56–0.93). However, public broadcasting (NHK) showed a non-significant relation between utilization and lower current health anxiety (OR: 0.85; 95% CI: 0.69–1.04). Moreover, there was a non-significant trend between utilization of Internet media and current strong health anxiety (OR: 1.56; 95% CI: 0.99–2.43) (Table 5).

Table 5. Multivariate logistic regression analysis with utilized media and current strong anxiety (forced/voluntary evacuees).

		Model 1			Model 2					
		Total Current Strong Anxiety (+/−)			Forced Evacuees Current Strong Anxiety (+/−)			Voluntary Evacuees Current Strong Anxiety (+/−)		
		(n = 219)			(n = 152)			(n = 67)		
		OR	(95% CI)	p-Value	OR	(95% CI)	p-Value	OR	(95% CI)	p-Value
Any local media	Yes	1.11	(0.90–1.36)	0.35	1.11	(0.86–1.44)	0.42	1.07	(0.72–1.57)	0.75
	No (Ref.)	1.00			1.00			1.00		
Any national media	Yes	1.01	(0.82–1.25)	0.90	1.04	(0.81–1.34)	0.74	0.89	(0.57–1.38)	0.60
	No (Ref.)	1.00			1.00			1.00		
Public broadcasting (NHK)	Yes	0.85	(0.69–1.04)	0.11	0.83	(0.65–1.05)	0.12	0.88	(0.59–1.31)	0.53
	No (Ref.)	1.00			1.00			1.00		
Any Internet media	Yes	1.11	(0.88–1.43)	0.36	0.96	(0.68–1.35)	0.81	1.56	(0.99–2.43)	0.05
	No (Ref.)	1.00			1.00			1.00		
Public relations from local government	Yes	0.76	(0.61–0.94)	0.01	0.72	(0.56–0.93)	0.01	0.89	(0.59–1.34)	0.57
	No (Ref.)	1.00			1.00			1.00		

Model 1: Adjusted for gender, age, education, and evacuation type. Model 2: Adjusted for gender, age, and education OR, odds ratio; CI, confidence interval.

4. Discussion

The present study aimed to clarify the association between media utilization (e.g., Internet media, public relations information from local government, and other traditional media) and current strong health anxiety at the time of answering the questionnaire in the context of the Fukushima nuclear disaster. As per the results, the present study found a significant association between the use of public relations information from local government and lower current health anxiety at the time of answering the questionnaire.

4.1. Utilization of Media Information

In a previous study that assessed media consumption after the Fukushima Daiichi nuclear disaster, over 95% of participants answered that they used television news as a common media source, whereas Internet news and personal Internet websites were used by less than 50% (39% and 14%, respectively) [12]. Although a simple comparison with our results is not possible due to differences in the survey items and methods, those findings are largely consistent with our present findings. On the other hand, the rate of use of any Internet media among voluntary evacuees was significantly higher than that among forced evacuees. In fact, the rate of Internet media usage was the highest among the media sources in the voluntary evacuees, while it was the lowest in the forced evacuees. When considering age, the Internet media utilization rate in the voluntary evacuees was 81.3% (13/16 respondents) among those aged 20–39 years (forced: 43.8%; χ^2 test, $p = 0.03$), 47.1% (16/34 respondents) among those aged 40–64 years (forced: 21.1%; χ^2 test, $p = 0.01$), and 5.3% (1/19 respondents) among those aged ≥65 years (forced: 1.6%; χ^2 test, $p = 0.36$) (Table 1 and Supplementary Tables S1 and S2). This suggests that younger generations use Internet media to the greatest extent among age groups, particularly among voluntary evacuees.

The utilization rate of public relations information from local government among forced evacuees was higher than that of voluntary evacuees. Compared by age group, the utilization rate among forced evacuees aged 40–64 years was significantly higher than that of the corresponding age group of voluntary evacuees (forced: 53.9%; voluntary: 17.6%; χ^2 test, $p < 0.01$), whereas the rates in those aged ≥65 years were similar between forced and voluntary evacuees (forced: 57.8%; voluntary: 52.6%; χ^2 test, $p = 0.69$) (Table 1 and Supplementary Tables S1 and S2). This result might be explained by differences in the age group composition of forced and voluntary evacuees.

4.2. Specific Aspects of Current Strong Health Anxiety

The proportion of respondents with current strong health anxiety due to radiation exposure at the time of answering the questionnaire was 20.3%. Among evacuees who experienced current strong health anxiety at the time of answering the questionnaire, more than 90% were concerned about the delayed effects, the genetic effects, and broadcasting about nuclear issues. In previous studies, specific anxiety was associated with the effects of radiation on the development of thyroid cancer [13,14], on the workplace environment [15], on expectant mothers and children [16], on the estimated occurrence of acute radiation syndrome (an acute illness caused by irradiation of the entire body by a high dose of radiation in a short period of time) [17], and on the reluctance to eat foods grown in the evacuation area [18]. Moreover, among the Fukushima nuclear disaster evacuees, concerns about radiation risks were associated with psychological distress [19]. Although risk perception or anxiety regarding the delayed and genetic effects due to radiation exposure decreased from 2012 to 2015 (delayed effects: 48.1% in 2012 to 42.8% in 2015; genetic effects: 60.2% in 2012 to 37.6% in 2015) [18,19], these rates of risk perception and anxiety were still over 30% among all evacuees, even four years after the disaster. Therefore, despite the gradual decrease in the risk perception of radiation exposure, anxiety regarding the delayed and genetic effects due to exposure was associated with current strong health anxiety.

During the nuclear emergency in Fukushima, the traditional media were found to provide a broad context, including frequent comparisons with previous nuclear accidents; however, the experts' technical vocabulary concerning radiation appeared incompletely translated for public understanding [20]. Therefore, our findings may show that, among evacuees who experienced current strong health anxiety at the time of answering the questionnaire, more than 90% had concerns about broadcasting regarding nuclear issues.

4.3. Association between Current Strong Health Anxiety and Utilization of Media Information: Considerations for Effective Disaster Communication

Among the responders, the proportion with current strong health anxiety due to radiation exposure at the time of answering the questionnaire was 20.3%. Current strong health anxiety at the time of answering the questionnaire was significantly lower among those who utilized public relations information from local government. The Public Relations Society of America (PRSA) stated that "Public relations is a strategic communication process that builds mutually beneficial relationships between organizations and their publics. It is thought that not providing information unilaterally but providing information promoting mutual-communication or useful information about lots of variety of consultation will lead to mutually beneficial relationships" [21]. In a previous report related to the Fukushima Daiichi Nuclear Power Plant accident, a unified approach was found no longer to be sufficient to address personal problems and anxiety as diverse information became available and people's perceptions developed. This led to the need for one-to-one or small-group communication [22]. Another study reported that attending radiation information seminars or programs helped to reduce anxiety and psychological distress in a post-Fukushima disaster setting [12,23]. The public relations information from local government in evacuation areas included several articles regarding the health effects of radiation exposure, as well as the maximum annual exposure dose. Other posted articles included records of decontamination processing, discussion records of the health risk communication promotion committee in evacuation areas, and articles providing information such as general health consultations and dialogue among evacuees and experts, as well as information including education regarding stress reactions and coping [24]. Therefore, utilizing public relations information from local government may be associated with lower current health anxiety at the time of answering the questionnaire.

Users of Internet media tended to feel anxiety toward perceived radiation health risks, but not to a significant degree. Several studies have examined the correlation between risk perception and anxiety and media/information after the Fukushima nuclear accident. Murakami et al. revealed that dread risk perception was greater among people who trusted direct information from online researchers or others than those who did not, but was lower among people who trusted central governmental information than among those who did not [25]. Sugimoto et al. surveyed 1560 residents of Soma City in July 2011 and found that health anxiety was high among those who relied on word-of-mouth or rumors as a means to obtain information [12]. Baseless rumors and conspiracy theories spread very quickly on the Internet, which may also explain the high levels of anxiety among those who mainly used the Internet as their information source. Any Internet media usage in this study did not include solely Internet news, but also the use of personal websites such as social networking sites (SNS), and information from these sources likely include word-of-mouth or rumors. This suggests a potential association between evacuees with strong anxiety and the use of any type of Internet media.

4.4. Limitations and Strengths

This study has several limitations. First, due to its cross-sectional design, causality could not be established. Second, our primary outcome, i.e., current anxiety regarding perceived radiation health risks, was a subjective response This could certainly be the case with actual and perceived health risks, leading to important differences in anxiety levels, without validated measures and reliability statistics such as a test–retest correlation, which is a critical limitation. Therefore, it would hardly be applicable to different settings without reliability. Further studies are needed to confirm the validity and reliability regarding current anxiety regarding perceived radiation health risks. Additionally, our definition of "current strong health anxiety" may be included as a bias. Those who responded to "Somewhat" (47.1% in both the forced and the voluntary evacuees, see Supplementary Table S3) as current health anxiety at the time of answering the questionnaire due to radiation exposure were categorized as the "no or weak health anxiety" group, although this could be in either group. However, this categorization was comparable to that of the Fukushima Health Management Survey report [26], which focused on high and extreme anxiety of health effects due to radiation exposure. The third limitation relates to sampling from non-evacuation areas. We could not grasp detailed enough information about the number of voluntary evacuations in advance. As a result, many residents had not experienced evacuation voluntary, and thus more than 600 respondents were later excluded from the analysis. Fourth, because respondents tended to be relatively older, our study population included fewer Internet users, in particular SNS users. Finally, depending on the three types of evacuation areas according to the spatial radiation dose rates, there may have been different perceived health risks, leading to important differences in anxiety levels. However, due to anonymous sampling, it was impossible to obtain the detailed information on whether subjects were living in one of the three types of evacuation areas. This is because the first-stage sampling was selected by municipality, not by each of the three area types.

Despite these limitations, we were able to show a positive association between the utilization of public relations information from local government and lower health anxiety due to radiation exposure, even after adjusting for age, gender, education, and evacuation type. Although we examined the association between utilization of media and current health anxiety after the 2011 nuclear disaster, further studies in other settings, such as that of the novel coronavirus pandemic, are needed.

5. Conclusions

The 2011 nuclear disaster in Fukushima was not only a health disaster, but also an information disaster. Our findings highlight the importance of public relations information from local government in terms of it being associated with lower current health anxiety at the time of answering the questionnaire related to disaster situations, and this could potentially aid in preparing for future disasters.

Supplementary Materials: The following are available online at http://www.mdpi.com/1660-4601/17/11/3921/s1, Table S1: Characteristics of media users relating to nuclear exposure (forced evacuees). Table S2: Characteristics of media users relating to nuclear exposure (voluntary evacuees). Table S3: Prevalence of current health anxiety due to radiation exposure.

Author Contributions: S.Y. designed the framed study and acquired funding. S.Y., T.N., M.S., C.N., and Y.K. contributed to designing the questionnaire. M.O., Y.K., N.M., H.I., T.H., and S.Y. investigated and administrated the survey. M.O. conducted data analysis and wrote the draft. All authors have read and agreed to the published version of the manuscript.

Funding: This study was supported by a grant from KAKENHI, Japan Society for the Promotion of Science (JSPS), as a Grant-in-Aid for Scientific Research (C) research (JSPS KAKENHI Grant Number: 15K08810).

Conflicts of Interest: The authors declare no conflict of interest.

References

1. Fukushima Prefectural Government. Fukushima Revitalization Station. 2017. Available online: http://www.pref.fukushima.lg.jp/site/portal-english/ (accessed on 17 May 2020).
2. Yamashita, S. Fukushima Nuclear Power Plant Accident and Comprehensive Health Risk Management—Global radiocontamination and information disaster. *Trop. Med. Healt.* **2014**, *42*, S14–S107.
3. Suzuki, Y.; Yabe, H.; Yasumura, S.; Ohira, T.; Niwa, S.; Ohtsuru, A.; Mashiko, H.; Maeda, M.; Abe, M.; Mental Health Group of the Fukushima Health Management Survey. Psychological distress and the perception of radiation risks: The Fukushima health management survey. *Bull. World Health Organ.* **2015**, *93*, 598–605. [CrossRef] [PubMed]
4. Gallego, E.; Cantone, M.C.; Oughton, D.H.; Perko, T.; Prezelj, I.; Tomkiv, Y. Mass Media Communication of Emergency Issues and Countermeasures in a Nuclear Accident: Fukushima Reporting in European Newspapers. *Radiat. Prot. Dosim.* **2017**, *173*, 163–169. [CrossRef] [PubMed]
5. Aitsi-Selmi, A.; Murray, V. The Chernobyl Disaster and Beyond: Implications of the Sendai Framework for Disaster Risk Reduction 2015–2030. *PLoS Med.* **2016**, *13*, e1002017. [CrossRef] [PubMed]
6. Jung, J.Y.; Moro, M. Multi-level functionality of social media in the aftermath of the Great East Japan Earthquake. *Disaster* **2014**, *38* (Suppl. 2), S123–S143. [CrossRef] [PubMed]

7. Pfefferbaum, B.; Newman, E.; Nelson, S.D.; Nitiéma, P.; Pfefferbaum, R.L.; Rahman, A. Disaster media coverage and psychological outcomes: Descriptive findings in the extant research. *Curr. Psychiatry Rep.* **2014**, *16*, 464. [CrossRef] [PubMed]
8. Bui, E.; Rodgers, R.F.; Herbert, C.; Franko, D.L.; Simon, N.M.; Birmes, P.; Brunet, A. The impact of internet coverage of the March 2011 Japan earthquake on sleep and posttraumatic stress symptoms: An international perspective. *Am. J. Psychiatry* **2012**, *169*, 221–222. [CrossRef] [PubMed]
9. Umeda, M.; Sekiya, Y.; Kawakami, N.; Miyamoto, K.; Horikoshi, N.; Yabe, H.; Yasumura, S.; Ohtsuru, A.; Akiyama, T.; Suzuki, Y. Reliability and validity of radiation anxiety scale developed for Fukushima community residents. In Proceedings of the 24th Annual Scientific Meeting of the Japan Epidemiological Association, Sendai, Japan, 23–25 January 2014. (In Japanese).
10. Fukasawa, M.; Kawakami, N.; Umeda, M.; Miyamoto, K.; Akiyama, T.; Horikoshi, N.; Yasumura, S.; Yabe, H.; Bromet, E.J. Environmental radiation level, radiation anxiety, and psychological distress of non-evacuee residents in Fukushima five years after the Great East Japan Earthquake: Multilevel analyses. *SSM Popul. Health* **2017**, *19*, 740–748. [CrossRef] [PubMed]
11. Nakayama, C.; Sato, O.; Sugita, M.; Nakayama, T.; Kuroda, Y.; Orui, M.; Iwasa, H.; Yasumura, S.; Rudd, R.E. Lingering health-related anxiety about radiation among Fukushima residents as correlated with media information following the accident at Fukushima Daiichi Nuclear Power Plant. *PLoS ONE* **2019**, *14*, e0217285. [CrossRef] [PubMed]
12. Sugimoto, A.; Nomura, S.; Tsubokura, M.; Matsumura, T.; Muto, K.; Sato, M.; Gilmour, S. The relationship between media consumption and health-related anxieties after the Fukushima Daiichi nuclear disaster. *PLoS ONE* **2013**, *8*, e65331. [CrossRef] [PubMed]
13. Hino, Y.; Murakami, M.; Midorikawa, S.; Ohtsuru, A.; Suzuki, S.; Tsuboi, K.; Ohira, T. Explanatory Meetings on Thyroid Examination for the "Fukushima Health Management Survey" after the Great East Japan Earthquake: Reduction of Anxiety and Improvement of Comprehension. *Tohoku J. Exp. Med.* **2016**, *239*, 333–343. [CrossRef] [PubMed]
14. Midorikawa, S.; Tanigawa, K.; Suzuki, S.; Ohtsuru, A. Psychosocial Issues Related to Thyroid Examination after a Radiation Disaster. *Asia Pac. J. Public Health* **2017**, *29*, 63s–73s. [CrossRef] [PubMed]
15. Takeda, S.; Orita, M.; Fukushima, Y.; Kudo, T.; Takamura, N. Determinants of intention to leave among non-medical employees after a nuclear disaster: A cross-sectional study. *BMJ Open* **2016**, *6*, e011930. [CrossRef] [PubMed]
16. Yoshii, H.; Saito, H.; Kikuchi, S.; Ueno, T.; Sato, K. Report on maternal anxiety 16 months after the great East Japan earthquake disaster: Anxiety over radioactivity. *Glob. J. Health Sci.* **2014**, *6*, 1–10. [CrossRef] [PubMed]
17. Orita, M.; Hayashida, N.; Nakayama, Y.; Shinkawa, T.; Urata, H.; Fukushima, Y.; Endo, Y.; Yamashita, S.; Takamura, N. Bipolarization of Risk Perception about the Health Effects of Radiation in Residents after the Accident at Fukushima Nuclear Power Plant. *PLoS ONE* **2015**, *10*, e0129227. [CrossRef] [PubMed]
18. Takebayashi, Y.; Lyamzina, Y.; Suzuki, Y.; Murakami, M. Risk Perception and Anxiety Regarding Radiation after the 2011 Fukushima Nuclear Power Plant Accident: A Systematic Qualitative Review. *Int. J. Environ. Res. Public Health* **2017**, *14*, 1306. [CrossRef] [PubMed]
19. Radiation Medical Science Center for the Fukushima Health Management Survey. Fukushima Medical University Fukushima Health Management Survey. Available online: https://www.pref.fukushima.lg.jp/site/portal/kenkocyosa-kokoro.html (accessed on 18 May 2020). (In Japanese).
20. Perko, T.; Mays, C.; Valuch, J.; Nagy, A. Mass and New Media: Review of Framing, Treatment and Sources in Reporting on Fukushima. *J. Mass Commun. Journalism.* **2015**, *5*, 252.
21. About Public Relations. Public Relations Society of America. Available online: https://www.prsa.org/all-about-pr/ (accessed on 18 May 2020).
22. Murakami, M.; Sato, A.; Matsui, S.; Goto, A.; Kumagai, A.; Tsubokura, M.; Orita, M.; Takamura, N.; Kuroda, Y.; Ochi, S. Communicating With Residents About Risks Following the Fukushima Nuclear Accident. *Asia Pac. J. Public Health* **2017**, *29*, 74S–89S. [CrossRef] [PubMed]
23. Imamura, K.; Sekiya, Y.; Asai, Y.; Umeda, M.; Horikoshi, N.; Yasumura, S.; Yabe, H.; Akiyama, T.; Kawakami, N. The effect of a behavioral activation program on improving mental and physical health complaints associated with radiation stress among mothers in Fukushima: A randomized controlled trial. *BMC Public Health* **2016**, *16*, 1144. [CrossRef] [PubMed]

24. Public Relations of Iitate, Iitate Village, Fukushima Prefecture, Japan. Available online: http://www.vill.iitate.fukushima.jp/life/5/19/73/ (accessed on 17 May 2020). (In Japanese).
25. Murakami, M.; Nakatani, J.; Oki, T. Evaluation of Risk Perception and Risk-Comparison Information Regarding Dietary Radionuclides after the 2011 Fukushima Nuclear Power Plant Accident. *PLoS ONE* **2016**, *11*, e0165594. [CrossRef] [PubMed]
26. Fukushima Prefectural Office. The Fukushima Health Management Survey. Available online: https://www.pref.fukushima.lg.jp/uploaded/attachment/350326.pdf. (accessed on 16 May 2020). (In Japanese).

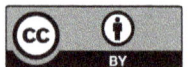

© 2020 by the authors. Licensee MDPI, Basel, Switzerland. This article is an open access article distributed under the terms and conditions of the Creative Commons Attribution (CC BY) license (http://creativecommons.org/licenses/by/4.0/).

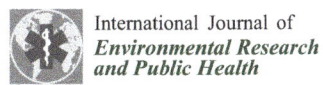
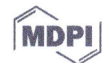

Article

Factors Associated with Urban Risk-Taking Behaviour during 2018 Typhoon Mangkhut: A Cross Sectional Study

Evan Su Wei Shang [1,2], Eugene Siu Kai Lo [1], Zhe Huang [1,2], Kevin Kei Ching Hung [1,3] and Emily Ying Yang Chan [1,2,3,4,*]

1. Collaborating Centre for Oxford University and CUHK for Disaster and Medical Humanitarian Response (CCOUC), The Chinese University of Hong Kong, Hong Kong, China; evanshang98@link.cuhk.edu.hk (E.S.W.S.); euglsk@cuhk.edu.hk (E.S.K.L.); huangzhe@cuhk.edu.hk (Z.H.); kevin.hung@cuhk.edu.hk (K.K.C.H.)
2. JC School of Public Health and Primary Care, The Chinese University of Hong Kong, Hong Kong, China
3. Accident & Emergency Medicine Academic Unit, The Chinese University of Hong Kong, Prince of Wales Hospital, Hong Kong, China
4. Nuffield Department of Medicine, University of Oxford, Oxford OX37BN, UK
* Correspondence: emily.chan@cuhk.edu.hk; Tel.: +852-2252-8702

Received: 18 May 2020; Accepted: 8 June 2020; Published: 10 June 2020

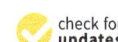

Abstract: Although much of the health emergency and disaster risk management (Health-EDRM) literature evaluates methods to protect health assets and mitigate health risks from disasters, there is a lack of research into those who have taken high-risk behaviour during extreme events. The study's main objective is to examine the association between engaging in high-risk behaviour and factors including sociodemographic characteristics, disaster risk perception and household preparedness during a super typhoon. A computerized randomized digit dialling cross-sectional household survey was conducted in Hong Kong, an urban metropolis, two weeks after the landing of Typhoon Mangkhut. Telephone interviews were conducted in Cantonese with adult residents. The response rate was 23.8% and the sample was representative of the Hong Kong population. Multivariable logistic regressions of 521 respondents adjusted with age and gender found education, income, risk perception and disaster preparedness were insignificantly associated with risk-taking behaviour during typhoons. This suggests that other factors may be involved in driving this behaviour, such as a general tendency to underestimate risk or sensation seeking. Further Health-EDRM research into risk-taking and sensation seeking behaviour during extreme events is needed to identify policy measures.

Keywords: typhoon; hurricane; cyclone; strong wind levels; natural disaster; Health-EDRM; urban; risk-taking behaviour; sensation seeking

1. Introduction

Asia is particularly at risk of tropical cyclones, also known as typhoons in the western Pacific, with around half of worldwide tropical cyclones recorded and more than 90% of cyclone-related deaths being from this region [1]. Typhoon Mangkhut, the fourth supertyphoon in the 2018 Pacific typhoon season, started east of Guam in September 2018 and caused devastating damage to the Philippines [2] and South China [3]. In Hong Kong, tropical cyclone warning signal No. 10 (the highest signal for Hong Kong) was hoisted for 10 h, with the highest wind speed exceeding 150 km/h, just lower than the respective records held by Typhoon York in 1999 and Typhoon Ellen in 1983 [4]. Although there were no deaths reported directly due to the typhoon, more than 60,000 trees had reportedly fallen and around 13,500 households experienced a power outage for more than 24 h in Hong Kong [5]. Record breaking storm surges coupled with high waves caused flooding in various coastal areas, despite not being at high tide, with hundreds of stranded or damaged vessels. These occurrences highlighted the increasing environmental hazards and potential health risks faced by coastal communities around the world as typhoons become more frequent and severe through climate change [6].

Health emergency and disaster risk management (Health-EDRM) is a field which involves the systematic analysis and management of health risks surrounding emergencies and disasters. By reducing risk and vulnerabilities and improving preparedness, response and recovery measures, the impact of disasters can be minimised [7]. Health-EDRM focuses on increasing the resilience of individuals, households and communities through education interventions, promotion of disaster risk reduction and supporting mechanisms in place to mitigate impacts of disasters [8]. These can include accessible disaster warning and information, protection of key health services and securing the basic needs of the population. By understanding the causes and factors in play regarding disaster risk, Health-EDRM provides evidence to drive future interventions and policy decisions.

A previous study on urban disaster preparedness in Hong Kong discovered that only 20.6% of respondents chose the correct action to take while major disaster warnings were in force (such as staying in a safe place until heavy rain has passed) [9]. However, few studies investigate individuals intentionally performing risk-taking behaviour during natural disasters. Research on 'storm chasers' (those who intercept severe convective storms for sport or for scientific research) [10] in the United States has examined individual perception of recreational storm chasing to dispel its myths [11], operational methods of storm chasing tour groups [12] and sensation seeking traits associated with tour participants [13]. There is a lack of research into such behaviour outside of the United States, especially in urban areas directly impacted by meteorological disasters. Various studies by Zuckerman on sensation seeking have identified its dimensions [14] and relationships to different aspects through the sensation seeking scale (SSS) [15]. A meta-analysis into sex differences in sensation seeking showed that men scored higher than women using Zuckerman's SSS-V and could be explained by evolutionary psychology and through a cultural socialisation perspective [16]. Furthermore, a review of behavioural and biological correlates of sensation seeking also found males significantly outscored females on total sensation seeking in different western countries and sensation seeking typically decreases with increasing age after adolescence [17]. Education and occupation were less associated with sensation seeking, particularly for females. The review also highlighted high sensation seekers perceived risks in the environment as less threatening compared to low sensation seekers and did not perceive engaging in high-risk behaviours would lead to negative consequences.

This article is an extension of the cross-sectional study investigating risk perception, household preparedness, and self-reported short-term impacts of typhoons after Typhoon Mangkhut [18]. Our previous published paper highlighted 16.0% of respondents reportedly left their homes when the warning signal was T8 or above, when the typhoon was at the height of strength. This behaviour will henceforth be referred to as risk-taking behaviour during typhoons (RBDT). Out of those respondents, a majority (74.7%) performed RBDT for non-essential reasons. The previous article also found that men and younger respondents were more likely to execute non-essential RBDT. Using the same dataset, the objectives of the current study are to expand on these findings and investigate other factors that may be related to RBDT, namely (1) to identify the sociodemographic characteristics of those who left their homes when the storm was at its height of strength (i.e., the warning signal was T8 or above); and (2) to explore the associations between sociodemographic factors other than age and gender, risk perception, household preparedness, and RBDT for non-essential purposes. The study findings will offer further insight into risk-taking behaviour during natural disasters to guide future interventions and policy on preventing such unnecessary high-risk behaviour.

2. Materials and Methods

A computerized digit dialling population-based household telephone survey was conducted from 17 September 2018 to 2 October 2018, right after the date of Typhoon Mangkhut landing in Hong Kong.

Random digit dialling and the last birthday method [19] (interviewer would seek the household member whose birthday was the closest to the interview date) were used to ensure randomization in the study. Hong Kong residents who understood Cantonese and were 18 years old or older were interviewed. In total, 2500 landline numbers were called, and 521 respondents were successfully recruited (Figure 1). The response rate was 23.8% (response rate: 521 (final sample size) /2188 (eligible persons)). Please refer to the previous published study for study design [18].

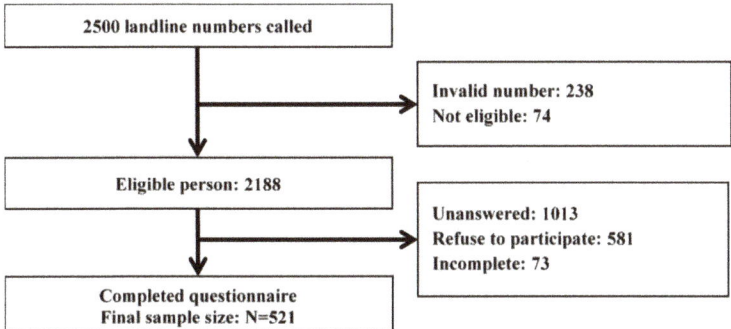

Figure 1. The recruitment details in the telephone survey.

This study investigates the associations between non-essential RBDT and the sociodemographic factors of education and income; indicators of risk perception including perception of Hong Kong being susceptible to disasters, perception of the impact of Typhoon Mangkhut compared to expectations and concern for the safety of oneself and family members; indicators of household preparedness including food and water reserves prepared routinely or specifically for Typhoon Mangkhut.

This paper considers the act of going outside during the strongest typhoon winds as risk-taking (RBDT) or high-risk behaviour, regardless of the reasoning. Those who go outside for work or emergency related purposes would be considered as engaging in socially acceptable or understandable risk-taking behaviour. This article focuses on active risk-taking behaviour, where individuals remove themselves from areas of safety to head into areas posing health risks, and does not investigate passive risk-taking behaviour, such as failure to act, evacuate or engage in other safety-seeking behaviour. This is because there are potentially different motivating factors, rationale and mechanisms involved in these two types of behaviour and research has found that passive risks are associated with a lower risk perception than equivalent active risks [20]. Previous literature has investigated passive risks associated with disasters and relevant methods to protect passive risk, but there is a lack of research into active risk-taking behaviour.

To clarify, the respondents were asked whether they left their homes to go outside during Typhoon Mangkhut while the typhoon warning signal T8 or above was in force. Those who left their home to address any perceived urgent and unexpected situations that required immediate action to prevent further deterioration, such as "due to injury or disease", were classified as having 'emergency' reasons. Those who did not have to manage such pressing issues or work-related duties but left their home for other reasons, such as "eating a meal or watching a movie", were categorized as having 'non-emergency' reasons. This paper will hence refer to RBDT due to 'non-emergency', also referred to as non-emergency and non-occupational reasons in our previous published paper, as non-essential reasons. Verbal informed consent was obtained at the beginning of the interview. The ethical approval of this study was obtained from the Survey Behavioural Research Committee at the Chinese University of Hong Kong (SBRE-18-075).

Descriptive chi-square (or X^2) tests were used to compare the study population and the respondents who reported going outdoors during Typhoon Mangkhut. We conducted univariate analyses to identify associations between sociodemographic characteristics, risk perception, disaster preparedness factors and the risk-taking behaviour. Multivariable logistic regression was performed to identify factors related to going outdoors during strong typhoon winds for 'non-emergency' reasons, using variables with at least marginal statistical association in the univariate analysis ($p < 0.10$). Age and gender were covariates for the multivariable model base. All odds ratios (OR) present in this paper were adjusted odds ratios from the multivariable models. Statistical analyses were performed using IBM SPSS 24 (International Business Machines Corporation, Armonk, NY, USA) [21] and statistical significance was set at $\alpha = 0.05$ two-sided.

3. Results

Data were collected from 17 September 2018 to 2 October 2018. The final sample size constituted 521 valid respondents (the response rate was 23.8% among eligible people called). The study population were comparable with the Hong Kong 2016 census data, except the study population were proportionally more middle age (age 45–64), more at the post-secondary education level and had higher income. Please refer to the previous paper [18] for further information and detailed analyses.

3.1. Description of the Study Population

For the descriptive comparison (Table 1), it was found that men were more likely to engage in non-essential RBDT ($p = 0.006$). There were no significant associations between RBDT and marital status, income, and respondents with chronic disease. Of the respondents with occupations which require emergency work while typhoon No. 8 or higher was in force, 72.2% reported staying home during Typhoon Mangkhut when the typhoon was at the height of strength. In addition, respondents who had occupations relating to "Sales and services" and "Elementary occupation" were more likely to leave their homes for emergency or work reasons. Respondents who participated in RBDT for emergency or work reasons were found to be more likely to obtain their weather-related information during this typhoon through television and newspapers and less likely through websites and mobile apps.

Table 1. Descriptive table of the study population.

Characteristics		Go Outdoor for Emergency/Work Reasons ($n = 21$)	Go Outdoor for Non-Essential Reasons ($n = 62$)	Did Not Go Outdoor ($n = 438$)	p-Value
Gender	Male	9 (42.9%)	38 (61.3%)	174 (39.7%)	0.006
	Female	12 (57.1%)	24 (38.7%)	264 (60.3%)	
Age	18–24	2 (9.5%)	14 (22.6%)	47 (10.7%)	
	25–44	9 (42.9%)	18 (29.0%)	127 (29.0%)	0.078
	45–64	9 (42.9%)	24 (38.7%)	191 (43.6%)	
	≥65	1 (4.8%)	6 (9.7%)	73 (16.7%)	
Education attainment	Primary or below	2 (10.0%)	5 (8.1%)	49 (11.3%)	
	Secondary	7 (35.0%)	18 (29.0%)	170 (39.2%)	0.407
	Post-secondary	11 (55.0%)	39 (62.9%)	215 (49.5%)	
Marital status	Single	8 (38.1%)	28 (45.2%)	176 (40.2%)	0.734
	Married	13 (61.9%)	34 (54.8%)	262 (59.8%)	
Income	<2000–9999	0 (0.0%)	5 (8.9%)	40 (9.9%)	
	10,000–19,999	2 (10.5%)	5 (8.9%)	66 (16.3%)	0.462
	20,000–39,999	6 (31.6%)	21 (37.5%)	133 (32.9%)	
	≥40,000	11 (57.9%)	25 (44.6%)	165 (40.8%)	
Occupation	Manager/Professional/Clerk	9 (45.0%)	24 (41.4%)	151 (35.4%)	
	Sales & Services	5 (25.0%)	2 (3.4%)	35 (8.2%)	
	Craft related/Machinery labour	0 (0.0%)	5 (8.6%)	20 (4.7%)	0.033
	Elementary occupation	3 (15.0%)	3 (5.2%)	23 (5.4%)	
	Housewives/Students	1 (5.0%)	14 (24.1%)	115 (26.9%)	
	Unemployed/Retired	2 (10.0%)	10 (17.2%)	83 (19.4%)	
Chronic disease	Yes	4 (19.0%)	10 (16.7%)	77 (17.7%)	0.965
	No	17 (81.0%)	50 (83.3%)	357 (82.3%)	
Routinely work during typhoon signal no.8	Yes	15 (83.3%)	4 (9.3%)	35 (13.4%)	<0.001
	No	3 (16.7%)	39 (90.7%)	227 (86.6%)	
Occupation involving mainly outdoor work	Yes	3 (17.6%)	10 (23.3%)	43 (16.8%)	0.591
	No	14 (82.4%)	33 (76.7%)	213 (83.2%)	
Channel of obtaining weather information	Television	12 (57.1%)	26 (41.9%)	236 (53.9%)	
	Radio	0 (0.0%)	6 (9.7%)	24 (5.5%)	0.015
	Website/Smartphone platform	6 (28.6%)	28 (45.2%)	168 (38.4%)	
	Newspaper or others	3 (14.3%)	2 (3.2%)	10 (2.3%)	
Disaster preparation immediately prior to the typhoon	No	0 (0.0%)	4 (6.5%)	28 (6.4%)	0.489
	Yes	21 (100.0%)	58 (93.5%)	410 (93.6%)	

3.2. Factors Associated with Non-Essential RBDT

In the multivariable logistic regressions (Table 2), the relationship between various sociodemographic details, the subject's perception and preparedness for the typhoon and non-essential RBDT was examined. As reported in the previous article, being male and younger were found to have higher odds in performing non-essential RBDT than those that did not go outside. All factors investigated in this article such as education, disaster risk perception or household preparedness were not found to have a statistically significant association with non-essential RBDT after adjusting for age and gender. Food and water reserves (both routine and specifically prepared for Typhoon Mangkhut) were also not found to be related.

Table 2. Chi-square comparison and multivariable logistic regressions of the associating factors towards non-essential RBDT.

Factors		χ^2 Test			Logistic Regression	
		Stayed Indoor	Non-essential RBDT	p-Value	OR (95% CI)	p-Value
Gender [a]	Male	174 (39.7%)	38 (61.3%)	0.001	Ref.	
	Female	264 (60.3%)	24 (38.7%)		0.435 (0.248–0.761)	0.004
Age [a]	18–24	47 (10.7%)	14 (22.6%)	0.041	Ref.	
	25–44	127 (29.0%)	18 (29.0%)		0.573 (0.260–1.263)	0.167
	45–64	191 (43.6%)	24 (38.7%)		0.527 (0.248–1.118)	0.095
	≥65	73 (16.7%)	6 (9.7%)		0.297 (0.106–0.833)	0.021
Education attainment [b]	Primary or below	49 (11.3%)	5 (8.1%)	0.144	Ref.	
	Secondary	170 (39.2%)	18 (29.0%)		0.799 (0.269–2.374)	0.687
	Post-secondary	215 (49.5%)	39 (62.9%)		1.110 (0.363–3.392)	0.854
Income [b]	<2000–9999	40 (9.9%)	5 (8.9%)	0.517	Ref.	
	10,000–19,999	66 (16.3%)	5 (8.9%)		0.465 (0.120–1.796)	0.267
	20,000–39,999	133 (32.9%)	21 (37.5%)		0.897 (0.28–2.784)	0.851
	≥40,000	165 (40.98)	25 (44.6%)		0.821 (0.264–2.555)	0.733
Perceived Hong Kong to be susceptible to disasters [b]	No	35 (8.0%)	4 (6.5%)	0.669	Ref.	
	Yes	402 (92.0%)	58 (93.5%)		1.474 (0.494–4.398)	0.486
Perceived impact of Typhoon Mangkhut compared to expectations [b]	Less than expected	118 (27.1%)	16 (25.8%)	0.919	Ref.	
	Same as expected	235 (54.0%)	33 (53.2%)		0.919 (0.477–1.773)	0.802
	Larger than expected	82 (18.9%)	13 (21.0%)		1.032 (0.462–2.303)	0.940
Concerned for the safety of oneself and family members [b]	No	159 (36.3%)	17 (27.4%)	0.171	Ref.	
	Yes	279 (63.7%)	45 (72.6%)		1.585 (0.860–2.922)	0.140
Practiced disaster preparedness immediately prior to the typhoon [b]	No	28 (6.4%)	4 (6.5%)	0.986	Ref.	
	Yes	410 (93.6%)	58 (93.5%)		1.077 (0.355–3.264)	0.896
Preparedness: routine food reserves [b]	No	81 (18.5%)	7 (11.3%)	0.163	Ref.	
	Yes	357 (81.5%)	55 (88.7%)		1.663 (0.717–3.857)	0.236
Preparedness: routine potable water reserves [b]	No	223 (50.9%)	32 (51.6%)	0.918	Ref.	
	Yes	215 (49.1%)	30 (48.4%)		0.842 (0.484–1.463)	0.541
Preparedness: food reserves specifically for Typhoon Mangkhut [b]	No	137 (31.3%)	25 (40.3%)	0.154	Ref.	
	Yes	301 (68.7%)	37 (59.7%)		0.666 (0.378–1.174)	0.160
Preparedness: potable water reserves specifically for Typhoon Mangkhut [b]	No	272 (62.1%)	39 (62.9%)	0.903	Ref.	
	Yes	166 (37.9%)	23 (37.1%)		0.894 (0.506–1.581)	0.700

[a] is the multivariable regression of age and gender; [b] is the logistic regression adjusted with age and gender.

4. Discussion

The current study is an extension of the previous published paper [18], which investigated risk perception, household preparedness, and self-reported short-term impacts of typhoons after Typhoon Mangkhut. This study aims to identify the sociodemographic characteristics of those who performed RBDT and investigate correlations between other sociodemographic characteristics apart from age and gender, risk perception and preparedness, and non-essential RBDT. There were no significant associations between RBDT and marital status, income, and respondents with chronic disease. Respondents who participated in RBDT for emergency or work reasons were more likely to watch television and read newspapers to obtain their weather-related information and less likely through websites and mobile apps. Education, income, risk perception and preparedness were found to be insignificantly associated with non-essential RBDT.

4.1. Comparison between Household Preparedness and Risk-Taking Behaviour

Household preparedness and risk-taking behaviour may be negatively associated, as household preparedness represents active protective behaviour, while non-essential RBDT involves potentially injurious active behaviour. Although this study did not find any significant negative association between higher educational level, higher risk perception and routine emergency preparedness with non-essential RBDT, the previous published paper [18] found a positive association of these factors with individuals who engaged in household preparedness. The results suggest these two behaviours may have different perceived levels of risk and/or involve separate rationale, such as respondents not considering non-essential RBDT as high-risk activity but performing household preparedness to ensure adequate supplies for family members. However, there is a lack of data in this study on the magnitude and severity of risk perceived from the typhoon to support this hypothesis. In addition, this study could not indirectly gauge the relative amount of risk respondents were willing to take for RBDT, which could be independent from perception of general risks of the typhoon and disasters.

4.2. Difference between Typhoon Risk Perception and Risk Perception of Non-Essential RBDT

Although there was no association between perceived impact of Typhoon Mangkhut compared to expectations and non-essential RBDT, 80.9% of all respondents thought the impact of the typhoon was similar or less than expected. This may suggest that fewer people underestimate the risks of typhoons, even after the recent typhoon influence, given that Typhoon Mangkhut was objectively one of the strongest typhoons in Hong Kong to date. The literature on sensation seeking involving demographics [17] has also shown that high sensation seekers have lower risk perception of activities they have not engaged in before and are less likely to perceive the negative consequences of risk-taking behaviour. Therefore, there may be a difference between the perceived risk of typhoons or the resulting impacts and non-essential RBDT which is an active behaviour. High sensation seekers may identify typhoons as events that cause harm but do not perceive the negative consequences of non-essential RBDT. As there is a lack of data directly investigating the reasons people performed non-essential RBDT, this study explores other inferred and documented possible rationale.

4.3. Other Reasons for Non-Essential RBDT

This study found food and potable water reserves, whether prepared regularly or specifically for this typhoon, were not associated with respondents going outside for non-essential reasons at the height of the storm. In addition to being markers of household preparedness, the reserves and the lack thereof may indicate situations of non-essential character, which could motivate individuals to leave their homes under the rationale of necessity. The results suggest that seeking these two necessities were not primary reasons for non-essential RBDT.

News outlets have documented a case of an elderly man in Hong Kong stranded at sea and requiring rescue after swimming during Typhoon Haima while the typhoon signal No. 8 was in force [22], highlighting an instance of RBDT which would have caused significant harm if rescue operations did not take place. As the man's motives were not interviewed and reported, the behaviour could have been due to an underestimation of the risk involved or due to sensation seeking. Despite warnings from the Hong Kong government [23] and Hong Kong Observatory [24] before and during Typhoon Mangkhut, people were reported participating in sensation seeking behaviour, such as 'experiencing the wind' and engaging in disaster photography [25,26]. High-risk behaviour during extreme weather has also been documented in the news, with 300 firefighters mobilised to rescue scores of 'frost chasers' and other hikers from Hong Kong's highest peak during the city's coldest day in six decades [27]. Although the news reports did not interview the individuals and verify their desire to seek novel and intense experiences, it is clear that the risk-taking behaviours reported were performed directly to experience aspects of the disasters.

4.4. Ethical Concerns in Rescue Operations

There is also an ethical argument on the duty of firefighters who bear personal risk and danger to help those engaging in sensation seeking behaviour. A fireman in Hong Kong died in 2017 after sustaining a cliff fall while rescuing a pair of hikers [28], highlighting the risk and peril involved even in normal conditions. While rescuers have a duty to respond to emergencies, in cases involving sensation seeking behaviour, this creates a moral issue posing unnecessary risks to the rescuers in such extreme weather events. Rescue operations may also hinder other emergency responses and invoke issues of justice and equitable resource allocation. In total, 160 firemen were involved in a 24 h operation to rescue a pair of hikers who were stuck on a hiking trail during Tropical Storm Pakhar, which struck Hong Kong only days after Typhoon Hato. The entire operation included a total of ten ambulances and thirty-one fire engines, with an estimated total cost of more than 344,000 HKD in staffing costs alone [29].

4.5. What Is the Gap Found in This Study?

One of the major gaps found in this study is that education, disaster risk perception and disaster preparedness were not found to be associated with whether respondents engaged in unexplained risky behaviour. Common understanding would suggest that those with better understanding of the risks presented and especially those concerned about the safety of themselves and their family members during the typhoon would practice less risk-taking or sensation seeking. This suggests that knowledge-based interventions may not be as effective in deterring individuals from engaging in non-essential RBDT.

4.6. Recommendations

As younger aged males were found to be more likely to engage in non-essential RBDT, health promotion targeting this group may be more effective, possibly through official government websites/apps or well-placed advertisements in social media platforms. Legislation limiting accessibility to areas of higher risk during typhoons, such as waterfronts and beaches, may also have a beneficial effect on warding off risk-taking behaviour. Numerous provinces and cities in the Philippines have imposed liquor bans during typhoons to prevent inebriated individuals from hindering relief operations [30–32], but the effectiveness of such legislation have not been investigated. Furthermore, legal restrictions of outdoor movement in the interests of public health may be more socially acceptable due to the experiences of social distancing amid COVID-19.

As some respondents were found to engage in RBDT for work purposes, the updated "Code of Practice in Times of Typhoons and Rainstorms", published by the Hong Kong Labour Department [33], is a crucial document in mitigating health risks to essential workers. Although the guidelines are not compulsory by law, employers and employees must discuss and clearly outline methods to protect the health of those working during extreme conditions. Interventions targeting this group may be more effective if broadcasted through television or newspapers. Thus, a multi-stakeholder approach should be adopted to promote work-related safety and reduce RBDT. This also has a global implication on preventable injury risk reduction, with international planning and discussions necessary in the near future before stronger natural disaster occur driven by climate change.

4.7. Limitations

The main limitation of the analysis is that the results do not demonstrate a causative effect since this study used descriptive analysis and logistic regression as a cross-sectional study. There may also be reporting bias as respondents may present with higher social desirability response bias due to telephone interviews [34]. In addition, analyses involving risk perception asked two weeks after may not correlate directly with risky actions performed during the disaster. This study is also unable to distinguish whether those who executed non-essential RBDT carried out high-risk behaviour due to perception of low-risk or for sensation seeking purposes. There may also be other reasons forcing individuals to remain outdoors during the typhoon, such as street sleepers unable to reach temporary shelters, unaccounted for due to the study design. Recruiting participants using the last birthday method also limits analysis on household preparedness as the recruited participant may not be the decision-maker for household preparedness [35], and thus, unfamiliar with the measures taken.

4.8. Future Research Directions

Future studies can directly investigate the reasons or rationale behind RBDT and explore the extent of such behaviour in detail. The sensation seeking trait and relevant factors could also be examined to determine its association and relevance to RBDT by using a modified version of the sensation seeking scale. Research into interpersonal perspectives through injunctive safety norms [36] and motivating factors for adaptation behaviour, such as descriptive norms [37], may also offer further insight into risk-taking behaviour during disasters. Future studies regarding disaster risk perception may also consider quantifying risk perception using balanced rating scales, as the degree of risk perceived is likely important when analysing risk-taking behaviour.

5. Conclusions

While age and gender were associated with risk-taking behaviour during natural disasters, other sociodemographic characteristics (such as education) and measures of disaster risk perception or disaster preparedness were not found to be correlated with non-essential RBDT. Despite the lack of literature investigating this phenomenon, media outlets in Hong Kong have reported several cases of sensation seeking behaviour during typhoons. Future studies are necessary to investigate the scope of risk-taking behaviour during disasters and the reasons driving this behaviour. Although there have been limited reports of injuries caused by risk-taking behaviour, relevant policy makers should begin to discuss and implement solutions to prevent any accidents and reduce potential extra burden on the emergency response system.

Author Contributions: Conceptualization, E.Y.Y.C.; methodology, E.Y.Y.C. and E.S.W.S.; validation, E.S.K.L. and Z.H.; formal analysis, E.S.K.L. and Z.H.; investigation, E.S.W.S., E.S.K.L., Z.H., E.Y.Y.C., K.K.C.H.; data curation, E.S.K.L. and Z.H.; writing—original draft preparation, E.S.W.S., E.S.K.L., Z.H.; writing—review and editing, E.S.W.S., E.S.K.L., K.K.C.H., E.Y.Y.C., Z.H.; visualization, E.S.K.L. and Z.H.; supervision, E.Y.Y.C.; funding acquisition, E.Y.Y.C. All authors have read and agreed to the published version of the manuscript.

Funding: This research paper was funded by the CCOUC Development Fund, Faculty of Medicine of The Chinese University of Hong Kong.

Conflicts of Interest: The authors declare no conflict of interest.

References

1. Doocy, S.; Dick, A.; Daniels, A.; Kirsch, T.D.; Hopkins, J. The human impact of tropical cyclones: A historical review of events 1980-2009 and systematic literature review. *PLoS Curr. Disasters* **2013**, *1*, 1–25. [CrossRef] [PubMed]
2. Republic of the Philippines National Disaster Risk Reduction and Management Council Situational Report No.57 re Preparedness Measures for TY OMPONG. Available online: http://www.ndrrmc.gov.ph/attachments/article/3437/SitRep_No_57_re_Preparedness_Measures_Effects_for_TY_OMPONG_as_of_0600H_06OCT2018.pdf (accessed on 10 January 2020).
3. A New Emergency Management Mechanism Would be Used to Respond to Typhoon "Mangkhut". Available online: http://www.cneb.gov.cn/2018/09/19/ARTI1537354136937520.shtml (accessed on 14 January 2020).
4. The Hong Kong Observatory Super Typhoon Mangkhut (1822). Available online: https://www.hko.gov.hk/en/informtc/mangkhut18/report.htm (accessed on 10 January 2020).
5. Hong Kong Legislative Council. *The Government's Preparations, Emergency Response and Recovery Efforts Arising from Super Typhoon Mangkhut*; Hong Kong Legislative Council: Hong Kong, China, 2018.

6. Tu, J.; Chou, C.; Chu, P. The abrupt shift of typhoon activity in the vicinity of Taiwan and its association with Western North Pacific–East Asian climate change. *J. Clim.* **2009**, *22*, 3617–3628. [CrossRef]
7. World Health Organization. Disaster Risk Management for Health Fact Sheets: Disaster Risk Management for Health Overview. Available online: http://www.who.int/hac/events/drm_fact_sheet_overview.pdf (accessed on 12 January 2020).
8. Chan, E.Y.Y.; Murray, V. What are the health research needs for the Sendai Framework? *Lancet* **2017**, *390*, e35–e36. [CrossRef]
9. Lam, R.P.K.; Leung, L.P.; Balsari, S.; Hsiao, K.H.; Newnham, E.; Patrick, K.; Pham, P.; Leaning, J. Urban disaster preparedness of Hong Kong residents: A territory-wide survey. *Int. J. Disaster Risk Reduct.* **2017**, *23*, 62–69. [CrossRef] [PubMed]
10. Glickman, T.S. *Glossary of Meteorology*; Leif, E.H., Ed.; American Meteorological Society: Boston, MA, USA, 2000.
11. Robertson, D. Beyond Twister: A Geography of Recreational Storm Chasing on the Southern Plains. *Geogr. Rev.* **1999**, *89*, 533. [CrossRef]
12. Cantillon, H.; Bristow, R.S. Tornado Chasing: An Introduction to Risk Tourism Opportunities. Available online: https://www.srs.fs.usda.gov/pubs/19699 (accessed on 10 January 2020).
13. Xu, S.; Barbieri, C.; Stanis, S.W.; Market, P.S. Sensation-seeking attributes associated with storm-chasing tourists: Implications for future engagement. *Int. J. Tour. Res.* **2011**, *14*, 269–284. [CrossRef]
14. Zuckerman, M. Dimensions of sensation seeking. *J. Consult. Clin. Psychol.* **1971**, *36*, 45–52. [CrossRef]
15. Zuckerman, M.; Kolin, E.A.; Price, L.; Zoob, I. Development of a sensation-seeking scale. *J. Consult. Psychol.* **1964**, *28*, 477–482. [CrossRef] [PubMed]
16. Cross, C.P.; Cyrenne, D.L.M.; Brown, G.R. Sex differences in sensation-seeking: A meta-analysis. *Sci. Rep.* **2013**, *3*, 2486. [CrossRef] [PubMed]
17. Roberti, J.W. A review of behavioral and biological correlates of sensation seeking. *J. Res. Pers.* **2004**, *38*, 256–279. [CrossRef]
18. Chan, E.; Man, A.; Lam, H.; Chan, G.; Hall, B.; Hung, K. Is urban household emergency preparedness associated with short-term impact reduction after a super typhoon in subtropical city? *Int. J. Environ. Res. Public Health* **2019**, *16*, 596. [CrossRef] [PubMed]
19. Binson, D.A.; Canchola, J.A.; Catania, J. Random selection in a national telephone survey: A comparison of the kish, next-birthday, and last-birthday methods. *J. Off. Stat.* **2000**, *16*, 53–59.
20. Keinan, R.; Bereby-Meyer, Y. Perceptions of active versus passive risks, and the effect of personal responsibility. *Pers. Soc. Psychol. Bull.* **2017**, *43*, 999–1007. [CrossRef] [PubMed]
21. Downloading IBM SPSS Statistics 24. Available online: https://www-01.ibm.com/support/docview.wss?uid=swg24041224 (accessed on 27 January 2020).
22. Elderly Man Swims While Typhoon No. 8 Signal is in Force, Gets Stranded at Sea. Available online: https://coconuts.co/hongkong/news/elderly-man-swims-while-typhoon-no-8-signal-force-gets-stranded-sea/ (accessed on 13 January 2020).
23. Lam, J.; Ng, N. Hong Kong Leader Carrie Lam Warns Residents Not to Take Any Chances as Super Typhoon Mangkhut Looms. South China Morning Post. Available online: https://www.scmp.com/news/hong-kong/politics/article/2164231/super-typhoon-mangkhut-dont-be-storm-chasers-carrie-lam (accessed on 13 January 2020).
24. Tropical Cyclone Warning Signals Leaflet. Available online: http://www.hko.gov.hk/publica/gen_pub/tcws.pdf (accessed on 13 January 2020).
25. Collier, H. Hong Kong Typhoon Mangkhut: Daredevils Risk Their Lives to Take Selfies in Deadly Storm. The Evening Standard. Available online: https://www.standard.co.uk/news/world/hong-kong-typhoon-mangkhut-daredevils-risk-their-lives-to-take-selfies-at-victoria-harbour-seafront-a3937121.html (accessed on 13 January 2020).
26. Huang, E. The Videos that will Make You Glad You weren't Outside in Hong Kong When Typhoon Hato Struck. Available online: https://qz.com/1060272/photos-and-videos-typhoon-hato-signal-t10-batters-hong-kong-macau/ (accessed on 13 January 2020).
27. Leung, C. Hong Kong Frost Chasers Ridiculed: Hospitalisations, Arguments with Police, 300 Firemen and 8 Helicopter Flights to Rescue Them. Available online: https://www.scmp.com/news/hong-kong/health-environment/article/1905267/hong-kong-frost-chasers-ridiculed-hospitalisations (accessed on 15 January 2020).

28. Lo, C.; Lau, C. Heroic Hong Kong Fireman Dies in Clifftop Rescue Drama. Available online: https://www.scmp.com/news/hong-kong/law-crime/article/2081110/hong-kong-fireman-coma-after-rescuing-hikers-ma-shan (accessed on 15 January 2020).
29. Hollingsworth, J.; Leung, C. Cost to Rescue Two Stranded Hikers in Hong Kong Runs into Hundreds of Thousands. Available online: https://www.scmp.com/news/hong-kong/health-environment/article/2108670/cost-rescue-two-stranded-hikers-hong-kong-runs (accessed on 15 January 2020).
30. Liquor Ban Policy Before and During Typhoon Disaster Prevention Measure. Available online: https://www.culionpalawan.gov.ph/?p=1028 (accessed on 16 January 2020).
31. Ilocos Norte Bans Liquor Consumption, Sale Amidst 'Ompong' Threats. Available online: https://pia.gov.ph/news/articles/1012683 (accessed on 16 January 2020).
32. Mallari, D.T., Jr. Quezon Town Mayor Imposes Liquor Ban as Typhoon Safety Measure. Available online: https://newsinfo.inquirer.net/1196920/quezon-town-mayor-imposes-liquor-ban-as-typhoon-safety-measure (accessed on 16 January 2020).
33. Code of Practice in Times of Typhoons and Rainstorms. Hong Kong Labour Department. Available online: https://www.labour.gov.hk/eng/public/wcp/Rainstorm.pdf (accessed on 12 January 2020).
34. Holbrook, A.L.; Green, M.C.; Krosnick, J.A. Telephone versus face-to-face interviewing of national probability samples with long questionnaires. *Public Opin. Q.* **2003**, *67*, 79–125. [CrossRef]
35. Hung, L.S. Married couples' decision-making about household natural hazard preparedness: A case study of hurricane hazards in Sarasota County, Florida. *Nat. Hazards* **2017**, *87*, 1057–1081. [CrossRef]
36. Pek, S.; Turner, N.; Tucker, S.; Kelloway, E.K.; Morrish, J. Injunctive safety norms, young worker risk-taking behaviors, and workplace injuries. *Accid. Anal. Prev.* **2017**, *106*, 202–210. [CrossRef] [PubMed]
37. Valkengoed, A.M.V.; Steg, L. Meta-analyses of factors motivating climate change adaptation behaviour. *Nat. Clim. Chang.* **2019**, *9*, 158–163. [CrossRef]

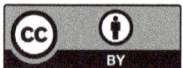

© 2020 by the authors. Licensee MDPI, Basel, Switzerland. This article is an open access article distributed under the terms and conditions of the Creative Commons Attribution (CC BY) license (http://creativecommons.org/licenses/by/4.0/).

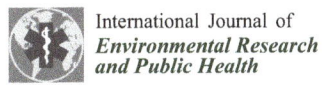

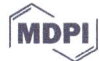

Article

Forecasting of Landslide Displacement Using a Probability-Scheme Combination Ensemble Prediction Technique

Junwei Ma [1], Xiao Liu [1,*], Xiaoxu Niu [1], Yankun Wang [2], Tao Wen [3], Junrong Zhang [2] and Zongxing Zou [1]

1. Three Gorges Research Center for Geo-Hazards of the Ministry of Education, China University of Geosciences, Wuhan 430074, China; majw@cug.edu.cn (J.M.); nxx@cug.edu.cn (X.N.); zouzongxing@cug.edu.cn (Z.Z.)
2. Faculty of Engineering, China University of Geosciences, Wuhan 430074, China; yankun_wang@cug.edu.cn (Y.W.); zjr@cug.edu.cn (J.Z.)
3. School of Geosciences, Yangtze University, Wuhan 430100, China; wentao200840@yangtzeu.edu.cn
* Correspondence: liuxiao@cug.edu.cn

Received: 9 June 2020; Accepted: 30 June 2020; Published: 3 July 2020

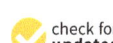

Abstract: Data-driven models have been extensively employed in landslide displacement prediction. However, predictive uncertainty, which consists of input uncertainty, parameter uncertainty, and model uncertainty, is usually disregarded in deterministic data-driven modeling, and point estimates are separately presented. In this study, a probability-scheme combination ensemble prediction that employs quantile regression neural networks and kernel density estimation (QRNNs-KDE) is proposed for robust and accurate prediction and uncertainty quantification of landslide displacement. In the ensemble model, QRNNs serve as base learning algorithms to generate multiple base learners. Final ensemble prediction is obtained by integration of all base learners through a probability combination scheme based on KDE. The Fanjiaping landslide in the Three Gorges Reservoir area (TGRA) was selected as a case study to explore the performance of the ensemble prediction. Based on long-term (2006–2018) and near real-time monitoring data, a comprehensive analysis of the deformation characteristics was conducted for fully understanding the triggering factors. The experimental results indicate that the QRNNs-KDE approach can perform predictions with perfect performance and outperform the traditional backpropagation (BP), radial basis function (RBF), extreme learning machine (ELM), support vector machine (SVM) methods, bootstrap-extreme learning machine-artificial neural network (bootstrap-ELM-ANN), and Copula-kernel-based support vector machine quantile regression (Copula-KSVMQR). The proposed QRNNs-KDE approach has significant potential in medium-term to long-term horizon forecasting and quantification of uncertainty.

Keywords: landslide displacement; predictive uncertainty; ensemble prediction; probability combination scheme; quantile regression neural networks (QRNNs); kernel density estimation (KDE)

---

1. Introduction

As one of the most common natural hazards in the world, landslides pose a significant threat to public health and safety. According to statistics, landslides have affected 4.8 million people and caused 18,275 deaths during the period of 2009–2019 [1]. Landslide displacement prediction, which provides the necessary information to determine the extent of ongoing hazard, has proven to be the most cost-saving risk reduction measure [2–4]. However, landslide displacement prediction is complex and remains a key challenge in natural hazard research. This challenge arises because landslides are nonlinear, dynamic systems, and the associated movements can be induced by different causes, such as geological factors [5], hydrological factors [6,7], morphological factors, and human activities [4,8].

A large number of efforts in the literature have focused on the precise prediction of landslide displacement [9]. Currently, approaches used for landslide displacement prediction are categorized as physical modelling approaches and data-driven approaches [10]. Physical models (also known as white-box models), which rely on detailed descriptions of landslide mechanism processes, can provide clear physical explanations of landslides. The commonly used physical models include the tertiary creep model [11], the Hayashi model [12], and the general creep model [13]. Those physical models require numerous expensive geotechnical characterizations of the materials involved in landslides and therefore may be applicable only in limited cases [14].

Data-driven models differ from physical models because a characterization of the actual landslide mechanism processes is not fully required. Thus, the data-driven models are also known as black-box models. The main advantage of data-driven models is that the trained models can be easily updated on the basis of new and more recent data.

Data-driven models include but are not limited to statistical methods, artificial neural networks (ANNs), support vector machines (SVMs) [15], and extreme learning machines (ELMs) [16]. Owing to their capacity to approximate arbitrary, nonlinear, and dynamic systems with high precision, data-driven models achieve good model performance in the prediction of landslide displacement.

Despite their widespread application, the output of most existing data-driven models is a single estimate for each prediction horizon. These single estimates, which provide deterministic values, are referred to as point predictions [3]. The defining characteristic of a point prediction is its accessibility with regard to understanding and operation. The main drawback of point prediction is that it only provides the prediction error, with no information regarding the associated predictive uncertainties, which limits the use of point prediction in decision-making applications.

The predictive uncertainties consisting primarily of input uncertainty, parameter uncertainty, and model uncertainty could be substantial. It is highly desirable to know the degree of uncertainty that is associated with a particular point prediction and convert the point prediction into informative resources for emergency landslide risk management [3,17]. Only limited studies have examined the quantification of uncertainty associated with landslide displacement prediction by constructing prediction intervals (PIs). The output of a PI is an interval composed of upper and lower bounds, where we expect the predictive value of the series to fall within some (prespecified) probability, which is deemed the PI nominal confidence (PINC). A hybrid approach based on an echo state network and mean-variance estimation was proposed by Yao et al. [18] to measure the uncertainty in landslide deformation prediction and perform interval prediction. A bootstrap-based approach was proposed by Ma et al. [4] to perform interval prediction of landslide displacement. Wang et al. [2] proposed a direct interval prediction using least squares support vector machines or the construction of PIs of landslide displacement. Kernel-based support vector machine quantile regression (KSVMQR) was utilized in [3] for quantification of the predictive uncertainty of landslide displacement.

However, the traditional methods have certain disadvantages in displacement prediction and quantification of predictive uncertainty. For example, the bootstrap-based approach requires significantly high computational costs, especially for large datasets [2]. Additionally, the performances of SVM-based approaches are sensitive to the choice of kernel type and parameter values [19]. Therefore, more efforts still need to be made for the improvement of prediction performance and quantification of the predictive uncertainty.

Ensemble prediction, a state-of-the-art artificial intelligence technique, aims to improve prediction robustness and accuracy and uncertainty quantification [20,21]. Ensemble prediction has been successfully applied in a variety of fields, including prediction performance improvement and uncertainty quantification of remaining useful life [22], bankruptcy [23], shear capacity of reinforced-concrete deep beams [24], residential electricity consumption [25], wind power [26], flood susceptibility [27,28], and landslide susceptibility [29].

In this study, a probability-scheme combination ensemble prediction that employs quantile regression neural networks and kernel density estimation (QRNNs-KDE) was proposed for robust and accurate prediction and uncertainty quantification of landslide displacement. The Fanjiaping landslide with long-term and near real-time monitoring data was selected as a case study to explore the performance of the QRNNs-KDE approach. The deformation characteristics were clarified for fully understanding the triggering factors.

2. Methodology

2.1. Description of Uncertainty Sources

Predictive uncertainty in data-driven models consists primarily of input uncertainty, parameter uncertainty, and model uncertainty [30–32].

The input uncertainty is related to the input data uncertainty and the input variable section uncertainty. The input data uncertainty is primarily due to measurement and sampling error and environmental noise. The input variable section uncertainty accounts for uncertainty inherent in the selection of input variables from the candidate data set. For physical models, the required inputs are pre-determined, being consistent with considered rheological models. However, for data-driven models, the selection of input variables is problem-dependent and cannot be determined in advance. Only major and relevant variables are selected as final inputs to train the data-driven model. The selection of the variables to include in a data-driven model from the original data set is inherently uncertain, especially when the input candidate pool is very large. For example, in data-driven models that utilize decomposition algorithms, only a portion of the decomposed sub-components are selected as input variables. The candidate input pool, which consists of sub-components, increases very quickly with the decomposition level and potentially increases the input variable selection uncertainty.

The parameter uncertainty refers to the uncertainty in the model parameter vector and mainly arises from the inability to identify a unique set of best parameters for the model [33].

Model uncertainty arises primarily from the model structure uncertainty and model error. Model structure uncertainty is associated with the specific model setting of learning algorithms, such as the polynomial order in polynomial regression models, the number of hidden nodes in an ANN or ELM, and the type of kernel function in an SVM. The input uncertainty may also account for model structure uncertainty, because different input variables "automatically" produce different model structures. Model error refers to the difference between two model estimates with respect to the corresponding target and is caused by the inability to reproduce the real processes.

2.2. Ensemble Prediction

Ensemble prediction is not a specific learning algorithm but a strategic combination of multiple predictions into a single output with a model combination process [21]. Based on the selection of the learning algorithm, ensemble prediction models can be further classified into homogeneous and heterogeneous ensemble models (Figure 1). A homogeneous ensemble model generates multiple learners with the same learning algorithm on different training datasets, which are produced by manipulating the original training data (schematic illustrated in Figure 1a). Bootstrap aggregation, also known as bagging for short, is the most straightforward and widely used method of manipulating the training dataset. By contrast, a heterogeneous ensemble model generates multiple learners with different learning algorithms on the same training data set (schematic illustrated in Figure 1b).

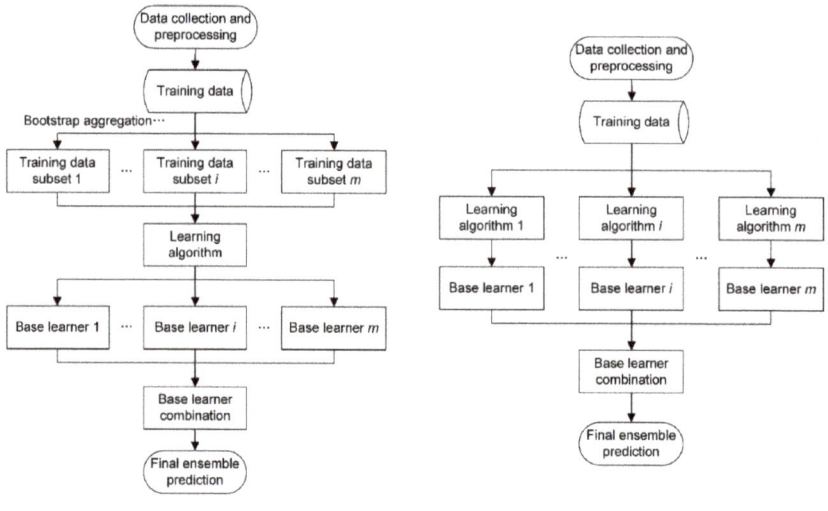

Figure 1. General framework for ensemble prediction models. (**a**) Homogeneous ensemble model and (**b**) heterogeneous ensemble model.

The base learner combination is the main step in the ensemble prediction model. Summation and averaging are simple combination schemes. A more general approach involves assigning a weight to each base learner. In the present study, a heterogeneous ensemble model was built based on QRNNs and KDE. QRNNs serve as base learning algorithms to produce multiple base learners, and the probability combination scheme based on KDE is used to combine the base learners into the final ensemble prediction.

2.3. Quantile Regression Neural Network

2.3.1. Quantile Regression

Quantile regression is a common statistical technique for conducting inferences concerning conditional quantile functions [34,35]. More formally, any real-valued random variable Y may be characterized by its distribution function as follows:

$$F(y) = \text{Prob}(Y \leq y) \tag{1}$$

whereas for any $0 < \tau < 1$,

$$Q(\tau) = \inf\{y : F(y) \geq \tau\} \tag{2}$$

is called the τth quantile of Y.

Given a data set $(x_i(t), Y(t))$ for $i = 1, 2, \cdots, I$ and $t = 1, 2, \cdots, N$, the linear quantile regression can be expressed as follows:

$$\hat{Y}_\tau(t) = \sum_{i=1}^{I} \theta_i x_i(t) + b \tag{3}$$

where $0 < \tau < 1$ is the quantile, and b is an error with zero expectation.

The estimated parameters θ_i can be approximated by minimizing a sum of the asymmetrically weighted absolute residual cost functions, which are expressed as follows:

$$E_\tau = \frac{1}{N}\sum_{t=1}^{N}\rho_\tau(Y(t) - \hat{Y}_\tau(t)) \qquad (4)$$

where $Y(t)$ is the observation at time t and ρ_τ is the check function, which is also known as the pinball loss function and is defined as follows:

$$\rho_\tau(x) = \begin{cases} \tau x & \text{if } x \geq 0 \\ (\tau - 1)x & \text{if } x < 0 \end{cases} \qquad (5)$$

2.3.2. Quantile Regression Neural Network

Given inputs $x_i(t)$ and an output $Y(t)$, the output from a QRNN is calculated as follows:

Consider a hidden-layer transfer function $h(\cdot)$; the output from the j-th hidden-layer node $g_j(t)$ is given by applying the hidden-layer transfer function to the inner product between $x_i(t)$ and hidden-layer weights $w_{ij}^{(h)}$ plus the hidden-layer bias $b_j^{(h)}$, which can be calculated as follows:

$$g_j(t) = h(\sum_{i=1}^{I} x_i(t)w_{ij}^{(h)} + b_j^{(h)}) \qquad (6)$$

An estimate of the conditional τ-quantile $\hat{y}_\tau(t)$ is

$$\hat{Y}_\tau(t) = f(\sum_{j=1}^{J} g_j(t)w_j^{(o)} + b^{(o)}) \qquad (7)$$

where $w_j^{(o)}$ are the output-layer weights, $b^{(o)}$ is the output-layer bias, and $f(\cdot)$ is the output-layer transfer function. The transfer function $h(\cdot)$ and $f(\cdot)$ are usually set as the hyperbolic tangent sigmoidal and linear function, respectively [36].

As an alternative method to prevent overfitting, weight delay regularization for the magnitude of the input-hidden layer weight can be applied by setting a penalty with a nonzero value.

2.4. Kernel Density Estimation (KDE)

Nonparametric density estimation is the process of fitting a parametric density model of a random variable without making the assumption that the density belongs to a particular parametric family [37,38]. Various methods have been proposed for nonparametric density estimation, e.g., k-nearest neighbors method, Parzen windows, histogram, and KDE [38]. In the domain of nonparametric density estimation, the K-nearest neighbors method has a very limited scope of practical applications due to its very poor performance. The Parzen windows method presents slightly better performance but also produces discontinuities (stair-like curves) that are quite annoying in practice [38]. A histogram is a simple form of the nonparametric density estimation. However, it suffers serious and noticeable drawbacks. First, the resulting visualization strongly depends on the choice of binning. Second, the natural feature of the histogram is discontinuity, which causes extreme difficulty if derivatives of the estimates are required.

Fortunately, those abovementioned drawbacks can be easily eliminated by using KDE [38,39]. In fact, KDE has been extensively studied and has become the most popular method in nonparametric density estimation. Given a random sample $Y_1, Y_2, \cdots, Y_m$, the value of the density at the point y estimated by the KDE method is given by the following:

$$\hat{f}(y,h) = \frac{1}{mh}\sum_{i=1}^{m} K(\frac{y-Y_i}{h}) \tag{8}$$

where h is the bandwidth with positive real value and $K(\cdot)$ is the kernel function. In this study, the most effective Epanechnikov kernel [38] was adopted and expressed as

$$K(y) = \frac{3}{4}(1-y^2)\mathbb{R}(|y| \leq 1) \tag{9}$$

where $\mathbb{R}(\cdot)$ is the indicator function, that is, $\mathbb{R}(y \in A) = 1$ for $y \in A$ and $\mathbb{R}(y \in A) = 0$ for $y \notin A$.

The selection of bandwidth parameter is a crucial issue in KDE. The bandwidth parameter influences the smoothness of the KDE curve and also determines the tradeoff between the bias and variance. In general, the smaller the bandwidth, the smaller the bias, and the larger the variance. A number of methods have been proposed to find the optimal bandwidth, such as Silverman's rule of thumb and the Sheather-Jones method. Silverman's rule of thumb bandwidth with a Gaussian kernel and Epanechnikov kernel can be computed as follows:

$$h^{optimal} \approx 1.06\hat{\sigma}n^{-\frac{1}{5}} \tag{10}$$

$$h^{optimal} \approx 2.34\hat{\sigma}n^{-\frac{1}{5}} \tag{11}$$

where $\hat{\sigma}$ is the estimation of σ (standard deviation of the input data) [38].

2.5. Ensemble Prediction Employing QRNNs and KDE

The proposed ensemble prediction employing QRNNs and KDE is shown in Figure 2. The QRNNs-KDE approach consists of four stages: (1) data splitting and normalization, (2) QRNN modelling, (3) probability density function (PDF) estimation by KDE, and (4) final ensemble prediction.

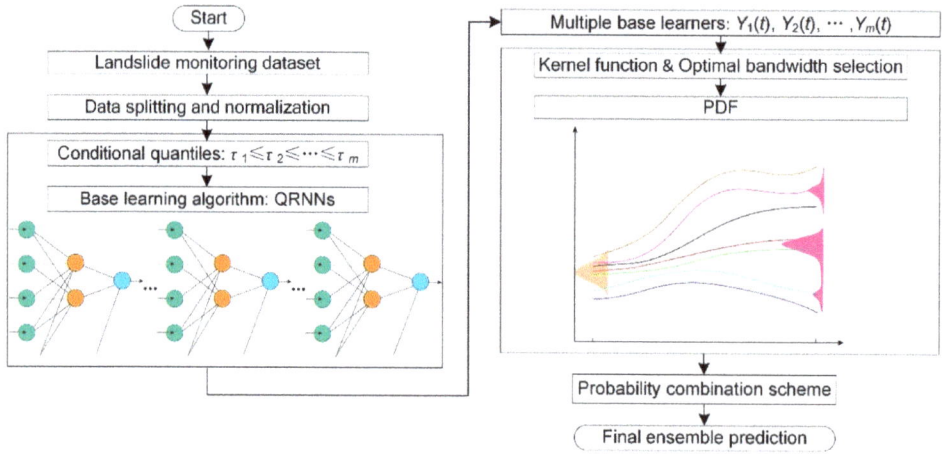

Figure 2. The overall flowchart of ensemble prediction based on the quantile regression neural networks and kernel density estimation (QRNNs-KDE) approach.

Data splitting and normalization: The original landslide monitoring dataset is divided into training data and testing data. The training data are used for model construction, and the testing data are used to evaluate the performance of the constructed model. To eliminate the influence of dimensional data, the training data and testing data are first normalized in the range of 0 to 1.

QRNNs modelling: QRNNs serve as base learning algorithms to generate multiple base learners $Y_1(t), Y_2(t), \cdots, Y_m(t)$ by applying a finite number of conditional quantiles $\tau_1 \leq \tau_2 \leq \cdots \leq \tau_m$ within the domain $0 < \tau < 1$, e.g., $\tau = 0.01, 0.02, \ldots, 0.98, 0.99$. The base learners of landslide displacement are obtained after renormalizing the outputs from the QRNNs approach. To avoiding overfitting in QRNNs modelling, a penalty parameter with nonzero value is applied.

PDF estimation by KDE: Multiple base learners from the QRNNs base model are treated as the input for KDE to estimate the probability density function (PDF) of the base learners. The kernel function and bandwidth influence the shape of the KDE curve. An appropriate kernel function and an optimal bandwidth should be chosen to best match the features of the original dataset.

Final ensemble prediction: In the present study, the final ensemble prediction was obtained through a probability combination scheme as follows:

$$u_t = \sum_{i=1}^{m} p_i(t) Y_i(t) \tag{12}$$

where $p_i(t)$ is the probability value of the i-th base learner and $Y_i(t)$ is obtained from the KDE for monitoring period t.

2.6. Evaluation Metrics and Uncertainty Quantification

In this study, five indices—coefficient of determination (R^2) MSE, RMSE, NRMSE, and MAPE—were applied to assess the performance of point prediction. R^2, MSE, RMSE, NRMSE, and MAPE are defined as

$$R^2 = \left[\frac{\sum_{t=1}^{N}(u_t - \overline{u})(\hat{u}_t - \overline{\hat{u}})}{\sqrt{\sum_{t=1}^{N}(u_t - \overline{u})^2 (\hat{u}_t - \overline{\hat{u}})^2}} \right]^2 \tag{13}$$

$$MSE = \frac{\sum_{t=1}^{N}(\hat{u}_t - u_t)^2}{N} \tag{14}$$

$$RMSE = \sqrt{\frac{\sum_{t=1}^{N}(\hat{u}_t - u_t)^2}{N}} \tag{15}$$

$$NRMSE = \sqrt{\frac{\sum_{t=1}^{N}(\hat{u}_t - u_t)^2}{\sum_{t=1}^{N} u_t^2}} \tag{16}$$

$$MAPE = \frac{1}{N}\left(\sum_{t=1}^{N}\left|\frac{\hat{u}_t - u_t}{u_t}\right|\right) \times 100\% \tag{17}$$

where $\hat{u}_t$ and u_t denote the t-th predictive value and observation, respectively, and $\overline{u}$ and $\overline{\hat{u}}$ denote the mean of the observation and the mean of the predictive value, respectively.

In the present study, the associated predictive uncertainties were quantified with PIs. After the above procedures, full PDFs of the future landslide displacement were achieved. An interval prediction with a $(1 - \alpha) \times 100\%$ confidence interval can be obtained from the $\alpha/2$ and $1 - \alpha/2$ quantiles of the obtained PDF. The α level, also called the significance level, ranges from 0 to 1 and is the probability of not capturing the value of the parameter. The predictive values of the $\alpha/2$ quantity and $1 - \alpha/2$ quantity are set as the upper bound ($U_t^{1-\alpha}$) and lower bound ($L_t^{1-\alpha}$), respectively. For example, a 90% central PI can be obtained from the 0.05 and 0.95 quantiles of the PDF. The upper bound and lower bound of the 90% confidence level correspond to the predictive values of the 0.95 and 0.05 quantiles of the obtained PDF.

The prediction interval coverage probability (PICP), normalized mean PI width (NMPIW), and coverage width-based criterion (CWC) are three indices for evaluating the correctness of the approximated PIs. The PICP reflects the degree of reliability of PIs and is defined as

$$\text{PICP} = \frac{1}{N}\sum_{t=1}^{N} I_t^{1-\alpha} \tag{18}$$

where $I_t^{1-\alpha}$ is defined as follows:

$$I_t^{1-\alpha} = \begin{cases} 1 & u_t \in [L_t^{1-\alpha}, U_t^{1-\alpha}] \\ 0 & u_t \notin [L_t^{1-\alpha}, U_t^{1-\alpha}] \end{cases} \tag{19}$$

NMPIW measures the width of the PI; it is defined as

$$\text{NMPIW} = \frac{1}{N\varsigma}\sum_{t=1}^{N}(U_t^{1-\alpha} - L_t^{1-\alpha}) \tag{20}$$

where ς is the range of the underlying targets.

For high-quality PIs, narrow PIs (smaller NMPIW) with a high coverage probability (large PICP close to 100%) have great value [40,41]. Theoretically, NMPIW and PICP are conflicting. Therefore, CWC, which is a new balance criterion between PICP and NMPIW [42], is proposed to give a comprehensive assessment of PIs. CWC is defined as

$$CWC = (NMPIW + \psi)e^{\frac{\gamma(PICP-\mu)}{2\delta^2}} \tag{21}$$

where ψ is a small positive value within the range of (0.1%, 0.5%), μ corresponds to the nominal confidence level associated with PIs that is usually set to $1 - \alpha$, and δ is a small positive value less than 1. γ is set to 1 during the training process; for testing, it is defined by the following step function:

$$\gamma = \begin{cases} 1, & PICP \geq \mu \\ 0, & PICP < \mu \end{cases} \tag{22}$$

3. Case Study: Fanjiaping Landslide

3.1. Features of the Fanjiaping Landslide

The Fanjiaping landslide is located on the southern bank of the Yangtze River and upstream of the Baishuihe landslide and downstream of the well-known Huangtupo landslide, which is approximately 56 km northwest of the Three Gorges Reservoir Dam (see Figure 3 for location). The Fanjiaping landslide is an ancient landslide [43,44] composed of two blocks: the Muyubao landslide and Fanjiaping landslide. The entire planar area of the landslide is approximately 1.96 million square meters, and the landslide volume is approximately 106 million cubic meters. The thickness of the Fanjiaping landslide ranges from 40 to 139.16 m. The Muyubao landslide is approximately 1500 m long and 1200 m wide. The average thickness of the Muyubao landslide body is approximately 50 m, and its estimated volume is 90 million m^3.

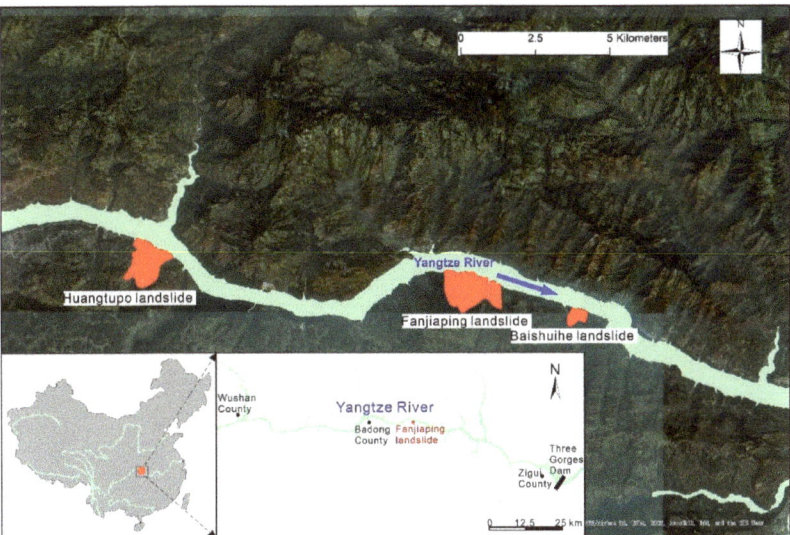

Figure 3. Location of the landslide site.

The Muyubao landslide extends from an elevation of 100 m at the toe to 520 m at the crown (Figure 4a,b). The slope surface consists of alternating gentle and comparatively steep landforms. The sliding direction of the landslide is 20°. The Tanjiahe landslide, located on the downstream of the Muyubao landslide, is approximately 1000 m long and 400 m wide. The average thickness of the Tanjiahe landslide body is approximately 40 m, and its estimated volume is 16 million m^3. The Tanjiahe landslide extends from an elevation of 135 m at the toe to 420 m at the crown (Figure 4c,d). The slope surface consists of alternating gentle and comparatively steep landforms. The sliding direction of the landslide is 345°.

The site-specific investigation shows that the landslide materials are arranged in two different layers: a colluvial deposit at the upper surface and highly disturbed sandstone at the lower surface. The cataclastic sandstone is underlaid by sandstone and mudstone of the Jurassic Xiangxi formation (J1x) with an average dip direction of 10–25° and a dip angle of 27–36° (Figure 4b,d). Soft coal layers are prevalent in the J1x formation, and many landslides have developed along the soft coal layers. The borehole data indicates that the landslide mass of the Muyubao and Tanjiahe landslide slide along a soft coal layer with a thickness ranging from 0.1 to 0.3 m. According to laboratory testing of sliding zone soil obtained from the borehole, the natural moisture content of the soil is 12.6%, and the natural density is 1.9 g/cm^3.

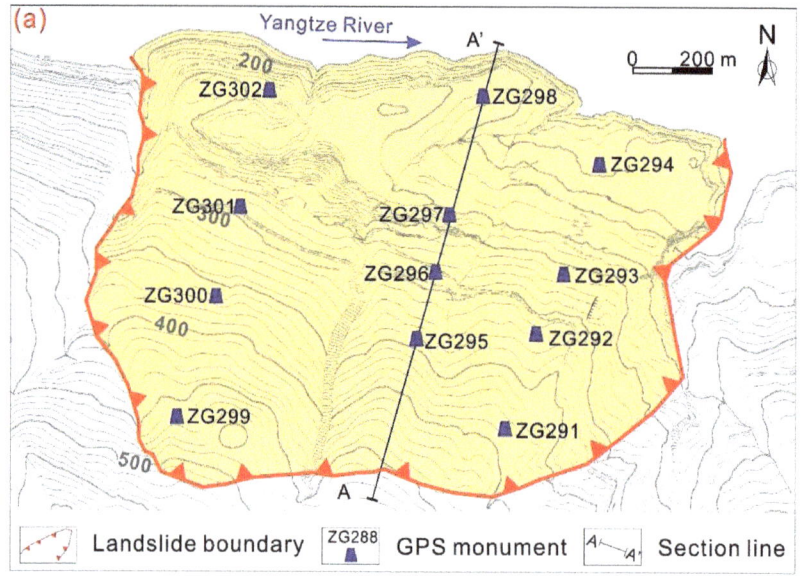
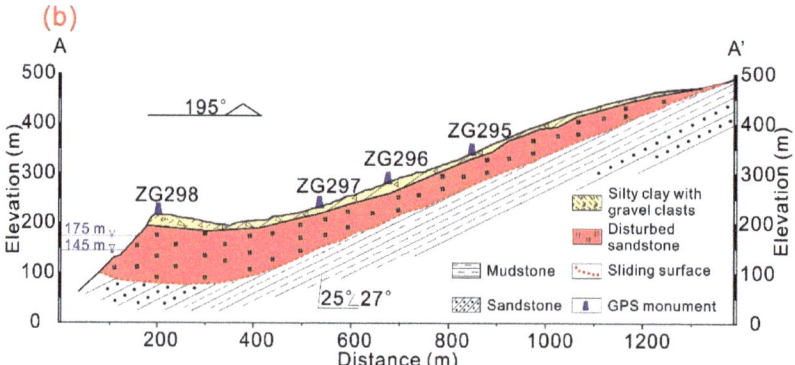

Figure 4. Cont.

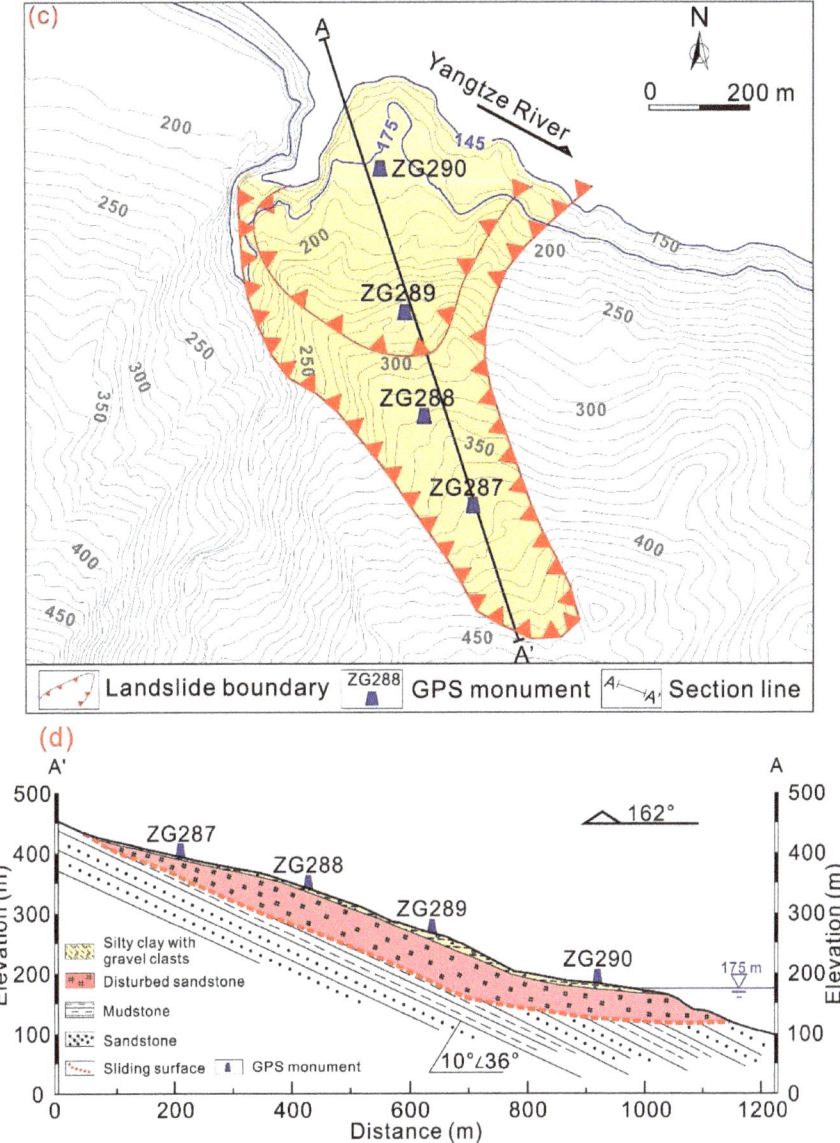

Figure 4. Topographic map and geological profile of the Fanjiaping landslide. (**a**) Topographic map of the Muyubao landslide. (**b**) Geological profile of the Muyubao landslide along sections A-A', as recorded with monitoring instruments. (**c**) Topographic map of the Tanjiahe landslide. (**d**) Geological profile of the Tanjiahe landslide along sections B-B', as recorded with monitoring instruments.

3.2. Input Data

A total of sixteen GPS beacons were installed on the landslide mass to monitor the landslide movements in September 2006 (see Figure 4 for the GPS locations): four on the Tanjiahe landslide and twelve on the Muyubao landslide. The GPS monuments were manually surveyed once a month. In April 2016, four GPS monitoring points, ZG295, ZG296, ZG297, and ZG298, were updated to near real-time monitoring. At most, thirteen years' worth of monitoring data were obtained. Figure 5 shows the monthly rainfall intensity obtained from the Shazhenxi Meteorological Station near the Fanjiaping landslide, the reservoir water level, and the displacement from GPS survey monuments over the thirteen-year period from October 2006 to March 2018. The available data indicate that the landslide was unstable and continuously deforming during the entire monitoring period. The landslide exhibits a step-like deformation behavior because of the periodic fluctuations in the reservoir water level and heavy precipitation. The monitoring data from both Muyubao and Tanjiahe show that larger displacements occurred in the upper middle part of the landslide mass. From the sequence of the surface cracks and displacement magnitude, we speculate that the movement occurred first at the rear part and progressed downslope. Based on a previous study on the relations between slip-surface geometry, material structures, and deformational structures [45,46], the observed kinematic behaviors are expected independent of the characteristics of the landslide material. However, more work is needed to confirm these findings.

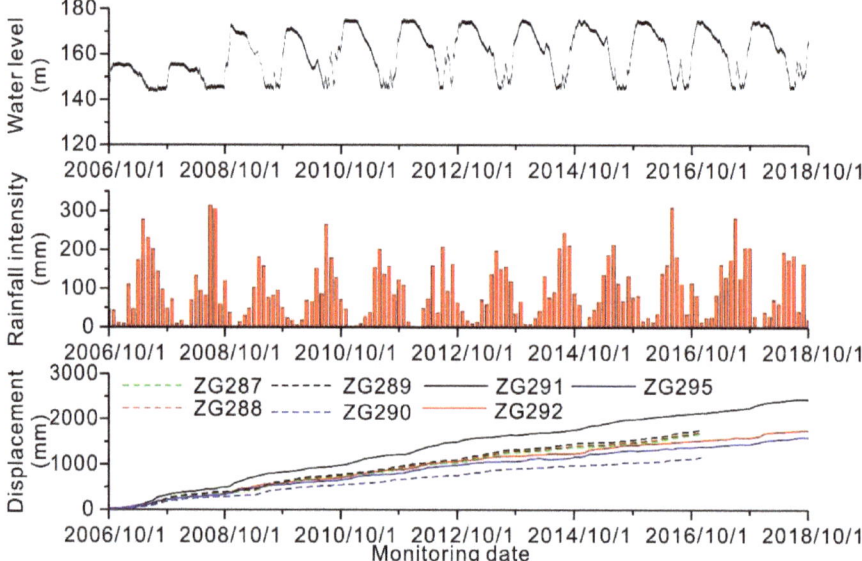

Figure 5. Reservoir water level, monthly rainfall intensity, and cumulative displacement from the Fanjiaping landslide area.

3.3. Triggering Factors of the Landslide Movements

Although the Fanjiaping landslide is one of the largest landslides in the TGRA, very few publications have reported detailed information on the triggering factors of the landslide movements. Fully understanding the triggering factors is critical for landslide mitigation and early warning. In this study, long-term and near real-time monitoring data were used to comprehensively analyze the landslide movements. The cumulative displacement at monitoring point ZG295, monthly rainfall intensity, and reservoir water levels in 2009, 2011, 2012, 2015 are shown in Figure 6a–d. The available data shows the following trends:

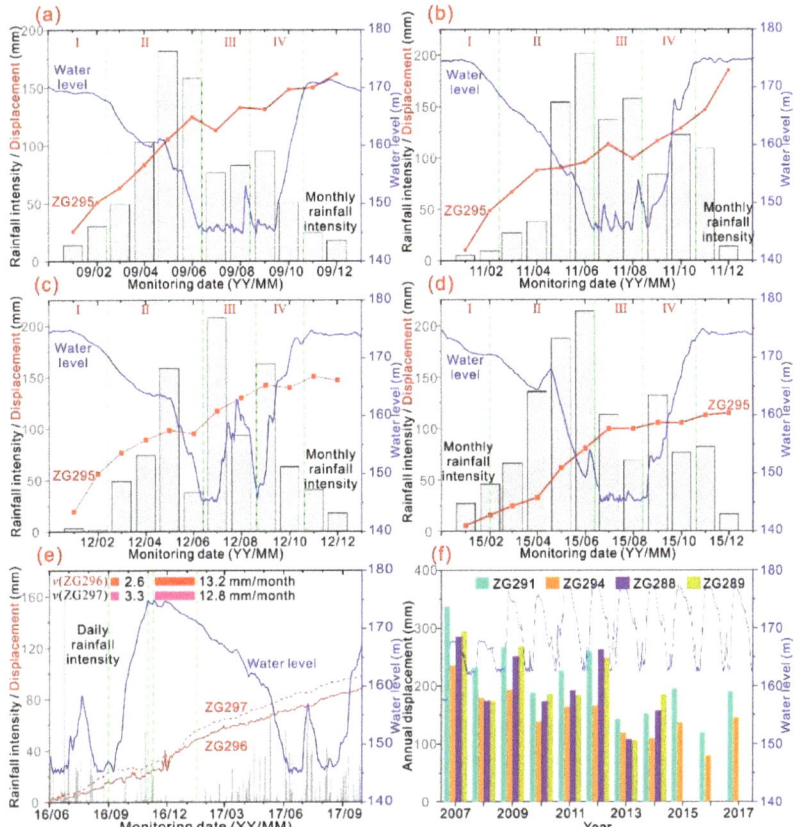

Figure 6. (**a–d**) Cumulative displacement at monitoring point ZG295, monthly rainfall intensity, and reservoir water level spanning the period of 2009, 2011, 2012, and 2015. (**e**) Cumulative displacement at monitoring points ZG296 and ZG297, daily rainfall intensity, and reservoir water level spanning the period of June 2016 to October 2017. (**f**) Annual displacement at monitoring point ZG291, ZG294, ZG288, and ZG289, and reservoir water level spanning the period of 2007 to 2017.

(1) When the reservoir water level first rose from 135 to 156 m at the end of 2006, a significant annual displacement of 330 mm occurred at monitoring point ZG291 in 2007. Similarly, an annual displacement of 260 mm occurred at monitoring point ZG291 in 2009 when the reservoir water level rose from 156 to 172 m at the end of 2008. After 2009, the annual displacements shows a decreasing trend (Figure 6f). The results of the above analysis suggest that landslide deformation occurred at the preliminary operation phase, and more significant movement is likely to occur when the reservoir water level reaches a new higher level.

(2) A large deformation occurred when the reservoir water level slightly dropped from 175 m to 170 m in November to February (I in Figure 6). During 2009 to 2015, the monthly deformation rate during this drawdown period was greater than 20 mm per month (Figure 6a–d). For example, when the reservoir water level dropped from 174 m to 172.21 m in January 2012 to February 2012, the displacements measured at monitoring points ZG295, ZG296, ZG297, and ZG298 were 38.98, 26.39, 35.12, and 41.78 mm, respectively (Figure 6c). However, when the reservoir water level significantly dropped from 170 m to 145 m in February to June (II in Figure 6), the monthly deformation rate decreased to less than 20 mm per month.

(3) When the reservoir level remained at 145 m in July to September (III in Figure 6) and the landslide area suffered a heavy rainfall event, the landslide deformation was likely to be suspended except for 2012. The maximum monthly rainfall intensity during those suspended activities was 158 mm. In July 2012, the landslide area suffered from a heavy rainfall event with a monthly rainfall intensity of 208 mm, and the monitoring point deformed at a high rate. From those comparative analyses, we can speculate than the minimum triggering threshold consists of episodes lasting one month with cumulative rainfall exceeding 158 mm.

(4) When the reservoir rose from 145 m to 175 m in September to November (IV in Figure 6), monthly deformation rate decreased to a small positive (less than 10 mm per month) or even negative value.

(5) The near real-time monitoring data also showed the abovementioned trends: when the reservoir water level rose from 147.25 to 174.42 m on August 31 2016 to October 27 2016, the monthly deformation rates for ZG296 and ZG297 were 2.6 and 3.3 mm/month, respectively. When the reservoir dropped from 174.45 to 171.18 m on November 9 2016 to January 16 2017, deformations of 24.07 and 26.46 mm occurred at ZG296 and ZG297, respectively. The corresponding monthly deformation rates were 12.8 and 13.2 mm/month, respectively.

From the above analysis we can conclude that landslide movement was especially pronounced under prolonged periods of dropping reservoir levels, especially during periods of slight dropdown at the highest reservoir level, and the minimum triggering threshold consisted of episodes lasting one month, with cumulative rainfall exceeding 158 mm.

3.4. QRNNs-KDE-Based Method for Ensemble Prediction

3.4.1. Data Splitting and Normalization

The available data (Figure 5) indicate that for the two active blocks, the largest displacements were observed at monitoring points ZG289 and ZG291, respectively. Therefore, monitoring points ZG289 and ZG291 were selected to establish a prediction model for the Fanjiaping landslide.

Previous correlation analysis in [3] revealed that weak to very strong correlations exist between landslide displacement and triggering and state variables. Therefore, based on triggering factor analysis and previous work on correlation analysis in [3], seven variables including four trigger variables and three state variables were selected as the inputs: rainfall intensity over the past month ($x_1(t)$), rainfall intensity over the past two months ($x_2(t)$), average reservoir water level in the current month ($x_3(t)$), variation in the reservoir water level in the current month ($x_4(t)$), displacement over the past one month ($x_5(t)$), displacement over the past two months ($x_6(t)$), and displacement over the past three months ($x_7(t)$). In addition, the displacement in the current month ($Y(t)$) was selected as the output. A data set $(x_i(t), Y(t)), i = 1, 2, \cdots, 7$ was generated based on the inputs and corresponding outputs. For the Tanjiahe landslide, the data from October 2006 to January 2015 with a size of 100 were treated as the training set, and the data from February 2015 to June 2015 with a size of 5 were used as the testing set. For the Muyubao landslide, the data from October 2006 to January 2015 with a size of 133 were treated as the training set, and the data from November 2017 to October 2018 with a size of 12 were used as the testing set.

3.4.2. QRNN Modelling

Two nonlinear models with a sigmoidal transfer function and linear transfer function for $\tau = 0.01$, 0.02, ... , 0.98, 0.99 with an interval of 0.01 were trained for monitoring points ZG289 and ZG291 to generate multiple base learners. The number of hidden nodes in the QRNNs model was set to 5. The penalty for weight delay regularization was set to 1 to prevent overfitting in QRNNs model construction. For each monitoring period, a total of 99 base learners were obtained at conditional quantities ranging from 0.01 to 0.99 based on the QRNNs. The main parameters applied in the modelling of QRNNs are shown in Table 1.

Table 1. The parameters utilized in the QRNNs modeling for the Fanjiaping landslide.

Parameter	Value	Parameter	Value
Maximum number of iterations	5000	Penalty for weight decay regularization	1
Number of quantiles	99	Number of input nodes	7
Number of repeated trials	5	Number of hidden nodes	5

3.4.3. PDF Estimation by KDE

The multiple base learners from QRNNs were employed as inputs of Epanechnikov KDE to estimate the PDF. The optimal bandwidths for PDF estimation were calculated based on Silverman's rule of thumb. The optimal bandwidths for PDF estimation of testing data at ZG289 were set to 7.98, 8.05, 5.66, 7.05, and 9.26. The optimal bandwidths for PDF estimation of testing data at ZG291 were set to 5.28, 8.61, 7.77, 5.62, and 5.30.

3.4.4. Final Ensemble Prediction

Final ensemble predictions for the Fanjiaping landslide were generated through a probability combination scheme. PIs were constructed from the obtained PDF to estimate the predictive uncertainty. For the purpose of aiding decision-making, it is preferable to have prediction information with high confidence levels to reduce risks. Therefore, PIs at a high PINC value of 90% were obtained and analyzed in the study.

4. Results

PDFs: The PDFs of predictive displacement at ZG289 and ZG291 constructed by the proposed QRNNs-KDE approach are shown in Figures 7 and 8. The fast movement is the main concern in landslide displacement prediction. Here, only a portion of the prediction describing the fast landslide is selected and shown. Figures 7 and 8 show that rather than a single estimate, the range and complete PDF of the predictive displacement are provided by the proposed approach. All landslide displacement observations are distributed in the middle of the PDFs with high probability in addition to the observations of May and June at ZG289, which appear at the tail of the probability density curve. The small fraction falling into the right tail follows the increase in the prediction period; here, there are more uncertainties associated with longer-term landslide predictions.

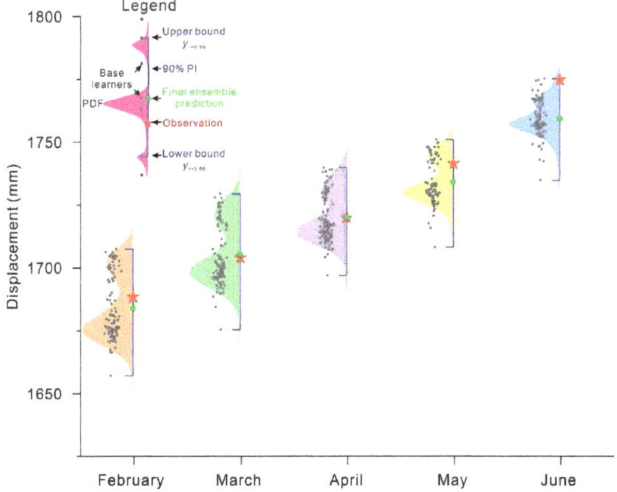

Figure 7. Probability density functions (PDFs) for the Fanjiaping landslide at ZG289 from February 2015 to June 2015.

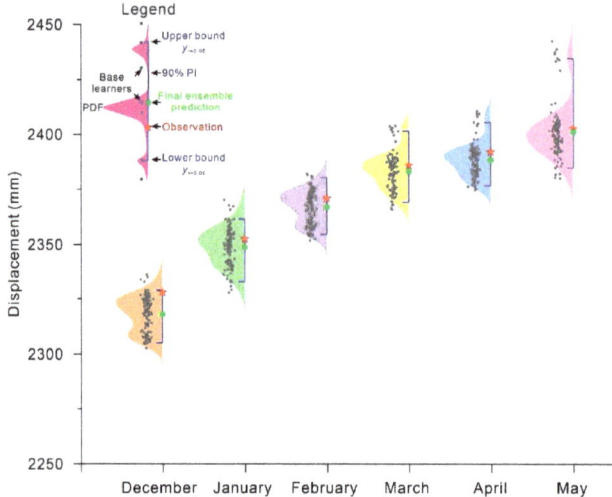

Figure 8. PDFs for the Fanjiaping landslide at ZG291 from December 2017 to May 2018.

Final ensemble prediction: Figure 9 shows the final ensemble predictions. As shown in Figure 9, the ensemble predictions obtained via the probability combination scheme showed a high degree of consistency in the landslide displacement observations, with coefficient of determination values of 0.999932 and 0.999944. To further evaluate the prediction performances of ensemble prediction based on the QRNNs-KDE, the evaluation metrics of the BP, RBF, ELM, and SVM approaches are shown in Table 2. As shown in Table 2, the final ensemble predictions using the QRNNs-KDE approach outperformed the persistence methods with the smallest MSE, RMSE, NRMSE, and MAPE and the largest R^2. Moreover, compared with predictions at monitoring point ZG289 using the Copula-KSVMQR approach in [3], the QRNNs-KDE approach provided more accurate prediction with smaller MAPE and RMSE.

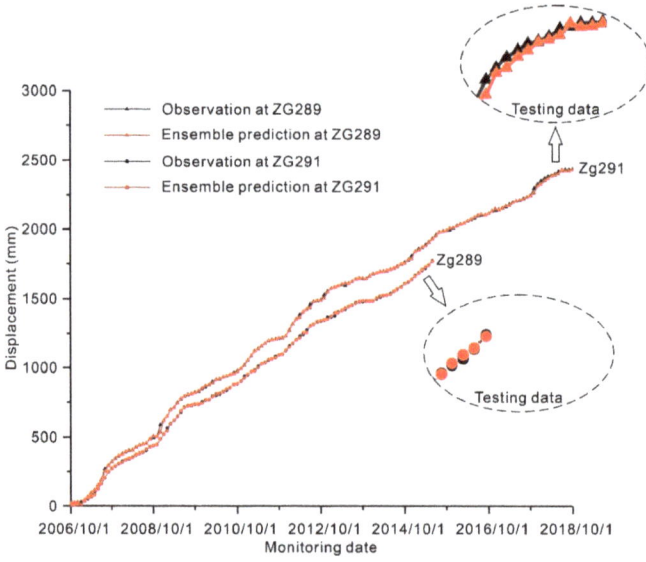

Figure 9. Comparisons of the final ensemble predictions and observations for the Fanjiaping landslide at ZG289 and ZG291.

Table 2. Comparisons of predictions obtained from QRNNs-KDE, BP, RBF, ELM, and SVM for the Fanjiaping landslide.

Monitoring Point	Model Index	BP	RBF	ELM	SVM	QRNNs-KDE
ZG289	R^2	0.99730	0.99992	0.99785	0.99993	*0.99997*
	MSE	3192.07	99.54	2538.74	78.12	*30.69*
	RMSE	56.50	9.98	50.39	8.84	*5.54*
	NRMSE	0.032263	0.005697	0.028772	0.005047	*0.003163*
	MAPE	2.74	2.00	1.57	1.27	*1.17*
ZG291	R^2	0.99991	0.99759	0.99991	0.99995	*0.99997*
	MSE	206.32	5684.98	215.41	119.75	*70.15*
	RMSE	14.36	75.40	14.68	10.94	*8.38*
	NRMSE	0.005953	0.031251	0.006083	0.004536	*0.003471*
	MAPE	3.97	1.96	2.59	2.33	*0.41*

Note: The most accurate prediction results are shown in bold italics.

Uncertainty quantification: Based on the PDFs shown in Figures 7 and 8, PIs at a high confidence level (90%) were constructed for ZG289 and ZG291 (Figure 10a,c, respectively). To evaluate the prediction performances based on the QRNNs-KDE approach, 90% PIs were constructed based on the bootstrap-ELM-ANN approach (Figure 10b,d). The corresponding evaluation metrics are shown in Table 3. As shown in Figure 10 and Table 3, the constructed PIs based on the QRNNs-KDE approach perfectly covered the observations with a high percentage, and the QRNNs-KDE approach outperformed the bootstrap-ELM-ANN approach with smaller NMPIW and CWC. For example, the performance indices NPIW and CWC of 90% PIs at ZG289 were 0.0215 and 0.1661, respectively, which were lower than those obtained using the bootstrap-ELM-ANN approach. The normalized mean PI width using the QRNNs-KDE approach was approximately 90% narrower than that for the bootstrap-ELM-ANN approach.

The experimental results show that the final ensemble predictions based on the QRNNs-KDE approach outperformed the traditional BP, RBF, ELM, SVM, and Copula-KSVMQR algorithms with regard to deterministic point prediction. The QRNNs-KDE approach was more informative than traditional algorithms because it provided the likely range of landslide displacement. The landslide observations were distributed in the middle of the prediction range with high probability. Moreover, regarding the aspect of uncertainty quantification, the QRNNs-KDE provided more satisfactory PIs than the bootstrap-ELM-ANN approach. Therefore, we believe that the final ensemble predictions based on the QRNNs-KDE approach have the advantages of accurate prediction and uncertainty quantification of landslide displacement.

Table 3. Comparisons of 90% PIs obtained from Bootstrap-ELM-ANN and QRNNs-KDE for the Fanjiaping landslide.

Monitoring Point	Index Model	PICP	NPIW	CWC
ZG289	Bootstrap-ELM-ANN	100%	0.27	0.2071
	QRNNs-KDE	*100%*	*0.0215*	*0.1661*
ZG291	Bootstrap-ELM-ANN	99%	0.024	0.143
	QRNNs-KDE	*99%*	*0.018*	*0.085*

Note: The prediction results with a narrower PI range are shown in bold italics.

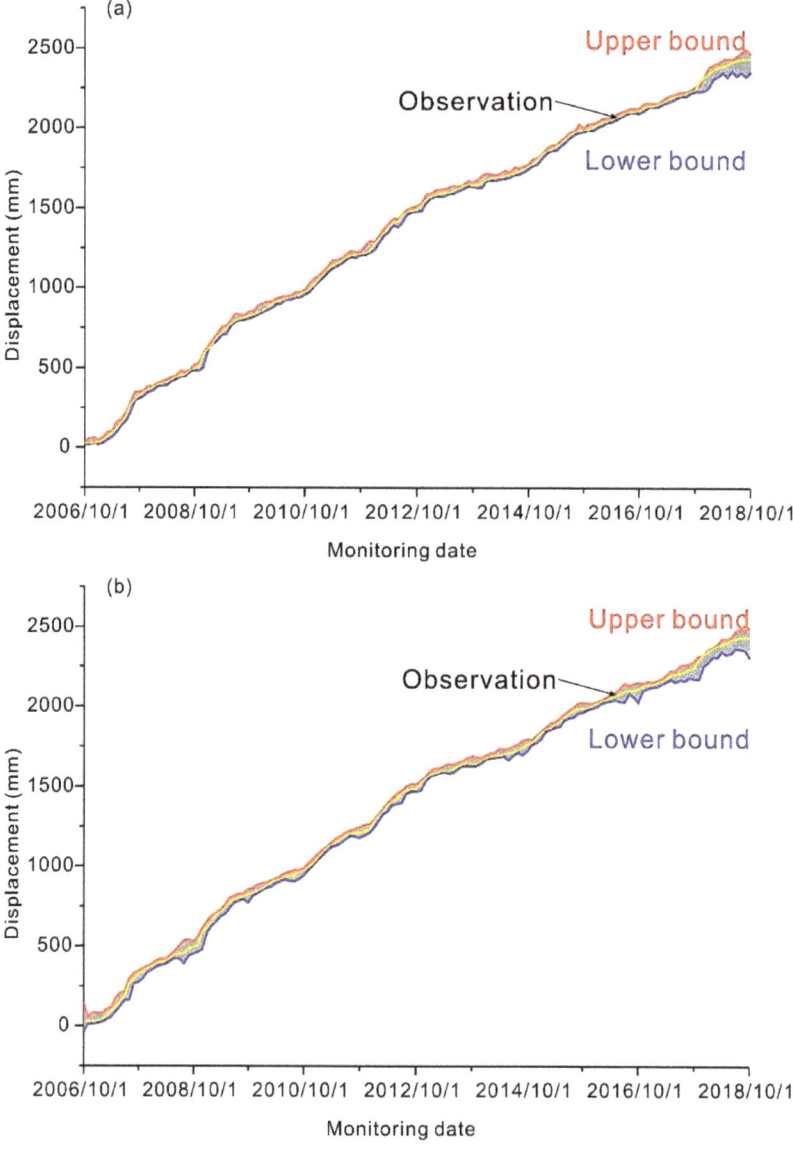

Figure 10. *Cont.*

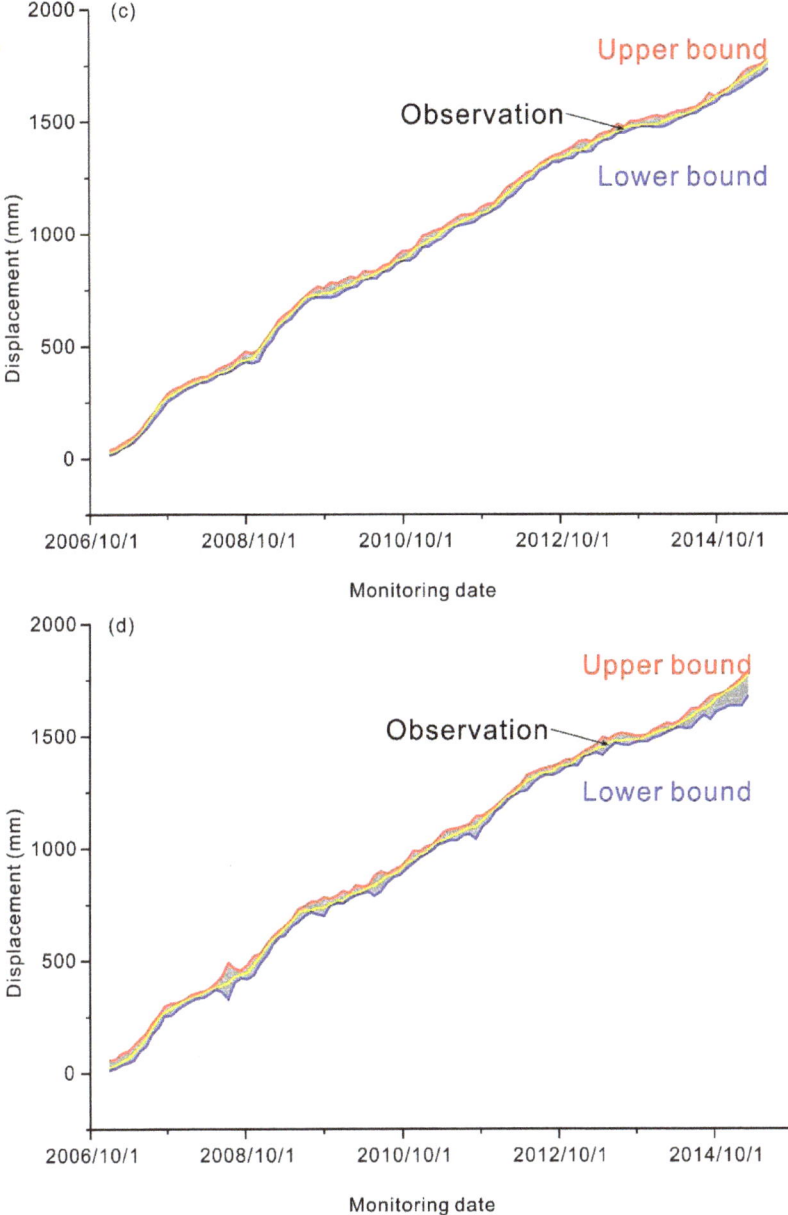

Figure 10. Comparisons of the observations and the constructed PIs at a 90% confidence level for the Fanjiaping landslide at ZG289 and ZG291 using QRNNs-KDE and bootstrap-ELM-ANN. (**a**) 90% PIs at ZG291 using QRNNs-KDE; (**b**) 90% PIs at ZG291 using bootstrap-ELM-ANN; (**c**) 90% PIs at ZG289 using QRNNs-KDE, (**d**) 90% PIs at ZG289 using bootstrap-ELM-ANN.

5. Discussion

In this study, with regard to point prediction, the probability-scheme combination ensemble prediction, which employs QRNNs-KDE, provided the best prediction. The fundamental reasons behind this can be explained from statistical, computational, and representational perspectives [47].

From a statistical perspective, the available training data set may not be able to provide sufficient information for training the true model (h^* in Figure 11). Constructing an ensemble model (h' in Figure 11) might not be better than the single best prediction model h^*, but it does reduce the risk of choosing a bad learner with poor generalizability (schematic in Figure 11a). From a computational perspective, in a single model the training algorithms might get stuck in lock optima by only performing a local search. Constructing an ensemble model by searching from different starting positions might be a better alternative (schematic in Figure 11b). From a representational perspective, it is possible that the searched hypothesis space might not contain the true model h^*. Constructing an ensemble model might expand the representable space (schematic in Figure 11c).

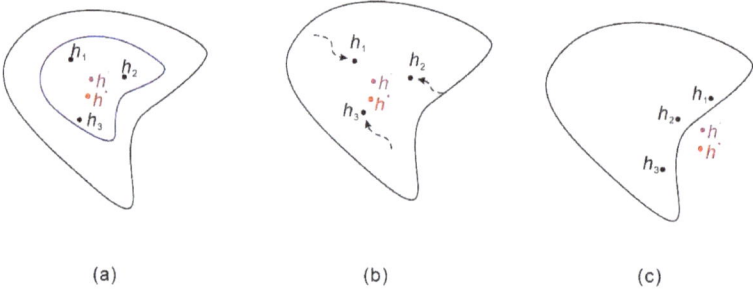

Figure 11. Schematic that shows the fundamental benefits of the ensemble prediction model from statistical (**a**), computational (**b**), and representational (**c**) perspectives. h^* is the true prediction model; h_1, h_2, and h_3 are single prediction models; and h' is the ensemble prediction model obtained by combining the single prediction models h_1, h_2, and h_3. The outer black curve is the hypothesis space of all possible models. The inner blue curve denotes the subset of hypotheses that give reasonable accuracy with the available training data (modified from [47]).

In the proposed QRNNs-KDE approach, the probability combination scheme is employed to combine 99 base learners into one final ensemble to improve the model performance. However, a concern about computational time may be associated with this ensemble strategy. The required computational time is highly related to the number of base learners. For the case of ZG 291, the required computation time is 191.85 s to train 99 base learners in RStudio Version 1.2.5042 on an Intel(R) Xeon(R) E-2176M @ 2.70 GHz CPU with 64 GB RAM. Thus, we believe that the proposed approach is computationally efficient.

Nevertheless, the probability-scheme combination ensemble prediction, which employ QRNNs and KDE, also holds inherent limitations associated with data-driven models, such as the lack of an explicit input-output relationship, and the requirement of large training data to maintain the model performance.

In practical applications, the main motivation for the construction of predictive range and complete PDF is to quantify the likely predictive uncertainty in the deterministic point predictions. Availability of range and complete PDF of the predictive displacement allows the researchers and practitioners to efficiently quantify the level of predictive uncertainty with the deterministic point predictions and to consider a multiple of solutions/scenarios for the best and worst conditions. Wide ranges are an indication of presence of a high level of uncertainty in the operation. This information can guide the researchers and practitioners to avoid the selection of risky actions under uncertain conditions. In contrast, narrow range means that decisions can be made more confidently with less chance of confronting an unexpected condition in the future, for example, if a sharp displacement increment with a wider range was predicted for the further. An alert should be carefully determined whether reaching tertiary creep stage by researchers and practitioners through comprehensive analysis. Under this circumstance, time-of-failure forecasting should be run in parallel, and a multiple of solutions/scenarios should be considered until either failure precursors are identified or the movements suspended.

The proposed QRNNs-KDE approach is suitable for medium-term to long-term horizon forecasting. Results from previous studies [2,48] have shown that the performance of data-driven models varies for landslides with different deformation behaviors. Usually, for landslides with drastic step-like deformation, the prediction accuracy is lower, and the corresponding prediction error is larger. Therefore, in practical applications of medium-term to long-term horizon forecasting, when predicting landslides with drastic deformation, the proposed QRNNs-KDE approach should be applied with caution. To achieve excellent performance, sufficient data are recommended and needed for model training.

6. Conclusions

In this study, a QRNNs-KDE approach was proposed to improve the prediction accuracy and uncertainty quantification of landslide displacement. The Fanjiaping landslide in the TGRA was selected as a case study to explore the performance of the QRNNs-KDE approach. The following conclusions from the study were obtained:

The movements of the Fanjiaping landslide was especially pronounced under prolonged periods of dropping reservoir levels, especially during periods of slight dropdown at the highest reservoir level, and the minimum triggering threshold consists of episodes lasting one month, with cumulative rainfall exceeding 158 mm.

The QRNNs-KDE approach achieves perfect performance and outperforms the traditional BP, RBF, ELM, SVM, bootstrap-ELM-ANN, and Copula-KSVMQR methods. Additionally, the proposed approach is more informative by providing the likely range and complete PDFs of landslide displacement. The landslide displacement observations are distributed in the middle of the prediction range with high probability.

In practical application, the proposed QRNNs-KDE approach is suitable for medium-term to long-term horizon forecasting. The range and complete PDF of the predictive displacement can supplement final point predictions for decision making.

Author Contributions: The work was carried out in collaboration between all the authors. J.M. and X.L. guided and supervised this research; X.N., Y.W., T.W., J.Z., and Z.Z. performed the field investigation; J.M. wrote the original draft; and J.M. and X.L. reviewed and edited the draft. All authors have contributed to, seen, and approved the manuscript. All authors have read and agreed to the published version of the manuscript.

Funding: This research was funded by the National Key R&D Program of China (Grant No. 2017YFC1501305), the National Natural Science Foundation of China (Grant Nos. 41702328 and 41572279), the Hubei Provincial Natural Science Foundation of China (Grant No. 2019CFB585), and the Huaneng Lancang River Hydropower Co., Ltd. (HNHJ18-H24).

Conflicts of Interest: The authors declare no conflict of interest.

References

1. CRED. EM-DAT: International Disaster Database. Available online: https://public.emdat.be/data (accessed on 9 June 2020).
2. Wang, Y.; Tang, H.; Wen, T.; Ma, J. Direct Interval Prediction of Landslide Displacements Using Least Squares Support Vector Machines. *Complexity* **2020**, *2020*, 7082594. [CrossRef]
3. Ma, J.W.; Niu, X.X.; Tang, H.M.; Wang, Y.K.; Wen, T.; Zhang, J.R. Displacement Prediction of a Complex Landslide in the Three Gorges Reservoir Area (China) Using a Hybrid Computational Intelligence Approach. *Complexity* **2020**, *2020*, 2624547. [CrossRef]
4. Ma, J.W.; Tang, H.M.; Liu, X.; Wen, T.; Zhang, J.R.; Tan, Q.W.; Fan, Z.Q. Probabilistic forecasting of landslide displacement accounting for epistemic uncertainty: A case study in the Three Gorges Reservoir area, China. *Landslides* **2018**, *15*, 1145–1153. [CrossRef]
5. Pinto, F.; Guerriero, L.; Revellino, P.; Grelle, G.; Senatore, M.R.; Guadagno, F.M. Structural and lithostratigraphic controls of earth-flow evolution, Montaguto earth flow, Southern Italy. *J. Geol. Soc. Lond.* **2016**, *173*, 649. [CrossRef]

6. Guerriero, L.; Diodato, N.; Fiorillo, F.; Revellino, P.; Grelle, G.; Guadagno, F.M. Reconstruction of long-term earth-flow activity using a hydroclimatological model. *Nat. Hazards* **2015**, *77*, 1–15. [CrossRef]
7. Hu, X.; Bürgmann, R.; Schulz, W.H.; Fielding, E.J. Four-dimensional surface motions of the Slumgullion landslide and quantification of hydrometeorological forcing. *Nat. Commun.* **2020**, *11*, 2792. [CrossRef]
8. Ma, J.W.; Tang, H.M.; Hu, X.L.; Bobet, A.; Zhang, M.; Zhu, T.W.; Song, Y.J.; Ez Eldin, M.A.M. Identification of causal factors for the Majiagou landslide using modern data mining methods. *Landslides* **2017**, *14*, 311–322. [CrossRef]
9. Corominas, J.; Moya, J.; Ledesma, A.; Lloret, A.; Gili, J.A. Prediction of ground displacements and velocities from groundwater level changes at the Vallcebre landslide (Eastern Pyrenees, Spain). *Landslides* **2005**, *2*, 83–96. [CrossRef]
10. Li, S.H.; Wu, L.Z.; Chen, J.J.; Huang, R.Q. Multiple data-driven approach for predicting landslide deformation. *Landslides* **2020**, *17*, 709–718. [CrossRef]
11. Saito, M. Forecasting the time of occurrence of a slope failure. In Proceedings of the 6th International Congress of Soil Mechanics and Foundation Engineering, Montreal, QC, Canada, 8–15 September 1965; pp. 537–541.
12. Hayashi, S.; Komamura, F.; Park, B.W.; Yamamori, T. On the forecast of time to failure of slope-Approximate forecast in the early period of the tertiary creep. *J. Jpn. Landslide Soc.* **1988**, *25*, 11–16. [CrossRef]
13. Federico, A.; Popescu, M.; Fidelibus, C.; Interno, G. On the prediction of the time of occurrence of a slope failure: A review. In Proceedings of the 9th International Symposium on Landslides, Rio de Janeiro, Brazil, 28 June–2 July 2004; pp. 979–983.
14. Ma, J.W.; Tang, H.M.; Liu, X.; Hu, X.L.; Sun, M.J.; Song, Y.J. Establishment of a deformation forecasting model for a step-like landslide based on decision tree C5.0 and two-step cluster algorithms: A case study in the Three Gorges Reservoir area, China. *Landslides* **2017**, *14*, 1275–1281. [CrossRef]
15. Wen, T.; Tang, H.M.; Wang, Y.K.; Lin, C.Y.; Xiong, C.R. Landslide displacement prediction using the GA-LSSVM model and time series analysis: A case study of Three Gorges Reservoir, China. *Nat. Hazards Earth Syst. Sci.* **2017**, *17*, 2181–2198. [CrossRef]
16. Huang, F.M.; Yin, K.L.; Zhang, G.R.; Gui, L.; Yang, B.B.; Liu, L. Landslide displacement prediction using discrete wavelet transform and extreme learning machine based on chaos theory. *Environ. Earth Sci.* **2016**, *75*, 1376. [CrossRef]
17. Zhang, J.; Wang, Z.P.; Zhang, G.D.; Xue, Y.D. Probabilistic prediction of slope failure time. *Eng. Geol.* **2020**, *271*, 105586. [CrossRef]
18. Yao, W.; Zeng, Z.G.; Lian, C. Generating probabilistic predictions using mean-variance estimation and echo state network. *Neurocomputing* **2017**, *219*, 536–547. [CrossRef]
19. Tehrany, M.S.; Pradhan, B.; Jebur, M.N. Flood susceptibility mapping using a novel ensemble weights-of-evidence and support vector machine models in GIS. *J. Hydrol.* **2014**, *512*, 332–343. [CrossRef]
20. Zhu, Y.J. Ensemble forecast: A new approach to uncertainty and predictability. *Adv. Atmos. Sci.* **2005**, *22*, 781–788. [CrossRef]
21. Wang, Z.Y.; Srinivasan, R.S. A review of artificial intelligence based building energy use prediction: Contrasting the capabilities of single and ensemble prediction models. *Renew. Sust. Energ. Rev.* **2017**, *75*, 796–808. [CrossRef]
22. Rigamonti, M.; Baraldi, P.; Zio, E.; Roychoudhury, I.; Goebel, K.; Poll, S. Ensemble of optimized echo state networks for remaining useful life prediction. *Neurocomputing* **2018**, *281*, 121–138. [CrossRef]
23. Kim, M.-J.; Kang, D.-K. Ensemble with neural networks for bankruptcy prediction. *Expert Syst. Appl.* **2010**, *37*, 3373–3379. [CrossRef]
24. Prayogo, D.; Cheng, M.-Y.; Wu, Y.-W.; Tran, D.-H. Combining machine learning models via adaptive ensemble weighting for prediction of shear capacity of reinforced-concrete deep beams. *Eng. Comput. Ger.* **2019**, *36*, 1135–1153. [CrossRef]
25. Chen, K.; Jiang, J.; Zheng, F.; Chen, K. A novel data-driven approach for residential electricity consumption prediction based on ensemble learning. *Energy* **2018**, *150*, 49–60. [CrossRef]
26. Lee, D.; Baldick, R. Short-Term Wind Power Ensemble Prediction Based on Gaussian Processes and Neural Networks. *IEEE Trans. Smart Grid* **2014**, *5*, 501–510. [CrossRef]

27. Choubin, B.; Moradi, E.; Golshan, M.; Adamowski, J.; Sajedi-Hosseini, F.; Mosavi, A. An ensemble prediction of flood susceptibility using multivariate discriminant analysis, classification and regression trees, and support vector machines. *Sci. Total Environ.* **2019**, *651*, 2087–2096. [CrossRef] [PubMed]
28. Chen, J.; Li, Q.; Wang, H.; Deng, M. A Machine Learning Ensemble Approach Based on Random Forest and Radial Basis Function Neural Network for Risk Evaluation of Regional Flood Disaster: A Case Study of the Yangtze River Delta, China. *Int. J. Environ. Res. Public Health* **2020**, *17*, 49. [CrossRef]
29. Di Napoli, M.; Carotenuto, F.; Cevasco, A.; Confuorto, P.; Di Martire, D.; Firpo, M.; Pepe, G.; Raso, E.; Calcaterra, D. Machine learning ensemble modelling as a tool to improve landslide susceptibility mapping reliability. *Landslides* **2020**. [CrossRef]
30. Srivastav, R.K.; Sudheer, K.P.; Chaubey, I. A simplified approach to quantifying predictive and parametric uncertainty in artificial neural network hydrologic models. *Water Resour. Res.* **2007**, *43*, W10407. [CrossRef]
31. Tiwari, M.K.; Chatterjee, C. Development of an accurate and reliable hourly flood forecasting model using wavelet-bootstrap-ANN (WBANN) hybrid approach. *J. Hydrol.* **2010**, *394*, 458–470. [CrossRef]
32. Kasiviswanathan, K.S.; He, J.; Sudheer, K.P.; Tay, J.-H. Potential application of wavelet neural network ensemble to forecast streamflow for flood management. *J. Hydrol.* **2016**, *536*, 161–173. [CrossRef]
33. Zhang, J.; Tang, W.H.; Zhang, L.M.; Huang, H.W. Characterising geotechnical model uncertainty by hybrid Markov Chain Monte Carlo simulation. *Comput. Geotech.* **2012**, *43*, 26–36. [CrossRef]
34. Cannon, A.J. Quantile regression neural networks: Implementation in R and application to precipitation downscaling. *Comput. Geosci. UK* **2011**, *37*, 1277–1284. [CrossRef]
35. Xu, Q.F.; Liu, X.; Jiang, C.X.; Yu, K.M. Quantile autoregression neural network model with applications to evaluating value at risk. *Appl. Soft Comput.* **2016**, *49*, 1–12. [CrossRef]
36. Donaldson, R.G.; Kamstra, M. Forecast combining with neural networks. *J. Forecast.* **1996**, *15*, 49–61. [CrossRef]
37. Charlton, T.S.; Rouainia, M. Probabilistic capacity analysis of suction caissons in spatially variable clay. *Comput. Geotech.* **2016**, *80*, 226–236. [CrossRef]
38. Gramacki, A. *Nonparametric Kernel Density Estimation and Its Computational Aspects*; Springer: New York, NY, USA, 2017.
39. Zhang, S.; Ma, J.W.; Tang, H.M. Estimation of Risk Thresholds for a Landslide in the Three Gorges Reservoir Based on a KDE-Copula-VaR Approach. *Geofluids* **2020**, *2020*, 8030264. [CrossRef]
40. Wan, C.; Xu, Z.; Pinson, P.; Dong, Z.Y.; Wong, K.P. Probabilistic forecasting of wind power generation using extreme learning machine. *IEEE Trans. Power Syst.* **2014**, *29*, 1033–1044. [CrossRef]
41. Wan, C.; Xu, Z.; Wang, Y.L.; Dong, Z.Y.; Wong, K.P. A hybrid approach for probabilistic forecasting of electricity price. *IEEE Trans. Smart Grid* **2014**, *5*, 463–470. [CrossRef]
42. Wang, Y.K.; Tang, H.M.; Wen, T.; Ma, J.W. A hybrid intelligent approach for constructing landslide displacement prediction intervals. *Appl. Soft Comput.* **2019**, *81*, 105506. [CrossRef]
43. Zhang, L.; Liao, M.S.; Balz, T.; Shi, X.G.; Jiang, Y.N. Monitoring landslide activities in the Three Gorges area with multi-frequency satellite SAR data sets. In *Modern Technologies for Landslide Monitoring and Prediction*; Scaioni, M., Ed.; Springer Berlin Heidelberg: Berlin/Heidelberg, Germany, 2015; pp. 181–208. [CrossRef]
44. Fan, J.H.; Qiu, K.T.; Xia, Y.; Li, M.; Lin, H.; Zhang, H.T.; Tu, P.F.; Liu, G.; Shu, S.Q. InSAR monitoring and synthetic analysis of the surface deformation of Fanjiaping landslide in the Three Gorges Reservoir area. *Geol. Bull. China* **2017**, *36*, 1665–1673.
45. Guerriero, L.; Coe, J.A.; Revellino, P.; Grelle, G.; Pinto, F.; Guadagno, F.M. Influence of slip-surface geometry on earth-flow deformation, Montaguto earth flow, southern Italy. *Geomorphology* **2014**, *219*, 285–305. [CrossRef]
46. Guerriero, L.; Bertello, L.; Cardozo, N.; Berti, M.; Grelle, G.; Revellino, P. Unsteady sediment discharge in earth flows: A case study from the Mount Pizzuto earth flow, southern Italy. *Geomorphology* **2017**, *295*, 260–284. [CrossRef]
47. Dietterich, T.G. Ensemble Methods in Machine Learning. In Proceedings of the Multiple Classifier Systems, Cagliari, Italy, 21–23 June 2000; pp. 1–15.
48. Du, J.; Yin, K.L.; Lacasse, S. Displacement prediction in colluvial landslides, Three Gorges Reservoir, China. *Landslides* **2013**, *10*, 203–218. [CrossRef]

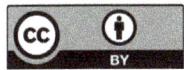

© 2020 by the authors. Licensee MDPI, Basel, Switzerland. This article is an open access article distributed under the terms and conditions of the Creative Commons Attribution (CC BY) license (http://creativecommons.org/licenses/by/4.0/).

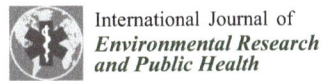 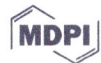

Article

Differences in Sense of Belonging, Pride, and Mental Health in the Daegu Metropolitan Region due to COVID-19: Comparison between the Presence and Absence of National Disaster Relief Fund

Young-Jae Kim, Jeong-Hyung Cho and E-Sack Kim *

Department of Physical Education, Chung-Ang University, Seoul 06974, Korea; yjkim@cau.ac.kr (Y.-J.K.); cheer1007@naver.com (J.-H.C.)
* Correspondence: dlaehkgg@naver.com; Tel.: +82-2-820-5386

Received: 15 June 2020; Accepted: 5 July 2020; Published: 7 July 2020

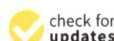

Abstract: Korea's Daegu Metropolitan City once had the second highest rate of COVID-19 infection after Wuhan in China. Following the outbreak, the government provided the first national disaster relief fund to citizens as financial aid. This study investigated whether the sense of regional belonging, pride, and mental health among 550 citizens of Daegu differed between the times before and after COVID-19, based on the presence or absence of the disaster relief fund. Frequency analysis, descriptive statistical analysis, and t-tests were conducted using the SPSS 25.0 program. Results showed that the sense of belonging was higher after COVID-19 than before, while pride was lower. Individuals who received the disaster relief fund showed higher levels of regional belonging and pride with statistical significance. The prevalence of melancholy and depression increased after COVID-19, but the presence or absence of the fund did not lead to a significant difference. Thus, in case of a future national disaster level, provision of the disaster relief fund can raise the sense of regional belonging and pride, in order to elicit communication among local residents toward overcoming difficulties. Furthermore, during challenging disaster situations, central and local governments should provide diverse programs for the citizens' mental health care.

Keywords: COVID-19; Daegu; sense of belonging; pride; mental health; disaster relief fund

1. Introduction

The high infectivity of COVID-19, first confirmed in China at the end of 2019, led to an exponential increase in the rates of incidence and infection [1]. COVID-19 has now spread across the world, adversely affecting the political, economic, psychological, and social states in each country [2].

The government of the Republic of Korea recently raised the COVID-19 national crisis level to "serious" [3], and the World Health Organization (WHO) has declared COVID-19 a global pandemic [4].

For a certain period in Korea, the COVID-19 incidence rapidly fell in comparison to other countries, and the daily lives of people seemed to return to normal [5]. However, the 31st patient confirmed to have COVID-19 on 18 February 2020, in Daegu Metropolitan City (Daegu) in Korea led to approximately 5300 additional confirmed patients within 15 days [6]. This spread of infection resulted in the United States raising the travel alert level to the highest phase, at 4, to prohibit trips to Daegu [7]. The rapid spread of COVID-19, however, turned out not just to be a situation in Daegu, Korea; the large number of confirmed cases in New York in the United States and the sudden rise in mortality paralyzed the city [8], and led to shortage of mortuaries in the city's hospitals [9].

Daegu in Korea was designated as a disaster area, due to the large-scale spread of COVID-19. For the first time, the city provided "disaster relief funds" to citizens after the outbreak of COVID-19 [10].

The funds were determined to prioritize the class that had difficulty receiving national welfare for COVID-19 [11].

However, the households that exceed the standard of the national health insurance premium by 100%, teaching staff and employees of public institutions are not eligible for disaster relief funds [12]. Daegu has offered prepaid cards, local currency, and gift cards that could only be used to help the financially distressed citizens and the local economy during the COVID-19 pandemic. This has been contributing to the revitalization of the local economy [13].

According to Park [14], overcoming regional economic difficulties is one of the ways of making citizens feel a sense of stability and a sense of belonging. Park [15] also stated that feeling proud of contributing to the restoration of a local market by using local currency leads to a sense of belonging to and affection for the community, and provides a chance to change the social atmosphere depressed by COVID-19 in a positive way.

The local residents of a city with a high number of confirmed COVID-19 cases may suffer from subsequent psychological trauma [16]. Such emotional damage could reduce residents' sense of regional belonging, as well as solidarity [17]. Thus, the basic data of the residents' sense of belonging and pride are necessary for those in regions, including Daegu, where COVID-19 incidence is high.

A terrifying aspect of COVID-19 is the ambiguity of the information regarding the factors related to the propagation, latency, geographical range, infection frequency, and actual mortality. In fact, an incorrect piece of information could induce anxiety and fear in people, which has a direct negative influence on mental health [18,19]. To understand the psychological and emotional impact of a pandemic, feelings like fear and rage have to be considered. The feeling of fear is a basic human psychological response to a potentially threatening incidence [20]. Nonetheless, continuing fear could exert harmful influence on mental health [21]. National disasters, such as the Ebola virus, severe acute respiratory syndrome outbreaks, and earthquakes, have been shown to have a negative influence on mental health [22–24]. When combating infectious diseases, fear increases the levels of anxiety and stress in healthy individuals, while aggravating the symptoms in those already suffering from a mental disorder, thus deteriorating their health further [25].

Quality of life and health are influenced by the balance between work and life, suggesting that quality of life could be enhanced when a healthy mind and lifestyle achieve harmony [26]. Hence, maintaining the quality of life at an adequate level is likely to improve the defense mechanism against stress and produce emotional stability [27].

A study on mental health among citizens of Hong Kong after the COVID-19 outbreak reported that mental health was influenced by COVID-19 [28]. The continuous spread of COVID-19 has resulted in a deterioration of the quality of life of Daegu citizens, and several people are experiencing reduced mental health [29]. Therefore, this study aimed to determine the necessary factors to aid people when a national disaster occurs, such as in the case of Daegu, while examining the needs of people during the spread of COVID-19. Furthermore, the sense of belonging, pride, and mental health as experienced by the citizens of Daegu was investigated, as Daegu is the city with the largest number of COVID-19 cases in Korea, and the differences based on the presence or absence of the national disaster relief fund was examined.

2. Materials and Methods

2.1. Study Design

This study analyzes the difference between the present and the past with group infection, based on the data of "Social Indices of Daegu in 2018" [30] and "Regional Health Statistics at a glance, 2008–2018" [31], published in the Daegu area before the COVID-19. A comparison between the presence and absence of national disaster relief fund. The data collection period was from 8 May to 13 May 2020.

2.2. Participants

A survey was conducted among Daegu residents aged 19–65 years, excluding adolescents and older adults. Convenience sampling was used, and a self-reported questionnaire was administered. The survey (550 sheets) was conducted online through EMBRAIN, the top survey company in Korea. Consent for participation was obtained from each participant using a preliminary question set, before conducting the survey. The study design was reviewed and approved by the Institutional Review Board at Chung-Ang University (1041078-202005-HRSB-119-01).

2.3. Measurement

To investigate the differences in pride, sense of belonging, and mental health among Daegu citizens with respect to COVID-19, the following measurement tools were used. The questionnaire required 10 min on average for completion.

2.3.1. Indicators of Sense of Belonging and Pride

To measure regional pride of Daegu citizens and its levels, a scale was developed, based on "Social Indices of Daegu in 2018" [30]. The sub-categories of a sense of belonging and pride were comprised of a total of two questions: one question about a sense of belonging as a Daegu citizen and one question about satisfaction. Based on the four-point Likert scale, the scale of a sense of belonging and pride contains four sentences regarding a sense of belonging: "Very strong sense of belonging", "A little sense of belonging", "Little no sense of belonging", and "No sense of belonging at all". There were also four sentences regarding pride: "Very strong sense of pride", "A little sense of pride", "Little no sense of pride", and "No sense of pride at all".

2.3.2. Indicators of Mental Health

Indicators of the mental health status of the citizens were based on the "Regional Health Statistics at a glance, 2008–2018" [31] survey conducted by the Ministry of Health and Welfare and the Korea Centers for Disease Control. The sub-category of mental health was comprised of one question on average daily sleep time and stress awareness, one question on the experience of the feeling of melancholy, and nine questions on the prevalence of depression. The sleep time diagnosis consisted of average daily sleep time was measured. The stress was composed of a four-point scale, and the degree of stress perceived by individuals was indicated. The melancholy experience was usually composed of yes or no, as a question about melancholy. Among the questions, the one regarding depression prevalence used the standardized Korean version of the nine-item Patient Health Questionnaire (PHQ-9), which is a screening tool for depression comprised of nine questions, based on the Diagnostic and Statistical Manual of Mental Disorders, 4th edition [32]. Based on the diagnosis of the prevalence of depression, 0 = "not at all", 1 = "several days", 2 = "more than half the days", and 3 = "nearly every day" were the criteria used to diagnose the prevalence of depression. The total score ranged 0 from 27, and a higher score means a higher incidence of depression [32]. The tool has been reported to have better sensitivity (88%) and specificity (88%) than the Self-Rating Depression Scale and Beck Depression Inventory, which are the most commonly used depression indicators. PHQ-9 has also been found to be valid, with a high level of reliability in the measurement of the severity of depression [33]. Despite the small number of questions that require less time for completion, the PHQ-9 has been reported as a more accurate diagnostic tool for depression in numerous recent studies [34]. This assumes significance in the present time, when almost half of the patients with depression remain undiagnosed, owing to insufficient consultation time in overcrowded outpatient clinics, or wherein most depression patients are examined primarily for physical symptoms like pain or reduced physical functions, rather than psychological ones [35]. In the present study, the Cronbach's alpha coefficient of the PHQ-9 was 0.88.

2.4. Data Analysis

All data in this study were analyzed using SPSS version 25.0 (IBM, Armonk, NY, USA), after a process of coding and data cleaning. For demographic factors, cross-analysis and descriptive statistical analysis were performed, and the results compared in order to analyze the mean and standard deviation from the "Social Indices of Daegu in 2018" and the "Regional Health Statistics at a Glance, 2008–2018". to ensure the required level of confidence in each tool, Cronbach's α values were computed. Lastly, in order to identify the differences according to provision of the national disaster relief fund, an independent t-test was carried out.

3. Results

Table 1 displays the characteristics of the participants. This study targeted 285 females (51.8%) and 265 males (48.2%), which means more females participated in the study. Also, 138 people in their 20s (25.1%) occupied the highest proportion of the subjects, and it was followed by 137 in their 40s (24.9%). There were statistically significant differences in age, monthly household income, and sense of pride depending on national disaster relief funds. Also, there were significant differences in national disaster relief funds depending on the PHQ-9 scores of the subjects.

Table 1. Demographic characteristics (n = 550).

Variable	Total	WDRF [1]	WODRF [2]	p-Value
n	550	264	286	
Gender				
Male, n (%)	265 (48.2)	128 (48.3)	137 (51.7)	0.891
Female, n (%)	285 (51.8)	136 (47.7)	149 (52.3)	
Age, mean (SD)	38.33 (10.64)	38.09 (10.66)	38.54 (10.64)	
20s, n (%)	138 (25.1)	69 (50.0)	69 (50.0)	
30s, n (%)	190 (34.5)	88 (46.3)	102 (53.7)	
40s, n (%)	137 (24.9)	73 (53.3)	64 (46.7)	0.017
50s, n (%)	66 (12.0)	21 (31.8)	45 (68.2)	
60–65 years n (%)	19 (3.5)	13 (68.4)	6 (31.6)	
Marital Status				
Single, n (%)	285 (51.8)	131 (46.0)	154 (54.0)	
Married, n (%)	249 (45.3)	123 (49.4)	126 (50.6)	0.365
Widowed or divorced, n (%)	16 (2.9)	10 (62.5)	6 (37.5)	
Education				
Under high school, n (%)	52 (9.5)	29 (55.8)	23 (44.2)	
College (2-year), n (%)	124 (22.5)	62 (50.0)	62 (50.0)	
University (4-year), n (%)	307 (55.8)	149 (48.5)	158 (51.5)	0.228
Master's degree, n (%)	54 (9.8)	20 (37.0)	34 (63.0)	
PhD degree, n (%)	13 (2.4)	4 (30.8)	9 (69.2)	
Monthly household income [a]				
Under ₩ 1,000,000, n (%)	22 (4.0)	17 (77.3)	5 (22.7)	
₩ 1,000,000–1,990,000, n (%)	32 (5.8)	23 (71.9)	9 (28.1)	
₩ 2,000,000–2,990,000, n (%)	118 (21.5)	68 (57.6)	50 (42.4)	
₩ 3,000,000–3,990,000, n (%)	90 (16.4)	47 (52.2)	43 (47.8)	0.000 *
₩ 4,000,000–4,990,000, n (%)	84 (15.3)	35 (41.7)	49 (58.3)	
₩ 5,000,000–5,990,000, n (%)	86 (15.6)	39 (45.3)	47 (54.7)	
₩ 6,000,000–6,990,000, n (%)	50 (9.1)	17 (34.0)	33 (66.0)	
₩ ≥ 7,000,000, n (%)	68 (12.4)	18 (16.5)	50 (73.5)	

Table 1. *Cont.*

Variable	Total	WDRF [1]	WODRF [2]	*p*-Value
Sleep time, mean (SD)	6.77(1.16)	6.77 (1.20)	6.76 (1.13)	0.946
Stress levels				
I feel a lot of stress frequently	57 (10.4	28 (49.1)	29 (50.9)	
I feel stress a lot	176 (32.0)	84 (47.7)	92 (52.3)	0.713
I feel stress a little	281 (51.1)	138 (49.1)	143 (50.9)	
I do not feel stress	36 (6.5)	14 (38.9)	22 (61.1)	
Melancholy				
Yes	104 (18.9)	55 (52.9)	49 (47.1)	0.268
No	446 (81.1)	209 (46.9)	237 (53.1)	
PHQ-9				
PHQ-9 score 0-4 (minimal)	266 (48.4)	117 (44.0)	149 (56.0)	
PHQ-9 score 5–9 (mild)	173 (31.5)	88 (50.9)	85 (49.1)	
PHQ-9 score 10–14 (moderate)	77 (14.0)	46 (59.7)	31 (40.3)	0.004
PHQ-9 score 15–19 (moderately severe)	23 (4.2)	5 (21.7)	18 (78.3)	
PHQ-9 score 20–27 (severe)	11 (2.0)	8 (72.7)	3 (27.3)	
Sense of belonging				
Very strong sense of belonging	68 (12.4)	36 (52.9)	32 (47.1)	
A little sense of belonging	282 (51.3)	141 (50.0)	141 (50.0)	0.174
Little no sense of belonging	163 (29.6)	75 (46.0)	88 (54.0)	
No sense of belonging at all	37 (6.7)	12 (32.4)	25 (67.6)	
Sense of pride				
Very strong sense of pride	41 (7.5)	27 (65.9)	14 (34.1)	
A little sense of pride	163 (29.6)	82 (50.3)	81 (49.7)	0.012
Little no sense of pride	259 (47.1)	124 (47.9)	135 (52.1)	
No sense of pride at all	87 (15.8)	31 (35.6)	56 (64.4)	

Notes: [1] WDRF: with disaster relief fund; [2] WODRF: without disaster relief fund; [a] South Korean 10.000 won (USD 1 = KRW 1203.00). The *p*-values were calculated from chi-square tests and *t*-tests, as appropriate. * Significant difference noted in the comparison between four groups ($p < 0.05$).

Table 2 includes a descriptive statistics analysis to determine the sleep time, stress level, melancholy and depression prevalence, sense of belonging, and sense of pride among Daegu citizens before and during COVID-19. Looking at the results, it was found that in 2016, the sleep time was at 6.6 h in 2016 and 6.8 h in the case of COVID-19. The stress level was 23.3% in 2018 and 42.4% with the current COVID-19. The depression was at 3.4% in 2018 and at 18.9% during COVID-19. The prevalence of depression was 1.9% in 2018 and 5.8% as of the emergence of COVID-19.

For the sense of belonging as a citizen of Daegu, "Very strong sense of belonging" was the lowest, at 5.9% in 2018—as of COVID-19, it was 12.4%. "A little sense of belonging" was at 47.2% in 2018, and 51.3% as of COVID-19. "Little no sense of belonging" was at 36.9% in 2012 and 2016, and 29.6% during COVID-19. "No sense of belonging at all" was at 2.0% in 2012, and 6.7% with COVID-19. Regarding pride, the "Very strong sense of pride" response was the lowest, at 5.6% in 2016 and currently at 7.5% during COVID-19. "A little sense of pride" was at 39.8% in 2018, and 29.6% during COVID-19. "Little no sense of pride" was at 43.0% in 2016, and COVID-19 responses were at 47.1%. Lastly, "No sense of pride at all" had 3.2% in 2012 and 15.8% with COVID-19.

Table 2. The mean and standard deviation (SD) of the mental health indicators, sense of belonging, and pride among Daegu citizens before and during COVID-19 (n = 550).

Items	2012	2014	2016	2018	COVID-19
Sleep time (hours), mean (SD)	6.7	6.7	6.6	6.7	6.8 (1.16)
Stress levels, % (n)	27.2	26.0	26.6	23.3	42.4 (233)
Melancholy, mean (SD)	5.6	5.4	4.9	3.4	18.9 (0.39)
Depression prevalence, mean (SD)				1.9	5.8 (5.05)
Sense of belonging					
Very strong sense of belonging, % (n)	9.9	8.3	7.1	5.9	12.4 (68)
A little sense of belonging, % (n)	51.2	49.2	50.8	47.2	51.3 (282)
Little no sense of belonging, % (n)	36.9	38.7	36.9	41.2	29.6 (163)
No sense of belonging at all, % (n)	2.0	3.8	5.2	5.8	6.7 (37)
Sense of pride					
Very strong sense of pride, % (n)	7.7	7.5	5.6	5.9	7.5 (41)
A little sense of pride, % (n)	47.2	43.0	45.8	39.8	29.6 (163)
Little no sense of pride, % (n)	42.0	45.5	43.0	48.0	47.1 (259)
No sense of pride at all, % (n)	3.2	4.1	5.6	6.3	15.8 (87)

Table 3 shows the independent t-test to determine whether each parameter showed differences according to provision of the disaster relief fund. It shows that all parameters exhibited differences between the presence and absence of the fund (sense of pride: t = 3.06, p = 0.002; sense of belonging: t = 2.01, p = 0.045).

Table 3. The differences between presence and absence of the national disaster relief fund (n = 550).

Items	Mean (SD)		Effect Size	t-Value	p-Value
	WDRF [1] (n = 264)	WODRF [2] (n = 286)			
PHQ-9, mean (SD)	1.85 (0.97)	1.74 (0.95)	0.12	1.40	0.163
Depression prevalence *	1.67 (0.57)	1.62 (0.55)	−0.09	1.01	0.312
Stress levels *	2.52 (0.76)	2.55 (0.78)	−0.04	−0.45	0.650
Melancholy *	1.79 (0.41)	1.83 (0.38)	−0.10	−0.10	0.269
Sense of belonging	2.76 (0.74)	2.62 (0.80)	0.17	2.01	0.045
Sense of pride	2.39 (0.83)	2.18 (0.80)	0.26	3.06	0.002

Notes: p-values were analyzed using the independent t-test. [1] WDRF: with disaster relief fund; [2] WODRF: without disaster relief fund. * Depression prevalence, stress levels, and melancholy each showed no significant difference.

The independent t-test to determine whether each parameter showed differences, according to provision of the disaster relief fund, showed that none of the parameters showed a difference between presence and absence of the fund, with the following results: depression prevalence, t = 1.01, p = 0.312; stress levels, t = −0.454, p = 0.650; and melancholy, t = −0.106, p = 0.269.

4. Discussion

This study aimed to investigate whether COVID-19 had led to differences in the sense of regional belonging, pride, and mental health among the citizens of Daegu, and to analyze the differences based on the presence or absence of the national disaster relief fund. The findings are discussed as follows.

First, the sense of regional belonging was found to have increased after COVID-19 when compared to the time before. Daegu was pointed out as the source of the explosive spread of COVID-19 by the general public, who criticized the citizens of Daegu and posted various expressions of hate on online portal sites and communities, holding them responsible for the COVID-19 outbreak incessantly [36]. Such accusations and discriminating behaviors from people in other regions are thought to have led to the increased sense of belonging among the people of Daegu. In the same context, as the people in other regions blamed the citizens of Daegu, the increased social sharing among the local residents enhanced the regional identity, and subsequently, the regional belonging. Daegu has endured a number of disasters in the past, such as a gas explosion and metro fire, and in each case, the disaster was overcome by the united efforts of the citizens [37]. This is presumed to be the reason behind the increased sense of regional belonging among the citizens of Daegu after COVID-19.

Individuals who received the national disaster relief fund were found to have higher awareness of regional belonging. Financial difficulties in households are being relieved by the disaster relief fund provided by the government [38]. It is thus presumed that the fund is financially aiding small business owners and socially disadvantaged groups to help them overcome the difficult time [39], and individuals who received the fund are consequently showing higher awareness of regional belonging [40]. The disaster relief fund was reported to have a positive influence on the quality of life of the working poor and people with disabilities, who are able to make less than half their original profits owing to the COVID-19 outbreak [41]. Thus, in a prolonged national disaster situation, as is the case of COVID-19, with consequently reduced social and economic activities, providing the national disaster relief fund to citizens, starting with small business owners and the socially disadvantaged, was found to have led to higher awareness of regional belonging among the citizens. Such an increase in regional belonging is likely to strengthen the solidarity among local residents, and the resulting social unity would help the citizens overcome the difficult situation, based on the strong confidence regarding the region, in case of a national disaster in the future.

The regional pride among the citizens of Daegu was shown to have decreased from 2018 after the arrival of COVID-19. This finding contradicts a previous study [42]. It has been reported that the number of additional confirmed patients have substantially decreased in Daegu, Korea—a city that had faced the first phases of COVID-19 outbreak outside China. In reality, however, Daegu is viewed by its citizens as a city where such a social difficulty or disaster may occur again at any time, even though might have overcome the COVID-19 situation, which consequently led to the fall in their regional pride.

This study shows that individuals who received national disaster relief funds had a higher level of pride. According to a previous study, the people of Daegu show high levels of unity, justice, and resourcefulness [43]. This is thought to have increased an already high level of regional pride among the citizens when the national disaster relief fund was provided. Thus, based on an already high level of regional pride, the sense of community among the citizens of Daegu is likely to have increased, and the fund is thought to have further increased their regional pride. Thus, the national disaster relief fund provided to the citizens of Daegu has led to trust towards the region, owing to regional characteristics like conservative ideas, loyalty, and exclusivity; such trust may serve as the basis for communication among local residents, which would help characterize Daegu as a city that can overcome any disaster in the future.

The rate of experiencing melancholy and depression among the citizens of Daegu after COVID-19 was shown to have increased. In addition, no significant difference was found for these parameters with respect to provisions of the disaster relief fund, based on the results of the *t*-test. This indicates that the presence or absence of the fund did not have a significant impact on people's mental health, and that COVID-19 itself is presumed to have had a negative influence on the mental health of the citizens. Hence, the reduced mental health compared to the past is thought to have resulted from the social isolation, staying indoors, and altered daily activities caused by COVID-19. Indicators such as melancholy, depression, and anxiety among the citizens of Hong Kong after COVID-19 showed far higher values than the time before, which is consistent with the results in this study [28]. The continuous increase in the level of melancholy due to COVID-19 among Daegu citizens has even led to coining of the term "Corona Blues", combining the coronavirus and melancholy (blues) [44]. The level of melancholy is thought to have increased in line with the increased anxiety among Daegu citizens, due to the rapid spread of COVID-19, which once led to as high as 741 confirmed patients a day. The social distancing from friends and family due to COVID-19 has led many people to suffer from melancholy [45]. In addition, the changed economic and social values and relationships after COVID-19 are exerting an influence on the psychological stress in people [46]. The findings of these previous studies were partially in agreement with those of the present study. Uncertain situations about COVID-19 have resulted in increased stress and anxiety about not maintaining daily life [47]. In the future, therefore, when a focused disaster situation occurs in a single city as in the case of Daegu, various methods should be sought to reduce the levels of melancholy and stress among the citizens for their mental health care through the use of different media, including phone and the internet, or through a national program developed for the emotional stability of the citizens.

This study has several limitations, as follows. First, the data of the study were gathered online with the use of a professional survey company. For this reason, the way of responding might be influenced by using a computer and computer skills. Second, this is a cross-sectional study, which means it is impossible to observe temporary changes in respondents' sense of belonging, pride, and mental health. Third, the study results cannot apply to other regions and groups in Korea for generalization. Fourth, although giving national disaster relief funds may influence a sense of belonging and pride, these can be boosted by more diverse psychological and social factors. That is why it is impossible to generalize the levels of a sense of belonging and pride revealed in this study.

5. Conclusions

This study examined the differences in the sense of regional belonging, pride, and mental health among the citizens of Daegu, due to COVID-19, between the times before and after COVID-19, and based on the presence or absence of the national disaster relief fund.

The level of regional belonging among the citizens increased after COVID-19, but the level of pride decreased. Regarding differences according to provision of the national disaster relief fund, all parameters of belonging and pride significantly increased among individuals who received the fund. This was thought to be due to the enhanced regional identity, based on the characteristics of Daegu citizens, which involve conservative ideas, local patriotism, loyalty, exclusivity, and faithfulness, combined with the social convention to overcome a difficult situation together. Therefore, in a challenging national situation, providing the disaster relief fund to the citizens is anticipated to raise the sense of regional belonging and pride to enhance regional identity and elicit communication among local residents, whereby the challenge can be overcome.

Furthermore, the citizens of Daegu were found to have experienced melancholy more frequently after COVID-19, and the depression prevalence was also higher compared to the time before COVID-19. In line with this, to protect the mental health of individuals in a national disaster, such as COVID-19, every local government should take initiatives to enhance the mental health of the citizens, and in a narrower sense, a way to enhance the mental health should be sought through the provision of aids to each household, so that the family members can acquire emotional stability.

Author Contributions: Conceptualization, Y.-J.K. and E.-S.K.; methodology, Y.-J.K., J.-H.C. and E.-S.K.; validation, Y.-J.K. and E.-S.K.; formal analysis, Y.-J.K., J.-H.C. and E.-S.K.; investigation, Y.-J.K. and E.-S.K.; data curation, Y.-J.K. and E.-S.K.; writing—original draft preparation, Y.-J.K.; writing—proofreading and editing, Y.-J.K., J.-H.C. and E.-S.K. Both authors have read and agreed to the published version of the manuscript. All authors have read and agreed to the published version of the manuscript.

Funding: This research received no external funding.

Conflicts of Interest: The authors declare no conflict of interest.

References

1. Ornell, F.; Schuch, J.B.; Sordi, A.O.; Kessler, F.H.P. "Pandemic fear" AND COVID-19: Mental health burden and strategies. *Braz. J. Psychiatry* **2020**, *42*, 232–235. [CrossRef]
2. Van Bavel, J.J.; Baicker, K.; Boggio, P.S.; Capraro, V.; Cichocka, A.; Cikara, M.; Drury, J. Using social and behavioural science to support COVID-19 pandemic response. *Nat. Hum. Behaviour.* **2020**, *4*, 460–471. [CrossRef] [PubMed]
3. Phase VI Pandemic, the Highest Alert Level, and the Second Declaration after the Swine Flu in 2009. Available online: http://www.donga.com/news/article/all/20200223/99833909/1 (accessed on 27 May 2020).
4. Grasselli, G.; Pesenti, A.; Cecconi, M. Critical care utilization for the COVID-19 outbreak in Lombardy, Italy: Early experience and forecast during an emergency response. *JAMA* **2020**, *323*, 1545–1546. [CrossRef] [PubMed]
5. "COVID-19 Will End Soon," says President Moon. Available online: https://news.joins.com/article/23705968 (accessed on 27 May 2020).
6. Choi, S.; Ki, M. Estimating the reproductive number and the outbreak size of COVID-19 in Korea. *Epidemiology and Health* **2020**, *42*, E2020011. [CrossRef]
7. Lee, H.S. "Travel Regulations May be Reinforced on 'Certain Countries' of High COVID-19 Incidence," said President Trump. Available online: http://news.chosun.com/site/data/html_dir/2020/03/03/2020030301684.html (accessed on 27 May 2020).
8. Yin, H.; Liu, Z.; Kammen, D.M. Impacts of Early Interventions on the Age-Specific Incidence of COVID-19 in New York, Los Angeles, Daegu and Nairobi. *medRxiv* **2020**. [CrossRef]
9. How South Korea Successfully Battled COVID-19 While the U.S. Didn't. Available online: https://www.healthline.com/health-news/what-south-korea-has-done-correctly-in-battling-covid-19 (accessed on 28 May 2020).
10. Daegu to Offer Emergency Aid to Virus-Battered Households, Businesses. The Korea Herald. Available online: http://www.koreaherald.com/view.php?ud=20200323000744 (accessed on 28 May 2020).
11. Businebusineyin-in-Battling-Covid-19s Angeles, Daeg Ohmynews. Available online: http://www.ohmynews.com/NWS_Web/View/at_pg.aspx?CNTN_CD=A0002621873 (accessed on 25 June 2020).
12. Daegu City Deciding to Give 500,000 to 900,000 Won to Recipients, Who Belong to Median-Income Households or Below. Available online: http://www.ohmynews.com/NWS_Web/View/at_pg.aspx?CNTN_CD=A0002625088 (accessed on 25 June 2020).
13. "The Emergency Relief Fund will be Provided in a Pre-Paid Card for Reviving the Local Economy" says the Mayor of Daegu. Available online: https://www.yna.co.kr/view/AKR20200326101400053 (accessed on 28 May 2020).
14. [Park Myeong Ho's Financial News Column] To Get Over the Corona Pandemic. Available online: https://www.idaegu.co.kr/news/articleView.html?idxno=309440 (accessed on 29 May 2020).
15. To Make a Meaningful Use of Chid Care Points and Disaster Relief Funds. Available online: http://www.ohmynews.com/NWS_Web/View/at_pg.aspx?CNTN_CD=A0002642483. (accessed on 25 June 2020).
16. Jung, S.J.; Jun, J.Y. Mental Health and Psychological Intervention Amid COVID-19 Outbreak: Perspectives from South Korea. *Yonsei Med. J.* **2020**, *61*, 271–272. [CrossRef] [PubMed]
17. Two Months with COVID-19 Shed Your Anxiety as Deep Sleep, Singing, Sun-Bathing are the Health Boosters. Available online: https://www.seoul.co.kr/news/newsView.php?id=20200318018003&wlog_tag3=naver. (accessed on 27 May 2020).
18. Malta, M.; Rimoin, A.W.; Strathdee, S.A. The coronavirus 2019-nCoV epidemic: Is hindsight 20/20? *EClinicalMedicine* **2020**, *20*, 100289. [CrossRef] [PubMed]
19. Cascella, M.; Rajnik, M.; Cuomo, A.; Dulebohn, S.C.; Di Napoli, R. Features, evaluation and treatment coronavirus (COVID-19). In *Statpearls*; StatPearls Publishing: Treasure Island, Finland, 2020.
20. Garcia, R. Neurobiology of fear and specific phobias. *Learn. Mem.* **2017**, *24*, 462–471. [CrossRef]
21. Shin, L.M.; Liberzon, I. The neurocircuitry of fear, stress, and anxiety disorders. *Neuropsychopharmacology* **2010**, *35*, 169–191. [CrossRef]
22. Shultz, J.M.; Baingana, F.; Neria, Y. The 2014 Ebola outbreak and mental health: Current status and recommended response. *JAMA* **2015**, *313*, 567–568. [CrossRef]

23. Zhang, Z.; Shi, Z.; Wang, L.; Liu, M. One year later: Mental health problems among survivors in hard-hit areas of the Wenchuan earthquake. *Public Health* **2011**, *125*, 293–300. [CrossRef]
24. Mak, I.W.C.; Chu, C.M.; Pan, P.C.; Yiu, M.G.C.; Chan, V.L. Long-term psychiatric morbidities among SARS survivors. *Gen. Hosp. Psychiatry* **2009**, *31*, 318–326. [CrossRef] [PubMed]
25. Shigemura, J.; Ursano, R.J.; Morganstein, J.C.; Kurosawa, M.; Benedek, D.M. Public responses to the novel 2019 coronavirus (2019-nCoV) in Japan: Mental health consequences and target populations. *Psychiatry Clin. Neurosci.* **2020**, *74*, 281. [CrossRef]
26. Sánchez-Hernández, M.I.; González-López, Ó.R.; Buenadicha-Mateos, M.; Tato-Jiménez, J.L. Work-Life Balance in Great Companies and Pending Issues for Engaging New Generations at Work. *Int. J. Environ. Res. Public Health* **2019**, *16*, 5122. [CrossRef]
27. Cook, L.H.; Shinew, K.J. Leisure, work, and disability coping: "I mean, you always need that 'in'group". *Leis. Sci.* **2014**, *36*, 420–438. [CrossRef]
28. Choi, E.P.H.; Hui, B.P.H.; Wan, E.Y.F. Depression and Anxiety in Hong Kong during COVID-19. *Int. J. Environ. Res. Public Health* **2020**, *17*, 3740. [CrossRef]
29. Panic Disorder, Claustrophobia . . . Citizens of Daegu Suffering from Concerns of Anxiety. Available online: https://www.hankookilbo.com/News/Read/202003011523782150 (accessed on 26 May 2020).
30. 2018 Daegu Community Survey Report. Available online: http://stat.daegu.go.kr/statsPublication/dgSocialSurvey.do (accessed on 10 May 2020).
31. 2008–2018 Regional Health Statistics at a Glance. Available online: https://chs.cdc.go.kr/chs/stats/statsMain.do (accessed on 10 May 2020).
32. Kroenke, K.; Spitzer, R.L.; Williams, J.B. The PHQ-9: Validity of a brief depression severity measure. *J. Gen. Intern. Med.* **2001**, *16*, 606–6132. [CrossRef]
33. Kim, S.R.; Shin, H.C.; Lee, D.C.; Kim, C.H.; Seong, E.J.; Lee, G.H.; Kim, J.Y. The Utility of PHQ-2/PHQ-9 Serial Test for the Screening of Major Depressive Disorder in Primary Health Care. *Korean Soc. Stress Med.* **2011**, *19*, 405–410.
34. Thibault, J.M.; Steiner, R.W. Psychiatric Briefs. *Prim. Care Companion J. Clin. Psychiatry* **2004**, *6*, 270.
35. Beck, A.T.; Ward, C.H.; Mendelson, M.; Mock, J.; Erbaugh, J. An inventory for measuring depression. *Arch. Gen. Psychiatry* **1961**, *4*, 561–571. [CrossRef] [PubMed]
36. Kim, J.S. "I am Disgusted at Anyone from Daegu" Hatred for the Region Brings More Horrors than Corona Virus. Available online: https://news.joins.com/article/23767330 (accessed on 28 May 2020).
37. [A Diary of a Corona Warrior] My 60-Year-Old Mum, Right Before retirement, Took Off Her Nurse Uniform to Put on the Armor. Available online: https://news.joins.com/article/23719357 (accessed on 29 May 2020).
38. 7 out of 10 Citizens Said, "Emergency Disaster relief Fund is Helpful.". Available online: http://www.ohmynews.com/NWS_Web/Event/Special/opinion_poll_2019/at_pg.aspx?CNTN_CD=A0002642570&CMPT_CD=P0010&utm_source=naver&utm_medium=newsearch&utm_campaign=naver_news (accessed on 26 May 2020).
39. Raschky, P.A.; Schwindt, M. On the Channel and Type of Aid: The Case of International Disaster Assistance. *Eur. J. Political Econ.* **2012**, *28*, 119–131. [CrossRef]
40. [LG Hello Vision] The Disaster Relief Fund has Revitalized the Markets. Available online: http://news.lghellovision.net/news/newsView.do?soCode=SC50000000&idx=276836 (accessed on 27 May 2020).
41. "We can Finally Breathe" A Month after Disaster Relief Fund. Available online: http://www.hani.co.kr/arti/politics/politics_general/944246.html#csidx200cbb47c3727c7b89d877092c9beb0 (accessed on 26 May 2020).
42. This South Korean City Once had the Biggest Coronavirus Outbreak Outside of China. Available online: https://www.weforum.org/agenda/2020/04/south-korean-daegu-china-coronavirus-covid19-cases-virus/ (accessed on 28 May 2020).
43. Yoon, S.G.; Kim, M.H. A Study on the Identity of the Citizens of Daegu Metropolitan and North Gyeongsang Regions. *Inst. East-West Thought* **2007**, *3*, 33–64.
44. Regular Briefing on the COVID-19 Response (10 April 2020). Available online: https://www.idaegu.co.kr/news/articleView.html?idxno=307979 (accessed on 27 May 2020).
45. Jiloha, R.C. COVID-19 and Mental Health. *Epidemiol. Int.* **2020**, *5*, 7–9. [CrossRef]

46. An Analysis on the Panic of Filipinos During COVID-19 Pandemic in the Philippines. Available online: https://www.researchgate.net/profile/Christian_Jasper_Nicomedes/publication/340081049_An_Analysis_on_the_Panic_of_Filipinos_During_COVID-19_Pandemic_in_the_Philippines/links/5e7606aa299bf1892cfc4dd3/An-Analysis-on-the-Panic-of-Filipinos-During-COVID-19-Pandemic-in-the-Philippines.pdf (accessed on 27 May 2020).
47. Li, S.; Wang, Y.; Xue, J.; Zhao, N.; Zhu, T. The Impact of COVID-19 Epidemic Declaration on Psychological Consequences: A Study on Active Weibo Users. *Int. J. Environ. Res. Public Health* **2020**, *17*, 2032. [CrossRef] [PubMed]

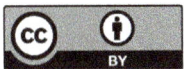 © 2020 by the authors. Licensee MDPI, Basel, Switzerland. This article is an open access article distributed under the terms and conditions of the Creative Commons Attribution (CC BY) license (http://creativecommons.org/licenses/by/4.0/).

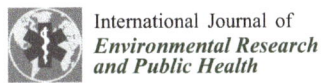 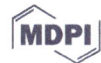

Communication

What Happened to People with Non-Communicable Diseases during COVID-19: Implications of H-EDRM Policies

Emily Ying Yang Chan [1,2,3,*], Jean Hee Kim [3], Eugene Siu Kai Lo [1,3], Zhe Huang [1,3], Heidi Hung [3], Kevin Kei Ching Hung [1,4], Eliza Lai Yi Wong [3], Eric Kam Pui Lee [3], Martin Chi Sang Wong [3] and Samuel Yeung Shan Wong [3]

1. Collaborating Centre for Oxford University and CUHK for Disaster and Medical Humanitarian Response (CCOUC), The Chinese University of Hong Kong, Hong Kong, China; Euglsk@cuhk.edu.hk (E.S.K.L.); huangzhe@cuhk.edu.hk (Z.H.); kevin.hung@cuhk.edu.hk (K.K.C.H.)
2. Nuffield Department of Medicine, University of Oxford, Oxford OX37BN, UK
3. JC School of Public Health and Primary Care, The Chinese University of Hong Kong, Hong Kong, China; JHKim@cuhk.edu.hk (J.H.K.); heidihung@link.cuhk.edu.hk (H.H.); lywong@cuhk.edu.hk (E.L.Y.W.); lkp032@cuhk.edu.hk (E.K.P.L.); wong_martin@cuhk.edu.hk (M.C.S.W.); yeungshanwong@cuhk.edu.hk (S.Y.S.W.)
4. Accident & Emergency Medicine Academic Unit, The Chinese University of Hong Kong, Prince of Wales Hospital, Hong Kong, China
* Correspondence: emily.chan@cuhk.edu.hk

Received: 18 June 2020; Accepted: 27 July 2020; Published: 3 August 2020

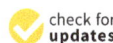

Abstract: People with existing non-communicable diseases (NCDs) are particularly vulnerable to health risks brought upon by emergencies and disasters, yet limited research has been conducted on disease management and the implications of Health-EDRM policies that address health vulnerabilities of people with NCDs during the COVID-19 pandemic. This paper reports the baseline findings of an anonymous, random, population-based, 6-month cohort study that aimed to examine the experiences of people with NCDs and their relevant self-care patterns during the COVID-19 pandemic. A total of 765 telephone interviews were completed from 22nd March to 1st April 2020 in Hong Kong, China. The dataset was representative of the population, with 18.4% of subjects reporting at least one NCD. Results showed that low household income and residence in government-subsidized housing were significant predictors for the subjects who experienced difficulty in managing during first 2 months of the pandemic (11% of the NCD patients). Of those on long-term NCD medication, 10% reported having less than one week's supply of medication. Targeted services for vulnerable groups during a pandemic should be explored to support NCD self-care.

Keywords: Health-EDRM; non-communicable disease; COVID-19; self-care; NCD management; home care; early phase of pandemic

1. Introduction

People with existing non-communicable diseases (NCDs) are particularly vulnerable to health risks brought upon by emergencies and disasters [1]. People who suffer from chronic diseases, such as cardiovascular disease, chronic lung disease, and diabetes, are more vulnerable to disruption and stress induced by disasters. A significant proportion of mortality in post-disaster phases results from the failure of health care services to cater to the needs of patients with chronic diseases [2].

The Health emergency and disaster risk management (Health-EDRM) framework emphasizes prevention and risk mitigation through hazard and vulnerability reduction, disaster preparedness, and response and recovery measures [3]. As the presence of NCDs are reported to be associated with worse outcomes of the COVID-19 disease, [4–6] strengthening NCD self-care and disease management during the pandemic could mitigate the health harm caused by COVID-19. In addition to the maintenance of healthy behaviours (e.g., regular exercise, personal hygiene), NCD patients should continue their regular medication and are recommended to stockpile at least one-month's supply of medication during the pandemic [7]. Ironically, some of the infection control measures, such as lockdowns, and the reallocation of healthcare resources to handle COVID-19 cases, have posed challenges for maintaining care among NCD patients.

The impact of COVID-19 on NCD management has caused global concerns, and the European WHO Regional Office has begun devising recommended actions for people with NCDs during this pandemic [8]. However, research on the status and disease management of NCD patients in the context of COVID-19 remains very limited. This study examines the situation of people with NCDs, their disease management difficulties, and household supply of medication during the early phase of the pandemic. The most vulnerable NCD patient subgroups were identified and discussed.

2. Materials and Methods

This is an anonymous, random, population-based, 6-month cohort study. This report highlights findings of the baseline data collection (22nd March to 1st April 2020). Participants were recruited through computerized random digit dialing (RDD). Stratified sampling was used to ensure that the dataset was representative of the Hong Kong general population in terms of age group, gender, and district of residence. Details of the methodology were reported in our previous study [9], which investigated the perception, attitude and preparation for the COVID-19 epidemic among the Hong Kong population. Data were collected in Hong Kong, a southern metropolis in China, and the health services delivery was in an urban setting.

The study population included those aged 18 years or above and residing in Hong Kong. Socio-demographic data (age, gender, household income, employment status, housing type) and details of NCD patients' disease management situation (presence and types of chronic condition(s), healthcare services utilization, routine care requirements) were collected by a standardized questionnaire. Participants were also asked about their past medical history and whether their family members had chronic condition(s). An NCD was defined as a self-reported, existing, chronic condition through the questions "Do you suffer from any form of chronic disease?" and "Which type of the chronic disease(s) are you diagnosed". Households reporting at least one member with an NCD were asked if they had at least one week's supply of NCD medications at home during the COVID-19 pandemic. In addition, they were further asked whether the COVID-19 pandemic had caused difficulty to their usual NCD care and the nature of these difficulties [9].

Differences between participants with and without perceived difficulty in their usual NCD care during the COVID-19 pandemic were examined by Chi-square tests and Fisher's exact tests ($\alpha = 0.05$). Respondents gave verbal informed consent and the study was approved by the Survey and Behavioral Research Ethics Committee at The Chinese University of Hong Kong (SBRE-19-498).

3. Results

Our telephone survey reached 765 households, and the final response rate was 44.0% (765/1738). Our sample was comparable to the Hong Kong general population [9]. Of all the households interviewed, 31.5% reported the presence of at least one person in the household diagnosed with an NCD, and among them, 9.1% reported not having at least one week's supply of NCD medications at the time of phone interview.

Of all the participants, 18.4% ($n = 141$) reported having at least one type of NCD, and approximately 5% (or 27% of these patients) reported more than one type of NCD. Approximately 44.7% of these NCD patients were aged 65 or above. The most commonly reported NCDs were hypertension (48.6%), diabetes (22.1%), cardiovascular diseases (16.4%), and hyperlipidemia (10.0%). Of NCD patients, nearly four-fifths ($n = 110$) had required medication(s) for their condition.

Around 11% of participants with NCDs reported difficulty in their routine NCD care, with the most common reasons being difficulty in getting to medical consultations/follow-up visits during the pandemic (62.5%) and difficulty in purchasing supplies, such as face masks and hand sanitizers, during this period (56.3%) (Figure 1). Among participants who reported difficulties in NCD management, those with lower income and those living in government-subsidized housing were more likely to perceive difficulties in NCD management (Table 1), while no statistically significant differences were noted for other demographic variables. The results also revealed no statistically significant difference between participants with different types of NCD or between patients with one NCD versus multiple NCDs.

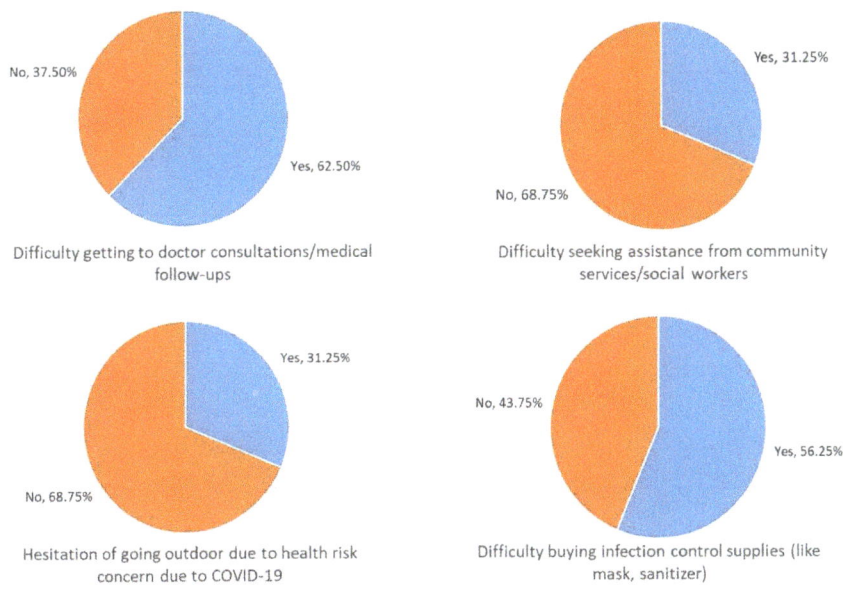

Figure 1. Difficulties reported by study samples for non-communicable diseases (NCD) management during COVID-19 pandemic ($n = 16$).

Table 1. Perceived difficulties for NCD management by sociodemographic factors during the COVID-19 pandemic.

	Perceived No Difficulty ($n = 125$)	Perceived Difficulty ($n = 16$)	p-Value
Gender			0.394
Male	48.8%	37.5%	
Female	51.2%	62.5%	
Age [a]			0.307
18–24	3.2%	0.0%	
25–44	7.2%	18.8%	
45–64	45.6%	31.3%	
65 or above	44.0%	50.0%	

Table 1. Cont.

	Perceived No Difficulty (n = 125)	Perceived Difficulty (n = 16)	p-Value
Education attainment [a]			0.087
Primary level or below	14.5%	18.8%	
Secondary level	54.0%	75.0%	
Tertiary level	31.5%	6.3%	
Living alone [a]			0.224
Not living alone	85.6%	100.0%	
Living alone	14.4%	0.0%	
Employment group [a]			0.289
White collar	24.2%	6.3%	
Blue collar	14.5%	31.3%	
Housewives	20.2%	25.0%	
Students	1.6%	0.0%	
Unemployment or retired	39.5%	37.5%	
Housing type [a]			0.012 *
Public housing	32.0%	18.8%	
Government subsidized housing	10.4%	31.3%	
Private housing	57.6%	43.8%	
Others	0.0%	6.3%	
Monthly household income (HK$) [a,b]			0.018 *
< 8000	22.8%	12.5%	
8000–19999	25.4%	62.5%	
20000–39999	20.2%	18.8%	
40000 or more	31.6%	6.3%	

[a] Fisher's exact test. [b] USD = 7.8 HKD. * $p < 0.05$.

4. Discussion

In our study, we found that around one-fifth of the Hong Kong population reported to have NCDs. Among those NCD patients, lower household income and residing in government-subsidized housing were found to be significantly associated with difficulty in NCD management during the first two months of the pandemic. In addition, households with NCD patients were reasonably well-prepared in terms of medication stockpiling during the COVID pandemic in Hong Kong, with over 90% possessing at least a week's supply of drugs. Moreover, all public outpatient clinics were open during COVID-19 with enhanced infection control measures, and allowed relatives/friends to obtain drugs for NCDs on the patients' behalf. Nonetheless, nearly one in ten NCD patients were insufficiently prepared with their medication supply.

Previous studies indicated that social distancing and quarantine could result in poor management of NCD behavioral risk factors, including various unhealthy lifestyle habits [10]. In particular, reduced social interaction, uncertainty in economic situations, and changes in the activities of daily living could further worsen disease management among NCD patients [8]. While only about 11% of the NCD patients in this study reported perceived difficulties in managing their NCD during the pandemic, the results indicate the pandemic disrupted access to NCD clinical care, possibly due to services/traffic interruption and difficulties arising from rescheduling of routine check-ups. NCD patients of lower income and those living in government-subsidized housing were significantly more likely to perceive difficulty in NCD management during the pandemic, indicating that material resources may be major barriers to care. A possible reason may be that since the willingness to wear face masks to prevent infection transmission in Hong Kong is high (e.g., around 90% of Hong Kong residents wore mask during the A/H5N1 avian influenza period in 2007 and A/H1N1 influenza period in 2009 [11]), it is not surprising that the most commonly reported difficulties for NCD care are getting to medical consultations/follow-up visits and purchasing medical supplies, given the soaring price of face masks in the first few months of the pandemic [12]. Thus, NCD patients should thereby receive more targeted services to facilitate their NCD self-care during a pandemic. Further studies, in particular on telemedicine, can investigate interventions to minimize such NCD management interruptions [13].

Health-EDRM concerns the analysis and management of health risks through reduction in hazard, exposure and vulnerability in every phase of the disaster management cycle [14]. Resilience-building is a key concept for minimizing the health risks of older people and chronic disease patients, and could be built through empowerment initiatives to improve their health outcomes. Self-care by the population concerned should also be promoted. For chronic disease patients, they should have adequate knowledge on how to use their medication (e.g., type of insulin used, insulin self-injection kit with instructions). For people with multiple drug prescriptions, it would be important for them to identify the critical, life-maintaining ones, and the key contraindications of their regular medications. In the event that health facilities and medical supplies are interrupted, it is important for chronic disease patients to stockpile, preferably, a 10–14 days' supply of medications [15]. Moreover, extensive effort is required to promote emergency preparedness among chronic disease patients, as a systematic review published in 2014 found that a considerable number of chronic disease patients lost their medication and medical aids during evacuation. Many did not bring prescriptions with them when evacuated, which made it difficult to fill in prescriptions, and that medication and prescription loss posed a significant burden on the medical relief teams [16]. Community partnership is crucial, and health care workers who are involved in disaster response and relief should be sensitive in choosing the most appropriate NCD health interventions (e.g., adverse drug interactions, unsuitable diets for people with diabetes [17]) to support patients during extreme events.

There were some limitations of this study. For the question of NCD medication stockpiling, since the interview could be answered by the patient's family members, the accuracy could be undermined by recall bias. In addition, the sample size of the chronic disease patients was very small and did not permit multivariable analysis. Although the results provided some initial insight into NCD healthcare needs and service gaps in a region that was affected by the early phase of the COVID-19 pandemic, the representativeness of the NCD subsample to the general population of NCD patients is unknown. The results should therefore be taken with caution, and future studies need to capture a larger, representative sample of NCDs patients for examination. In order to capture a representative sample of NCD patients with high quality data, a future study should be conducted by randomly sampling NCD patients from patient lists (which provides investigators with documentation of the clinical diagnoses and prescribed medications). These patients can be followed periodically during the epidemic in order to track changes in their healthcare needs and service gaps in the early and later phases. The time effect of self-reported disease management patterns will be examined in the second phase of data collection. Future studies should also examine the impacts of large-scale pandemics and public health emergencies on long-term NCD management.

5. Conclusions

This study examines the disease management difficulties faced by NCD patients during the early phase (first 2 months) of the COVID-19 pandemic and identified the most vulnerable NCD patient subgroups in an urban context. Study findings indicated low household income and residence in government-subsidized housing were found to be significant predictors among the 11% who reported difficulty in managing during first 2 months of the pandemic. Of those on long-term NCD medication, 10% reported having less than one week's supply of medication. Targeted services for vulnerable groups during a pandemic should be explored to facilitate resilience-building in Health-EDRM and to enable better self-care for people with NCDs.

Author Contributions: Conceptualization, E.Y.Y.C., E.L.Y.W., S.Y.S.W., and K.K.C.H.; methodology, J.H.K., E.K.P.L., E.S.K.L. and Z.H.; validation, J.H.K., M.C.S.W., H.H.; formal analysis, E.S.K.L. and Z.H.; investigation, E.Y.Y.C.; resources, E.Y.Y.C.; data curation, E.S.K.L. and Z.H.; writing—original draft preparation, J.H.K. and H.H.; writing—review and editing, E.Y.Y.C., J.H.K., E.L.Y.W., E.K.P.L., M.C.S.W. and S.Y.S.W.; supervision, K.K.C.H. and J.H.K.; project administration, E.S.K.L. and Z.H.; funding acquisition, E.Y.Y.C. All authors have read and agreed to the published version of the manuscript.

Funding: This research was fully funded by CCOUC development fund.

Conflicts of Interest: The authors declare no conflict of interest.

References

1. Chan, E.Y.Y. *Public Health Humanitarian Responses to Natural Disasters*; Routledge: Abingdon, UK, 2017.
2. World Health Organization. United Kingdom Health Protection Agency & Partners. Disaster Risk Management for Health: Non-Communicable Diseases. Available online: http://www.who.int/entity/hac/events/drm_fact_sheet_non_communicable_diseases.pdf?ua=1 (accessed on 18 June 2020).
3. World Health Organization. Health Emergency and Disaster Risk Management (Health-EDRM) Framework. Available online: https://www.who.int/hac/techguidance/preparedness/health-emergency-and-disaster-risk-management-framework-eng.pdf?ua=1 (accessed on 18 June 2020).
4. Guan, W.-J.; Liang, W.-H.; Zhao, Y.; Liang, H.-R.; Chen, Z.-S.; Li, Y.-M.; Liu, X.-Q.; Chen, R.-C.; Tang, C.-L.; Wang, T.; et al. Comorbidity and its impact on 1590 patients with COVID-19 in China: A nationwide analysis. *Eur. Respir. J.* **2020**, *55*, 2000547. [CrossRef] [PubMed]
5. Yang, J.; Zheng, Y.; Gou, X.; Pu, K.; Chen, Z.; Guo, Q.; Ji, R.; Wang, H.; Wang, Y.; Zhou, Y. Prevalence of comorbidities and its effects in coronavirus disease 2019 patients: A systematic review and meta-analysis. *Int. J. Infect. Dis.* **2020**, *94*, 91–95. [CrossRef] [PubMed]
6. Richardson, S.; Hirsch, J.S.; Narasimhan, M.; Crawford, J.M.; McGinn, T.; Davidson, K.W.; Barnaby, D.P.; Becker, L.B.; Chelico, J.D.; Cohen, S.L.; et al. Presenting Characteristics, Comorbidities, and Outcomes Among 5700 Patients Hospitalized With COVID-19 in the New York City Area. *JAMA* **2020**, *323*, 2052. [CrossRef] [PubMed]
7. World Health Organization. COVID-19 and NCD: Information note on COVID-19 and noncommunicable diseases. Available online: https://www.who.int/docs/default-source/inaugural-who-partners-forum/covid-19-and-ncds---final---corr7.pdf?sfvrsn=9b65e287_1&download=true (accessed on 18 June 2020).
8. Kluge, H.H.P.; Wickramasinghe, K.; Rippin, H.L.; Mendes, R.; Peters, D.H.; Kontsevaya, A.; Breda, J. Prevention and control of non-communicable diseases in the COVID-19 response. *Lancet* **2020**, *395*, 1678–1680. [CrossRef]
9. Chan, E.Y.Y.; Huang, Z.; Lo, E.S.K.; Hung, K.; Wong, E.L.-Y.; Wong, M.C. Sociodemographic Predictors of Health Risk Perception, Attitude and Behavior Practices Associated with Health-Emergency Disaster Risk Management for Biological Hazards: The Case of COVID-19 Pandemic in Hong Kong, SAR China. *Int. J. Environ. Res. Public Health* **2020**, *17*, 3869. [CrossRef] [PubMed]
10. Ryan, D.H.; Ravussin, E.; Heymsfield, S. COVID 19 and the Patient with Obesity—The Editors Speak Out. *Obesity* **2020**, *28*, 847. [CrossRef] [PubMed]
11. Chan, E.Y.Y.; Cheng, C.K.Y.; Tam, G.; Huang, Z.; Lee, P. Knowledge, attitudes, and practices of Hong Kong population towards human A/H7N9 influenza pandemic preparedness, China, 2014. *BMC Public Health* **2015**, *15*, 943. [CrossRef] [PubMed]
12. World Health Organization. Shortage of Personal Protective Equipment Endangering Health Workers Worldwide. Available online: https://www.who.int/news-room/detail/03-03-2020-shortage-of-personal-protective-equipment-endangering-health-workers-worldwide (accessed on 9 July 2020).
13. Wu, C.; Liu, Y.; Ohannessian, R.; Duong, T.; Odone, A. Global Telemedicine Implementation and Integration Within Health Systems to Fight the COVID-19 Pandemic: A Call to Action. *JMIR Public Health Surveill.* **2020**, *6*, e18710. [CrossRef]
14. Chan, E.Y.Y.; Hung, H. Key Public Health Challenges for Health-EDRM in the Twenty-First Century: Demographic and Epidemiological Transitions. In *Disaster Risk Reduction*; Springer Science and Business Media LLC: Berlin, Germany, 2020; pp. 19–38.

15. Arrieta, M.I.; Foreman, R.D.; Crook, E.D.; Icenogle, M.L. Insuring Continuity of Care for Chronic Disease Patients After a Disaster: Key Preparedness Elements. *Am. J. Med. Sci.* **2008**, *336*, 128–133. [CrossRef] [PubMed]
16. Ochi, S.; Hodgson, S.; Landeg, O.; Mayner, L.; Murray, V. Disaster-Driven Evacuation and Medication Loss: A Systematic Literature Review. *PLoS Curr.* **2014**, *6*. [CrossRef] [PubMed]
17. Chan, E.Y.Y.; Sondorp, E. Medical Interventions following Natural Disasters: Missing out on Chronic Medical Needs. *Asia Pac. J. Public Health* **2007**, *19*, 45–51. [CrossRef] [PubMed]

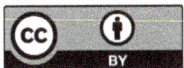

© 2020 by the authors. Licensee MDPI, Basel, Switzerland. This article is an open access article distributed under the terms and conditions of the Creative Commons Attribution (CC BY) license (http://creativecommons.org/licenses/by/4.0/).

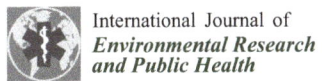

Review

Narrative Review on Health-EDRM Primary Prevention Measures for Vector-Borne Diseases

Emily Ying Yang Chan [1,2,3,4,5,*], **Tiffany Sze Tung Sham** [3,4], **Tayyab Salim Shahzada** [3,4], **Caroline Dubois** [4], **Zhe Huang** [1,3], **Sida Liu** [1,4], **Kevin K.C. Hung** [1,3,5], **Shelly L.A. Tse** [3], **Kin On Kwok** [3], **Pui-Hong Chung** [3], **Ryoma Kayano** [6] **and Rajib Shaw** [7]

1. Collaborating Centre for Oxford University and CUHK for Disaster and Medical Humanitarian Response (CCOUC), The Chinese University of Hong Kong, Hong Kong SAR, China; huangzhe@cuhk.edu.hk (Z.H.); sida.liu@gxfoundation.hk (S.L.); kevin.hung@cuhk.edu.hk (K.K.C.H.)
2. Nuffield Department of Medicine, University of Oxford, Oxford OX37BN, UK
3. JC School of Public Health and Primary Care, Faculty of Medicine, The Chinese University of Hong Kong, Hong Kong SAR, China; tiffany.sham@link.cuhk.edu.hk (T.S.T.S.); tayyabshahzada@link.cuhk.edu.hk (T.S.S.); shelly@cuhk.edu.hk (S.L.A.T.); kkokwok@cuhk.edu.hk (K.O.K.); chungpuihong@cuhk.edu.hk (P.-H.C.)
4. GX Foundation, Hong Kong SAR, China; caroline.dubois@gxfoundation.hk
5. Accident & Emergency Medicine Academic Unit, The Chinese University of Hong Kong, Prince of Wales Hospital, Hong Kong SAR, China
6. World Health Organization Centre for Health Development, Kobe 651-0073, Japan; kayanor@who.int
7. Graduate School of Media and Governance, Keio University, Fujisawa 252-0882, Japan; shaw@sfc.keio.ac.jp
* Correspondence: emily.chan@cuhk.edu.hk; Tel.: +852-2252-8850

Received: 15 July 2020; Accepted: 13 August 2020; Published: 18 August 2020

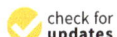

Abstract: Climate change is expanding the global at-risk population for vector-borne diseases (VBDs). The World Health Organization (WHO) health emergency and disaster risk management (health-EDRM) framework emphasises the importance of primary prevention of biological hazards and its value in protecting against VBDs. The framework encourages stakeholder coordination and information sharing, though there is still a need to reinforce prevention and recovery within disaster management. This keyword-search based narrative literature review searched databases PubMed, Google Scholar, Embase and Medline between January 2000 and May 2020, and identified 134 publications. In total, 10 health-EDRM primary prevention measures are summarised at three levels (personal, environmental and household). Enabling factor, limiting factors, co-benefits and strength of evidence were identified. Current studies on primary prevention measures for VBDs focus on health risk-reduction, with minimal evaluation of actual disease reduction. Although prevention against mosquito-borne diseases, notably malaria, has been well-studied, research on other vectors and VBDs remains limited. Other gaps included the limited evidence pertaining to prevention in resource-poor settings and the efficacy of alternatives, discrepancies amongst agencies' recommendations, and limited studies on the impact of technological advancements and habitat change on VBD prevalence. Health-EDRM primary prevention measures for VBDs require high-priority research to facilitate multifaceted, multi-sectoral, coordinated responses that will enable effective risk mitigation.

Keywords: health-EDRM; primary prevention; vector-borne disease; biological hazards; climate change; narrative review

1. Introduction

Vector-borne diseases (VBDs) are viral, parasitic and bacterial illnesses transmitted to humans through vectors such as mosquitoes, sand flies and ticks. Common VBDs affecting human health include malaria, yellow fever, dengue, Zika, chikungunya, Lyme disease, tick-borne encephalitis, leishmaniasis and African trypanosomiasis [1]. The complacency towards and reduced emphasis on vector control [2] and the redirection of health resources, together with population growth, urbanisation and globalization, have contributed to the increased frequency of VBD outbreaks in tropical areas of the world in the past decade [2]. With the impact of climate change on ecological and human living environment, the burden of VBDs has expanded from tropical and subtropical areas to temperate regions, placing 80% of the world's population at risk [3]. This shift in the human vulnerability profile has been attributed to rising temperatures, which favour the migration and geographical expansion of disease vectors [4]. Furthermore, altered precipitation patterns favour larval breeding and have accelerated VBD spread [5]. Contact patterns between humans and pathogens, vectors or hosts may also be altered by climate change in an unpredictable manner [4]. Increased occurrences of natural hazards, such as floods and cyclones, pose a further risk of VBD outbreaks [4]. Geographical areas that were previously unaffected are now facing growing risks [6,7], but are often underequipped in disaster prevention, preparedness and response capacities.

The World Health Organization (WHO) estimates that VBDs currently account for over 17% of the global burden of infectious diseases [1]. As indicated in the Global Burden of Disease Study [8], VBDs have substantial disability weights [9] and can be detrimental to the socioeconomic development of communities. Malaria is a disease which accounts for more than 50% of total deaths caused by VBD [10], and high-risk countries have on average a gross domestic product per capita growth that is over five times lower than countries not affected by the disease [11]. The economic burden of VBDs stems from increased household expenditure on disease prevention and management, lost income from minimised productivity due to sickness or care for the ill [3], damages to crops and livestock by disease vectors [2], and other impacting factors. The United Nations Sustainable Development Goals (SDG) emphasise good health and well-being (SDG 3) [12]. Collaborative initiatives and investments prioritising prevention and treatment research by international bodies in recent decades, such as efforts by the Global Fund [13], have contributed to the alleviation of the global disease burden induced by VBDs [10].

The WHO health-emergency and disaster risk management (health-EDRM) framework was developed in 2018 as an integrated approach for the utilisation and management of resources in addressing current and emerging risks to public health, with the aim of promoting joint action and coherence in implementing other global strategies such as the International Health Regulations (2005), the Sendai Framework for Disaster Risk Reduction 2015–2030, the Paris Agreement on Climate Change, and the Sustainable Development Goals 2015–2030 [14]. Overall, the framework guides the structured analysis and management of health risks brought on by emergencies and disasters, focusing on risk mitigation through hazard and vulnerability reduction, preparedness, response, and recovery measures [14,15]. Health-EDRM emphasises the significance of community involvement to mitigating and counteracting the potential negative impacts of hazardous events such as VBD outbreaks, which are considered biological hazards [14].

The concept of prioritising health in disaster risk management policies was already recognised in the Sendai Framework for Disaster Risk Reduction 2015–2030 [16]. Health actors at all levels have engaged with each other and the WHO in the implementation and monitoring of disaster risk reduction. WHO offices at the regional level, and country governments, have incorporated disaster risk management policies in the health sector, which is an important step in contextualising actions for implementation [17]. The Sendai Framework has been crucial in highlighting health as a core dimension of disaster risk management, and has paved the way for the establishment of the WHO Health-EDRM Research Network, strengthening research and knowledge-sharing globally, allowing for the enhancement of evidence-based policies and practices [17]. There is a crucial need for multi-sectoral, coordinated approaches between the countries' governments, health systems and other stakeholders, especially in the area of recording and reporting against the framework [17]. Additionally, systems need to reinforce the recognition of prevention and recovery within disaster management [17].

The health-EDRM framework outlines a hierarchisation of health risk prevention into primary, secondary and tertiary prevention [14,18]. Primary prevention mitigates against the onset of disease through health promotion targeted at behavioural modification and health risk reduction. Secondary prevention involves inhibiting disease progression through strategies such as screening and early detection. Tertiary prevention focuses on treatment and rehabilitation in order to minimise disabilities and complications [18,19]. Taking into consideration financial, clinical and infrastructural costs, primary prevention can effectively alleviate the burden of VBDs in a community, if necessary through measures that address a wide spectrum of VBDs, such as targeting diseases transmittable through multiple vectors [20] or focusing on vectors that are capable of transmitting multiple diseases [1]. Primary prevention measures often offer the most cost-effective outcomes and enhance health protection through increased community resilience against diseases where treatment is unavailable or access to healthcare is complicated. Secondary and tertiary prevention measures require significant human resources and health infrastructural support, and may therefore be costly, with higher programmatic risks, causing further economic stress on impacted communities.

There is a large amount of available evidence and research concerning clinical treatment approaches to some VBDs, such as Malaria. However, other VBDs, such as dengue, chikungunya, tick-borne encephalitis, Japanese encephalitis, yellow fever and leishmaniasis, lack standardised or straightforward treatments, and rely primarily on therapeutic interventions built on symptom management [21]. There are ongoing clinical trials in these areas, such as vaccine development for Zika and chikungunya, research into rapid malaria tests, as well as drug trials for chikungunya [22].

This narrative literature review examines published evidence on health-EDRM primary prevention measures for VBD risk mitigation, maps the contextual effectiveness or limitations of each preventive measure, and aims to identify areas of research that need be strengthened in order to develop effective strategies for VBD prevention. The strength of the available scientific evidence is evaluated for each of the prevention measures. Based on the health-EDRM framework, which emphasises the context-based determination of intervention efficacy, analysis of enabling and limiting factors is also included for each measure [14].

2. Materials and Methods

A keyword search-based narrative literature review was conducted using the databases PubMed, Google Scholar, Embase, Medline and ScienceDirect. The search was conducted in May 2020 and included English language-based international peer-reviewed articles, online reports, electronic books and press releases, as well as grey literature by institutions such as the WHO, the United Nations, the Global Fund, the United Nations Children's Fund, the International Energy Agency, the World Bank, the United States Centres for Disease Control and Prevention, the U.S. Food and Drug Administration, and the Hong Kong Centre for Health Protection, published between January 2000 and May 2020. The snowballing search methodology was also applied. Specific keywords and phrases used can be found in Appendix A. The emergence, primary prevention, associated risk factors and management of VBDs were reviewed in order to generate 10 core primary prevention measures for discussion.

With reference to the Oxford Centre for Evidence-Based Medicine (OCEBM) 2009 Levels of Evidence (Figure 1) criteria, the identified papers were categorised into their respective levels according to strength of evidence based on the study design and methodology [23]. Reviewed literature that could not be categorised using the OCEBM Levels of Evidence was classified as 'Others', which includes, but is not limited to, news articles or releases, books, textbooks, position papers, guidelines, case reports and organisational reports.

Level	Therapy/Prevention, Aetiology/Harm
1a	Systematic Review (SR) (with homogeneity) of Randomised Controlled Trials (RCTs)
1b	Individual RCT (with narrow Confidence Interval)
1c	All or none
2a	SR (with homogeneity) of cohort studies
2b	Individual cohort study (including low quality RCT; e.g., <80% follow-up)
2c	'Outcomes' Research; Ecological studies
3a	SR (with homogeneity) of case-control studies
3b	Individual Case-Control Study
4	Case-series (and poor-quality cohort and case-control studies)
5	Expert opinion without explicit critical appraisal, or based on physiology, bench research or 'first principles'

Figure 1. The Oxford Centre for Evidence-Based Medicine (OCEBM) 2009 Levels of Evidence (adapted from www.cebm.net) [23].

3. Results

The search identified 134 relevant publications, all of which were included in the results analysis.

Using the identified research, 10 core bottom-up primary prevention measures were proposed and discussed based on the health-EDRM framework. Five personal protection practices (wear protective clothing when outdoors, avoid heading outdoors to vector-prone areas and during peak biting conditions, apply insect repellent, sleep under bed nets, receive prophylactic vaccinations and chemoprophylaxis), three environmental management practices (use insect-killing traps, manage stagnant water appropriately, manage waste appropriately), and two customary household practices (minimise household entry points, cover exposed foodstuffs) were included. Tables 1 and 2 (personal), Table 3 (environmental) and Table 4 (customary household) highlight relevant health risk, desired behavioural change, potential co-benefits, enabling and limiting factors, alternatives, and strength of evidence available in published literature with regard to these primary prevention measures. Table 5 categorises all 134 reviewed publications according to the OCEBM Levels of Evidence [23]. Of note, a number of the reviewed articles report an assessment of more than one primary prevention measure. The review results indicate that approximately 60% of the studied literature relate to personal protection, 24% to environmental management, and merely 16% focus on customary household practices. Measures such as outdoor avoidance, sleeping under bed nets and receiving prophylactic vaccinations and chemoprophylaxis are amongst the most commonly reported studies. Details on the precise breakdown of each reviewed reference can be found in Table S1.

Table 1. Personal Protection Practices as Health Emergency and Disaster Risk Management (Health-EDRM) Primary Prevention Approaches against Vector-borne Diseases (VBDs) (Part 1).

Parametres	Wear Protective Clothing When Outdoors	Avoid Heading Outdoors to Vector-Prone Areas and During Peak Biting Conditions	
		Vector-Prone Areas	Peak Biting Conditions
Risk	• Disease vectors have landing preferences for exposed skin over fabric. This is evident in studies on the Human Landing Catch (HLC) technique—HLC participants wear protective clothing to limit the area of exposed skin that attracts vectors [24]. • There is often a greater risk of VBD transmission outdoors compared to indoors, as seen for malaria [25], chikungunya [26], and tick-borne disease transmission [27].	• Specific locations such as secondary forests and rubber plantations are at a high risk of VBD transmission, such as dengue and Japanese encephalitis [28].	• The time of the day and weather influence VBD exposure risk. Mosquitoes infected with *Plasmodium*, the parasite that causes malaria, are most active from dusk to dawn [29–31]. • There are positive correlations between temperature and the number of dengue [32] and tick-borne encephalitis [33] transmission incidences, as well as between temperature, humidity, rainfall and the number of malaria transmission incidences [34].
Behavioural Change	• Wear protective clothing, long-sleeve tops, and long trousers to minimise skin exposure and create a physical barrier against bites from vectors such as mosquitoes [31] and ticks [35]. • Wear light-coloured clothing [21]. • Wear loose-fitting and tightly-woven clothes to avoid vector bites through the clothing when it is pulled tight to the skin [36]. • Tuck trousers into socks and boots to further reduce skin exposure. Seal clothing junctions with adhesive tape as an additional precaution under extreme infestation pressure [36].	• Avoid vector-prone or VBD-endemic areas if possible [21,31,36,37].	• Avoid or minimise outdoor activities during hot and humid seasons, unless necessary [37]. • Avoid or minimise outdoor activities during specific periods of a day, such as from dusk to dawn in malaria-endemic areas if possible [21,31,36].
Co-benefit(s)	• Protects skin from sun exposure and lowers risk of sunburn [38,39]. • Protects skin from scratches and infections [39].	• Reduces hazardous risks such as tiger [40] and bear [41] attacks in rubber plantations and secondary forests respectively.	• Protects individuals from heat exhaustion and further progression to heat stroke under exposure to high temperatures [42,43]. • Protects individuals from health risks such as increased cardiovascular disease mortality under exposure to high humidity [44]. • Protects individuals from fall-related injuries, which are more prevalent during the rainy season [45].
Enabling Factor(s)	• Availability and affordability of protective clothing [46]. • Suitability of the weather—cool and dry weather is favourable where additional clothing is unlikely to cause discomfort.	• Ability and flexibility to stay indoors for long periods without great discomfort; adequate household space is favourable. • Ability to make informed decisions on specific local habitats and conditions to avoid; the risk variability of different environments and the non-exhaustive list of prone areas and peak biting conditions above should be noted.	

Table 1. *Cont.*

Parametres	Wear Protective Clothing When Outdoors	Avoid Heading Outdoors to Vector-Prone Areas and During Peak Biting Conditions	
		Vector-Prone Areas	Peak Biting Conditions
Limiting Factor(s) and/or Alternative(s)	• Lack of protective clothing [46]. • Presence of fabric holes in clothing; The holes serve as entry points for disease vectors to come into contact with skin. Holes may develop under the attack by fabric pests such as clothes moth larvae [47]. • Unfavourable circumstances: In scorching areas and for labour-intensive occupations, heavy protective clothing may cause discomfort or impair human body heat exchange with the environment and cause heat stress [46,48].	• Unfavourable circumstances: Staying indoors for long periods in poor, crowded living environments such as slums [49] may cause great discomfort. • Occupational limitations: Those such as farmers and rubber plantation workers do not have the flexibility to avoid prone areas.	• Unfavourable circumstances: Staying indoors for long periods in poor, crowded living environments such as slums [49] may cause great discomfort. • Occupational limitations: Those with night shifts such as security guards and police officers do not have the flexibility to avoid heading outdoors at night. • Unfavourable circumstances: For populations in areas which are typically sultry (hot and humid), such as the tropics [50], risk mitigation is more challenging.
Strength of Evidence	• The effectiveness of wearing protective clothing as a physical barrier against vector bites is well-supported by evidence. • While light-coloured clothing may enhance tick detection [37], it may also attract more ticks [51] and increase tick-borne disease risk. Findings on vector landing preferences on this matter are dated and inconsistent.	• The positive correlation between larvae breeding and the extent of vegetation cover [52] is well-supported by evidence. • The assertion that rubber latex collection cups in plantations are potential breeding sites for common vectors, especially during the rainy season [53], is well-researched.	• The negative correlation between humidity and mosquito desiccation risk, as well as the positive correlations between temperature and larvae breeding, adult vector development and virus replication, are well-supported by evidence [54,55]. • The relationship between temperature, humidity, rainfall, and vector transmission incidences is well-supported by evidence. • Research on the relationship between time of the day and peak biting conditions is limited to malaria-transmitting mosquitoes. Minimal evidence is available on other VBDs and disease vector types such as ticks and sand flies.

Table 2. Personal Protection Practices as Health-EDRM Primary Prevention Approaches against VBDs (Part 2).

Parametre	Apply Insect Repellent	Sleep Under Bed Nets	Receive Prophylactic Vaccinations and Chemoprophylaxis
Risk	• Vector landing rate is an indication of human biting rate of disease vectors [36], which is positively correlated with the risk of vector bites and subsequently VBD transmission.	• Specific mosquito species tend to have higher biting rates at night [30]. • An overwhelming majority of malaria vector bites occur when people are in bed [57].	• The immune status of a population largely influences its sensitivity to diseases [58]. • Immunologically-unprotected populations are particularly susceptible to infectious diseases [58].
Behavioural Change	• Apply insect repellent on exposed surfaces (skin or clothing, but not on both simultaneously) in vector-prone areas, especially when outdoors [21,31,36,37]. • Use repellent containing DEET, a common active ingredient that repels mosquitoes [59,60] and ticks [61], thus minimising their chance of landing. • Apply permethrin, another common active ingredient, to clothing. The chemical retains its effectiveness for up to six washings [62]. • Use roll-on repellents as opposed to sprays [63]; the former minimises repellent dispersion to nearby foodstuffs and more effectively concentrates the repellent.	• Sleep under bed nets in vector-prone areas [21,37]. • Use bed nets, which offer an immediate physical barrier, to prevent disease vector entrance. Some bed nets are treated with insecticides, creating an additional chemical barrier to repel vectors. • Ensure that the net fabric is not in contact with the user and no entry points are available for vectors [36]. • Check the bed nets for holes, which may severely reduce their efficacy [64–66]. • Select quality bed nets, which is essential to successfully prevent VBD transmission. Compared to conventionally-treated bed nets made by regularly dipping into insecticides [67], long-lasting insecticide-treated bed nets manufactured in factories have high efficacy and durability. Thus, the latter is recommended for long-term usage in vector-prone areas [67,68].	• Receive the appropriate and up-to-date vaccine for those living in or travelling to vector-prone areas [21,57]. Vaccination is a form of active immunisation achieved through exposing an unimmunised individual to a pathogenic agent. The immune system is stimulated, and long-term immunity is achieved through triggering cell- or antibody-mediated immunity [69]. • Receive the appropriate chemoprophylaxis recommended for those living in or travelling to vector-prone areas. Chemoprophylaxis is 'the administration of a drug to prevent the development of a disease' [70].
Co-benefit(s)	• No other health co-benefits to note beyond its intended use.	• Protects individuals from household pests such as rodents and cockroaches during sleep [64,71]. • Prevents dust from landing on bed sheets and coverings [64]. • Provides a sense of security through a closed sleeping environment, in particular for individuals living in open shelters.	• Provides individuals with the opportunity to interact with health workers, access health services, and receive health education when visiting healthcare units for prophylaxis, in particular for remote, rural populations living in endemic areas.
Enabling Factor(s)	• Availability and affordability of insect repellents. • Proper education on the correct use of insect repellents.	• Availability and affordability [72] of bed nets and related equipment for bed net hanging; Specific materials such as ropes and sticks [73] may be required to set up the bed nets. • Availability of space to hang the bed net. • Proper education on the correct use of bed nets [72].	• Availability and affordability of vaccinations and chemoprophylaxis. • Awareness and acceptance towards vaccinations and chemoprophylaxis. • Accessibility of adequate and appropriate healthcare services.

Table 2. *Cont.*

Parametre	Apply Insect Repellent	Sleep Under Bed Nets	Receive Prophylactic Vaccinations and Chemoprophylaxis

Limiting Factor(s) and/or Alternative(s)	• Lack of access to insect repellents: In resource-deprived areas, other potentially effective natural alternatives include eucalyptus-based repellents [74,75], neem [74] and citronella [74].
	• Potential health hazards: The active ingredients of insect repellents may cause allergy [76].
		• Lack of access to quality insecticide-treated bed nets: In resource-deprived areas, basic untreated bed nets, although not to the same extent, still offer significant protection from vectors as a physical barrier [77]. They may be constructed at home using mesh-like materials.
		• Physical deterioration [64–66]: Damaged bed nets have significantly reduced efficacies. Proper maintenance of bed nets is important.
		• Thermal discomfort [78,79]: Bed nets may attenuate airflow and cause discomfort to users, especially in hot and humid areas—this can be overcome with better designs.
		• Inconvenience: The hanging [72,80] and washing [80] of bed nets may be considered troublesome.
		• Complacency: People may underestimate the local severity and danger of VBDs [80], thus hold a complacent attitude towards the need for bed nets.
			• Vaccination hesitancy:
			  ○ People may lack confidence in and be fearful towards vaccines (e.g., needle phobia), especially with the misunderstanding that vaccines pose a risk of infection [81].
			  ○ Vaccination may go against traditions and beliefs in specific social contexts or religions [81], such as in ultra-orthodox Jewish communities [82].
			  ○ People may underestimate the local severity and danger of VBDs, thus hold a complacent attitude towards the need for prophylaxis [81].
			  ○ People may have a preference for community-perceived alternatives to vaccines, such as alcohol, religious prayers and traditional remedies [81].
			• Lack of access [83] to prophylactic strategies: Inadequate vaccine supply, poor road terrain and inconvenient transport to immunisation centres, limited service delivery points, and insufficient health workers may hamper vaccination rates in developing countries [84]. Mobile immunisation campaigns may be preferred to reach poorly accessible areas [81].
			• Proper health educational interventions [81] and extensive vaccination programmes are crucial to enhance prophylaxis.

Table 2. *Cont.*

Parametre	Apply Insect Repellent	Sleep Under Bed Nets	Receive Prophylactic Vaccinations and Chemoprophylaxis
Strength of Evidence	• Compared to other active ingredients in commercially-available insect repellents, DEET is well-supported to have a longer duration of efficacy [85]. • Research on the safety of DEET has yielded conflicting findings. While some studies demonstrate potential harms such as the pro-angiogenic properties of DEET [86], others suggest that DEET imposes minimal to no evident health risks under proper usage [87], even when applied on vulnerable groups such as children and pregnant women [88]. • Recommendations on the appropriate DEET concentration are inconsistent across international organisations and governments. Limited studies suggest that a higher DEET concentration indicates a longer duration of effectiveness, yet does not necessarily indicate higher insect-repelling ability [60,88]. More extensive research is necessary to establish a uniform DEET concentration recommendation across institutions. • The strength of evidence available to support the efficacy of local natural alternatives is variable and may be conflicting, as in the case of citronella [74,85]. • Local natural alternatives may also be subject to less stringent safety testing, as in the case of neem, which may cause dermatitis if used undiluted [74].	• The strength of evidence available to support the efficacy of bed nets is strong. • Bed nets demonstrate high potential for vector bite prevention in [89] vector-prone areas, such as for dengue and Japanese encephalitis [7,79]. The introduction of insecticide-treated bed nets has contributed to the substantial reduction in malaria transmission across sub-Saharan Africa [90]. • Regarding bed net coverage, studies demonstrate that insecticide-treated bed net use in nearby compounds had a protective effect for child mortality and other health hazards in compounds lacking the bed nets, which suggests that high coverage of bed net use not only provides protection to individuals, but also has an area-wide effect on the mosquito population [91]. There is also evidence of the importance of widespread bed net coverage in the whole population for equitable community-wide benefits of protecting vulnerable target groups, such as young children and pregnant women, rather than merely exclusive bed net coverage amongst the vulnerable [92]. • Bed net efficacy may be compromised under improper usage, such as incomplete net tucking and bed net sharing [64]. There is also evidence [64,93] of instances of mosquitoes biting through insecticide-treated bed nets, especially when users are in physical contact with the net fabric. There may further be a reduction in irritancy and toxicity of insecticide-treated nets to mosquitoes after they feed on insecticide-treated bed net users [93], although further research is necessary to fully support this possibility.	• The strength of evidence available to support the efficacy of VBD prophylaxis is variable. • Some VBDs such as yellow fever [94,95], tick-borne encephalitis [96,97] and Japanese encephalitis [98,94] have highly efficacious vaccines that are well-supported by evidence. • Some VBDs have limited prophylactic strategies available: ○ RTS,S, the only vaccine against malaria shown to be protective in young children, has been demonstrated to prevent 4 out of 10 cases of malaria in clinical trials [83]. Although RTS,S only offers partial protection and is a supplementary primary prevention strategy [83], pilot vaccination programmes have been or will be launched in three countries in sub-Saharan Africa [83,100]. ○ Malaria chemoprophylaxis, especially under long-term usage, may be associated with health risks, rare fatalities, adverse drug reactions and inadequacies [101,102], thus excluding chemoprophylaxis as a safe option for long-term travellers and populations in malaria-endemic locations and limiting its recommended use to short-term travellers [103]. Individualised strategies, such as sequential regimens with different medications for chemoprophylaxis, will have to be recommended instead [103]. Besides, vivax malaria relapses cannot be prevented with current first-line chemoprophylactic regimens [103]. ○ Dengvaxia, the only U.S. Food and Drug Administration (FDA)-approved vaccine against dengue fever [104], demonstrated poor efficacy [105], and may increase the risk of severe dengue symptoms in seronegative patients infected for the first time after vaccination, since it acts like a first dengue infection [105].

Table 3. Environmental Management Practices as Health-EDRM Primary Prevention Approaches against VBDs.

Parametre	Use Insect-Killing Traps	Manage Stagnant Water Appropriately	Manage Waste Appropriately
Risk	• VBDs are transmitted to humans via living organisms such as mosquitoes, sand flies, and ticks [2].	• Water bodies and still water are the most common mosquito larval habitats [53]; their prevalence increases the risk of disease transmission, as noted for VBDs such as Zika [106], chikungunya [107], and malaria [108]. • Specific disaster occurrences may also increase VBD health risks. Under climate change, extreme weather events such as flooding and heavy rainfall may increase habitats for common vectors [20].	• Accumulation and decomposition of solid waste attracts common houseflies, especially in areas with no centralised waste management systems and with open dumpsites [109]. • Improper waste disposal augments the risk of VBD outbreaks.

171

Table 3. *Cont.*

Parametre	Use Insect-Killing Traps	Manage Stagnant Water Appropriately	Manage Waste Appropriately
Behavioural Change	• Use insect-killing traps in areas with high-vector density [36]. Traps work by attracting and killing vectors. • Select the appropriate trap for the context. Traps eliminate vectors by different mechanisms, such as emitting blue UV-light irradiation to increase reactive oxygen species production and damage DNA structures [110], and electrocuting insects on a high voltage grid. • Dispose of dead insect bodies with care and proper hygiene such as thorough handwashing with soap and water after waste handling as they may carry VBDs and be hazardous.	• Practice long-term habitual draining and elimination of stagnant water in containers inside and outside of households [2,3]. • Take note of disaster-associated VBD health hazards in disaster-prone areas. • Ensure that drinking water is stored in proper, sealed environments which are free of breeding potential.	• Practice long-term habitual proper disposal of waste [21]. • Practice specific waste management strategies such as the separation of organic and inorganic waste and the disposal of solid waste in open dumpsites away from water bodies, which are potential larval breeding grounds [111]. • Microbial pathogens are prevalent in accumulated solid waste, and unprotected handling may result in infected wounds and sepsis [109,112]. Protect hands with gloves and/or use assistive tools such as clamps or tongs when handling waste. Wash hands thoroughly with clean water and soap after waste handling to minimise infection risk.
Co-benefit(s)	• UV-light traps serve as an alternative light source due to their luminescent property.	• Reduces the hazardous risk of slipping due to stagnant water on flooring [113]. • Reduces the risk of mould development which has respiratory repercussions [114].	• Encourages the separation of household waste which eases landfill burdens and reduces health hazards such as respiratory diseases and congenital abnormalities associated with proximity to landfills [15]. • Reduces the arbitrary disposal of hazardous household waste [15]. • Reduces surface water and groundwater pollution, air contamination, and greenhouse gas emissions (e.g., methane) from open waste dumping sites [16].
Enabling Factor(s)	• Availability and affordability of insect-killing traps. • Proper education on the correct use of insect-killing traps.	• Availability of direct household water supply. • Availability and affordability of tightly-sealed water containers.	• A well-coordinated waste management system [117]. • Availability and affordability of waste bags and bins.
Limiting Factor(s) and/or Alternative(s)	• Lack of electricity: Insect-killing traps often rely on electricity to function. Taking the case of sub-Saharan Africa, nearly 600 million people have no access to electricity [118]. Passive non-electricity-requiring traps using fipronil-laced honey or toxic honey baits [119] to kill mosquitoes can potentially serve as alternatives. • Lack of access to insect-killing traps: In resource-deprived areas, cheaper alternatives such as sticky paper traps with adhesive killing mechanisms can be used. However, their insect-trapping efficacy may be limited to closed environments such as greenhouses only [120].	• Lack of water supply: It would be a challenge to avoid stagnant water accumulation in communities that lack direct household water supply—for these communities, it is common to store collected water from community standpipes and rivers [121]. Under such circumstances, tightly-sealed water containers are recommended for water storage. • Lack of tightly-sealed water containers: For communities with only open plastic bottles or buckets available for water storage, larvicides can be added to the stagnant water. It is important to monitor the safety of the practice and educate people on the proper usage of larvicides [122].	• Lack of a well-coordinated waste management system: Insufficient waste collection points and inadequate waste bins around the community, especially in developing countries [116] and resource-deprived areas, serve as barriers to proper waste disposal [123].

Table 3. *Cont.*

Parametre	Use Insect-Killing Traps	Manage Stagnant Water Appropriately	Manage Waste Appropriately
Strength of Evidence	• A comparatively large amount of evidence on the working mechanisms and efficacy of insect-killing traps is available. A variety of attractants are used in insect-killing traps, such as blue UV-light [124], carbon dioxide [125], octenol [126] and heat [127], all of which are scientifically proven to draw insects. • Studies have shown that different commercial insect-killing traps have varying efficacies in trapping and killing vectors such as the *Aedes* species, which can transmit chikungunya and Zika viruses [128]. Some traps can potentially target sand flies in addition to mosquitoes [129]. • On the safety of different killing mechanisms, limited studies have demonstrated that the UV light in traps is non-hazardous to humans [130], whereas the electrocution of insects may potentially release bacteria and viruses [131]. • Studies on whether or not pathogens remain in the infected dead insects' bodies, and evidence-based guidelines on the proper disposal of dead insect bodies, are limited.	• A comparatively large amount of evidence on the effectiveness of proper stagnant water management on VBD risk reduction is available. The aquatic characteristics of larval habitats are well-evidenced, and extensive research has been conducted regarding areas that are prone to stagnant water accumulation. Numerous studies demonstrate that household water containers, holes and furrows in discarded tyres [132], mud pots [116], and blocked drainage systems [109] are common larval breeding grounds. • Case studies that evaluate the VBD outbreak risk associated with disaster occurrences that favour water accumulation are abundant. Taking the case of Djibouti, the country was suffering from pre-existing malaria and chikungunya outbreaks; studies reflect that heavy rain and floods in late 2019 further exacerbated the situation and exposed those affected to VBD risks [133].	• A comparatively large amount of evidence on VBD prevalence in areas with improper solid waste accumulation is available. Items such as tyres, porcelain, plastic materials, and open coconut shells are commonly suggested to 'provide breeding sites, burrows and food for vectors' [134,135]. Such studies often link back to the favourability of larval breeding under stagnant water accumulation in waste materials [116,132]. • There is also extensive research on how open dumping sites exacerbate VBD risks [116,134]. • Evidence of the effectiveness of putting proper waste management into practice in communities and its relation to VBD risk reduction is minimal.

Table 4. Customary Household Practices as Health-EDRM Primary Prevention Approaches against VBDs.

Parametre	Minimise Household Entry Points		Cover Exposed Foodstuffs
	Wall Cracks	Door and Window Openings	
Risk	• Household entry points such as wall cracks as well as open doors and windows provide opportunities for vector entrance, contributing to the risk of indoor infestation. • A significant number of vectors may accumulate in the cracks if they remain unrepaired [140].	• Entry points through open doors and windows have large surface areas and are more prone to the entrance of disease vectors [141].	• Common vectors such as flies are attracted to odours and chemicals released by exposed foodstuffs, such as the volatile fermentation products [136] of ripe fruits associated with the breeding of yeast in the fruit [137]. • Disease vectors may contaminate exposed foodstuffs in open containers via direct contact or droppings, which contribute to health hazards such as a high incidence of diarrhoea in children under six [138]. • If uncooked food with pathogens such as *Salmonella* and *E. Coli* are left uncovered, houseflies may serve as vectors and expose humans to the risk of food-borne pathogenic infections [139].

Table 4. *Cont.*

Parametre	Minimise Household Entry Points		Cover Exposed Foodstuffs
	Wall Cracks	Door and Window Openings	
Behavioural Change	• Household improvements to minimise entry points are effective in reducing infestation from vectors such as *Aedes aegypti*, which transmit the Zika and chikungunya viruses [142]. The risk of malaria transmission from the *Anopheles* mosquito is similarly reduced [143]. • Repair cracks to seal potential vector entry points [21].	• Install door and window screens and close windows in the early evening to reduce indoor disease vector density [21,36,144,145].	• Practice the covering of exposed foodstuffs with food covers or nets to prevent food contamination by flies [111], especially in contexts without refrigerators.
Co-benefit(s)	• Protects individuals from household pests such as rodents [146,147] and cockroaches [148]. • Reduces water leakage [150], such as during heavy rainfall.	• Enhances household safety, such as decreasing the risk of theft or burglary [151].	• Protects exposed foodstuffs from household pests such as rodents [149].
Enabling Factor(s)	• Availability and affordability of crack-repairing materials. • Knowledge about crack-repairing, or accessibility to professional services.	• Availability and affordability of door and window screens. • Knowledge about door and window screen installation, or accessibility to professional services.	• Availability and affordability of food covers.
Limiting Factor(s) and/or Alternative(s)	• Contextual limitations: Household modifications do not apply to the homeless and the impoverished living in open, unstable shelters. • Universal applicability: Household modification recommendations may not apply to all settings due to housing differences [152]. • Professional requirement: Crack-repairing and door and window screen installation using modern methods often require professional tools and skills as well as long-term maintenance strategies. • Lack of access to modern crack-repairing materials: In resource-deprived areas, mud and lime mixtures may serve as alternatives, although they may be more costly in the long-term [153]. Less well-off populations that cannot afford modern building materials [154] may use other locally-available alternatives.	• Lack of access to door and window screen installation services: The installation of door and window screens involves significant renovation work that is often costly and unaffordable for impoverished populations [155].	• Lack of access to quality food covers: In resource-deprived areas, clean pieces of cloth, lids, or any materials that can serve as physical barriers should be used as alternatives for covering exposed foodstuffs.

Table 4. *Cont.*

Parametre	Minimise Household Entry Points		Cover Exposed Foodstuffs
	Wall Cracks	Door and Window Openings	
Strength of Evidence	• While there is available evidence on the effects of crack-repairing on VBD risk reduction, studies on the detailed evaluation of different crack-repairing methods remain limited. • Materials such as cement, modern crack-fillers, and a mixture of mud and lime are scientifically proven to be efficacious in reducing indoor vector density. • There are few studies on other more cost-effective alternatives for populations in resource-deprived areas. Mud is a locally-available alternative, but there are limited studies on whether crack-repairing with mud alone is potentially correlated with an increased risk of vector entrance [56].	• A comparatively large amount of evidence on the efficacy of proper door and window screen installation, as well as the closing of windows, in reducing indoor vector density is available. • Given that variations exist in screening designs, further research on their specific efficacies is necessary [141].	• A comparatively large amount of evidence of the potential health risks associated with disease vectors if foodstuffs are exposed and not covered or stored well is available. • Research on the efficacy of the use of food covers, and that of potential alternatives in resource-deprived areas, is limited.

Table 5. Overview of Health-EDRM Primary Prevention Approaches against VBDs in the Reviewed Articles, Categorised by the Oxford Centre for Evidence-Based Medicine (OCEBM) Levels of Evidence. (Please see Table S1 for details.).

Category	Intervention	Number of Reviewed Articles under Each Category in the OCEBM Levels of Evidence										
		1a	1b	1c	2a	2b	2c	3a	3b	4	5	Others *	Total
Personal Protection Practices	Wear Protective Clothing When Outdoors	0	2	0	0	0	0	0	1	4	4	3	14
	Avoid Heading Outdoors to Vector-Prone Areas and During Peak Biting Conditions	0	0	0	0	0	0	0	0	3	16	4	23
	Apply Insect Repellent	0	1	0	0	0	0	0	0	2	9	5	17
	Sleep Under Bed Nets	2	2	0	0	2	0	1	0	5	7	3	22
	Receive Prophylactic Vaccinations and Chemoprophylaxis	1	0	0	1	0	0	1	0	3	8	6	20
Environmental Management Practices	Use Insect-Killing Traps	0	1	0	0	0	0	0	0	0	8	5	14
	Manage Stagnant Water Appropriately	0	0	0	0	2	0	0	0	1	11	1	15
	Manage Waste Appropriately	0	0	0	1	1	0	0	0	1	4	2	9
Customary Household Practices	Minimise Household Entry Points	1	3	0	1	1	0	0	1	6	3	2	18
	Cover Exposed Foodstuffs	0	0	0	0	1	0	0	1	2	2	1	7
Total		4	9	0	3	7	0	2	3	27	72	32	159 **

* 'Others' includes but is not limited to news articles or releases, books, textbooks, position papers, guidelines, case reports and organisational reports. ** Of the 134 publications reviewed, some included findings on more than one primary prevention measure, and are counted more than once in Table 5.

4. Discussion

VBDs are classified as biological hazards under the WHO health-EDRM framework [14] and their associated health risks should be managed according to the disaster management cycle (prevention, mitigation, preparedness, response and recovery), which encompasses both top-down and bottom-up interventions [157,158]. Top-down interventions require well-driven bottom-up initiatives to achieve effective primary prevention and to modify community health risk reduction-related measures [159]. Both the WHO health-EDRM framework [14] and the WHO global vector control response 2017–2030 framework [3] emphasise community engagement and mobilisation in enhancing protection against VBDs. The scientific effectiveness and feasibility of the community-level implementation of the 10 proposed primary prevention measures in this review can each be influenced by distinctive external factors, particularly with regards to access to financial or material resources.

Health promotion enables people to have more control over the improvement of their health outcomes, and is done through enhancing health literacy, encouraging behavioural change, and developing supportive policies [160]. There are numerous models which explore behavioural change as a result of education-based health promotion, one of which is the 'knowledge, attitudes, practices model', which prompts behavioural changes through knowledge enhancement [160]. In the case of vaccinations and chemoprophylaxis, it is critical for health interventions to enhance individual knowledge and awareness on why and how to receive prophylaxis as a primary prevention mechanism against VBDs, particularly in addressing misconceptions which underestimate the danger of VBDs [81]. Behaviour can be changed through addressing attitudes, such as misunderstandings [81], perception of social norms, cultural traditions and religious beliefs, for example in the case of ultra-orthodox Jewish communities who do not practice vaccination [81,82]. Finally, the behavioural change theory should consider how to promote practice. The viability and efficacy of the practice itself is favoured or limited by a variety of factors; policies will have to address barriers to accessing, and augmenting motivation in, the community [159].

The enabling and limiting factors that impact the effective uptake of primary prevention measures are closely interlinked. This review identified a number of determinants of success, including adequate resources, risk awareness, and well-coordinated supportive systems. A number of primary prevention measures rely on the availability and affordability of material resources, such as insect repellents, protective clothing, UV lamps, household building materials and bed nets (which additionally require space and equipment to set up [73]). Resource-deprived communities, which are at a higher risk of facing vulnerability, may lack the necessary material or financial resources. Materials must be accompanied by knowledge of their appropriate use. Inadequate information can lead to the improper maintenance of vector-prevention commodities, subsequently compromising their efficacy. For example, damaged bed nets with holes and improper bed net usage have been shown to lead to outcomes worse than no usage at all [64–66]. Some measures may also be affected by other health conditions, such as allergic reactions to insect repellent active ingredients [76], while others may be limited by cultural concerns, as demonstrated in the case of vaccination hesitancy in certain religious communities [81,82]. The feasibility of certain measures, such as the avoidance of outdoors, is dependent on an individual's personal, professional and socioeconomic situation. Avoidance of going outdoors into vector-prone areas and during peak biting conditions can be impractical, such as in farming populations that need to spend long periods outdoors, and in tropical areas where the climate is 'peak-biting'—hot and humid—all year long [50]. Similarly, there may be cases where access to a fully enclosed shelter or household improvements are not feasible, such as for those who are homeless or living in temporary shelters. Beyond resource access, proper education and personal circumstances, some primary prevention measures rely heavily on infrastructural and systemic support. Ensuring community access to vaccinations and chemoprophylaxis requires functioning health systems able to provide the necessary services, including an adequate supply of vaccines or medicine, trained health workers for administration and education, and an established clinic (fixed or mobile) from where the vaccine or drug can be distributed. Health system infrastructure is a critical enabling factor lacking in many rural or resource-poor contexts [84]. The environmental management of vectors also requires a robust and coordinated top-down waste management system [109,117], with multi-sectoral collaboration [161] between the health, environmental and civil engineering sectors, as well as other local and national-level authorities. Authorities should ensure the sufficiency of waste collection points such as waste bins [123], which can affect proper waste disposal, and the supply of electricity [118], which can affect the use of insect-killing traps, particularly in developing contexts [116]. Therefore, the success or failure of a community's uptake of primary prevention measures is shaped by the availability of material resources and information, supportive health and civil infrastructure, policy formulation, geographical climate, individual or professional flexibilities, and social contexts. Nonetheless, it should always be noted that each measure offers its contribution towards VBD prevention, and the measures serve as an alternative to one another. When one measure cannot be carried out, the practice of other measures is not necessarily impeded.

In comparing the strength of evidence of the reviewed literature (Table 5, please see Table S1 for details), the largest proportion (45%) fell into Level 5 classification, which covers a wide range of study designs and methodologies, such as entomological studies, observational exploratory studies, experimental studies, modelling studies, qualitative studies, and expert opinions. 20% of the reviewed literature was categorised into 'Others', which includes but is not limited to news releases, reports by international organisations like the WHO, and textbooks. Level 4 publications, such as cross-sectional mixed method studies, behavioural surveys, household surveys, questionnaires, interventional studies and case series studies contributed a relatively large portion (17%), with many addressing the knowledge, perceptions, acceptance and opinions of populations with regards to VBD-prevention measures. Regarding individual primary prevention measures, evidence is most lacking at all levels with regard to the practices of covering exposed foodstuffs (4%) and proper waste management (6%). The literature relevant to sleeping under bed nets and minimising household entry points was significantly stronger in study design. There is published evidence on the risk reduction relating to wearing protective clothing and the management of stagnant water; however, while a multitude of studies emphasised the impact of primary prevention measures on VBD health risk reduction, a limited number of studies focused on the impact of the measure itself on disease prevention efficacy or outcome. For instance, many studies demonstrate the potential VBD-related health risks of exposed foodstuffs [136–139] and household entry points [140,141]; however, there are limited studies that demonstrate the effectiveness of covering food or household crack-repairing on disease incidence reduction within a community [156]. Similarly, for solid waste management, while evidence on the health risks [134,135] associated with improper solid waste accumulation is available, there is a lack of in-depth comparative studies between different waste management system models and their strengths and weaknesses.

The methodology used for this review is limited in that it does not include non-English-based literature, non-electronically-accessible literature, grey literature outside of those areas deliberately searched, any publications before 2000, or any publication not identified due to incompatibility with the keywords used for the literature search. Notably, publications documenting experiences from low-resource VBD-endemic settings that are not readily accessible via mainstream databases or online platforms may not have been included in this review.

Certain areas were found to be lacking in the updated evidence. On the efficacy of light-coloured clothing, while the WHO provides recommendations for protective wear against VBDs [21], the search generated no clear evidence, that had been updated within the past two decades, to support the rationale behind vector landing preferences on darker surfaces, and vice versa. Recommendations concerning the appropriate concentration of DEET in insect repellent are often inconsistent across international organisations and governments. More extensive research is needed to better establish the correlation between DEET concentration, repellent strength and duration of efficacy. In addition, while there are various observational studies on the correlation between modern technological advancements, such as air conditioning, and decreased disease vector bites [162–165], there is limited updated scientific evidence available on the precise impacts of such advancements on changes to vector habitat. Addressing these research gaps will facilitate better-grounded and more evidence-based institutional guidelines.

The best available evidence is always evolving, requiring the continuous updating of guidelines and recommendations. The ongoing research on VBD prophylactic strategies is very active, as well as that on the development of insecticide resistance regarding insecticide-treated bed nets [166,167] and insect repellents [168]. In light of the many different designs, parameters, sample sizes and investigation methods used, it is often difficult to evaluate and compare related studies, thus resulting in a lack of standardisation in guidelines. For instance, a variety of attraction and killing mechanisms, as well as door and window screen designs [141], are used in different studies to evaluate insect-killing trap and household modification efficacies. Efforts to achieve increased consistency in the methodology of published research are crucial to making comparative analyses between studies on different VBD-prevention commodities possible [169–172].

Three areas are particularly lacking in the published evidence. Firstly, there has been minimal research done on available alternatives to the proposed practices. Taking the case of insect repellents, numerous studies are available to prove the efficacy [59–61,85] and explore the potential safety concerns [86–88] of DEET. However, the strength of research supporting the repellence of natural alternatives like plant oils is variable [74]. For instance, limited and conflicting findings on citronella efficacy were identified [74,85], and potential health hazards, like dermatitis under high-concentration neem-oil use, are indicated, with less stringent safety testing conducted compared to DEET [74]. Secondly, limited research is available on other disease vectors such as sand flies and ticks. A bulk of the literature identified in this analysis focuses on mosquitoes—the discussions on common vector breeding grounds [52,106–108] and the efficacy of insect-killing traps seldom involve other disease vectors [128]. There is a need for research into effective methods to better understand the breeding habitat ecology of sand flies in immature stages, which will facilitate the development of targeted control strategies such as source reduction, which are not yet possible as sand fly larvae can be difficult to detect, in contrast to other vectors such as mosquitoes [173–175]. Similarly, in the case of insect-killing traps, only limited studies demonstrate their potential in targeting sand flies in addition to mosquitoes [129], and evidence on tick elimination by the traps is lacking entirely. Thirdly, research on the spectrum of VBDs is disproportionately distributed; studies are oftentimes skewed towards more prevalent VBDs, such as malaria. While consideration is given to other VBDs such as Zika or tick-borne encephalitis, this literature review occasionally extrapolates the primary prevention measures proposed for the more extensively-researched diseases so as to apply them to other VBDs as well—for example, the determination of the time of day with peak biting conditions was based on *Plasmodium*-infected (malaria) mosquitoes being active from dusk to dawn [29–31]. Further research on these three areas is necessary in order to develop comprehensive and informed guidelines or policies that can be implemented in varying contexts to mitigate against the risk and alleviate the disease burden of VBDs.

This review has identified major research gaps in the current published literature relating to health-EDRM primary prevention measures for VBDs (Table 6). Strengthening the available evidence in these areas will create a scientific basis on which governments, policy-makers and community stakeholders can develop effective, targeted and achievable strategies for protecting at-risk populations against VBDs. Aspects of the WHO health-EDRM framework can be applied to address these research gaps. Increasing capacities for information and knowledge management can support collection, analysis and dissemination across multiple sectors, allowing for the comparative evaluation of available evidence, as well as the development of consistent guidelines and recommendations [14]. This is particularly important for any research undertaken in resource-poor contexts, which will provide necessary evidence towards developing effective and targeted VBD prevention measures in such contexts. The framework highlights the need for more multifaceted and multisectoral approaches, the lessons of which will lead to the further development of evidence-based strategies [14].

Table 6. Major Research Gaps in Current Published Literature Relating to Health-EDRM Primary Prevention Measures for VBDs.

	Research Gaps
1	Current studies on health-EDRM primary prevention measures for VBDs mostly focus on health risk reduction practices, yet efficacy evaluation on actual disease reduction is lacking.
2	Available literature is mostly classified as cross-sectional studies. Evidence on efficacy of the prevention measure based on randomised controlled studies or extensive cohort studies is limited.
3	Comparative evaluations for variations of certain primary prevention measures, such as efficacy of different insect-killing mechanisms or household modification materials, are limited.
4	Research outcomes are skewed towards certain vectors (e.g., mosquitoes). Research evidence on other vectors such as sand flies or ticks is limited.
5	Research outcomes are skewed towards certain VBDs (e.g., malaria). Research evidence on other VBDs such as Zika, chikungunya, or tick-borne encephalitis is limited.
6	Research and evidence on available alternatives to the proposed practices (e.g., using natural substitutes as opposed to chemical-based insect repellents) is limited.
7	Updated research on evidence relating technological advancements and the rapid change of ecological and human living environments to behavioural practices against VBDs is limited.
8	Consistency in recommendations from research papers, policies, and frontline international agencies (e.g., as in DEET concentration recommendations) is lacking.
9	Literature highlighting the effectiveness of multi-faceted, multi-sectoral and coordinated responses in enabling effective risk mitigation for population-level protection is lacking.

All 10 primary prevention measures require sustainable, continuous implementation and maintenance in order to be truly effective in preventing VBDs. Primary prevention measures focusing on stagnant water, waste management and the covering of exposed foodstuffs offer the long-term co-benefit of mitigating risks arising from other biological hazards under the health-EDRM framework [14], such as water-borne and food-borne diseases [139]. Practising continuous primary prevention is particularly necessary as long as certain VBDs do not have standardised effective treatment options, and if vector-elimination is not feasible. Some preventive measures face more complex challenges in practise without adequate health or governance infrastructure. Others are more easily implemented, but are nonetheless reliant on materials such as insect repellents or bed nets, which can be an obstacle in resource-poor settings where the population is already facing vulnerability to impoverishment or disease. It is crucial for policymakers to ensure that systems are able to identify and assess needs, and provide the necessary support for the sustainable and fair distribution of resources. Empowering bottom-up initiatives requires well-coordinated top-down policies [83] that effectively disseminate resources and information, especially in resource-deprived, rural, or health-illiterate populations. A strong, accessible health system is key to providing materials and education to the at-risk population. Centralised, coordinated and well-regulated infrastructure, such as a uniform waste management system [176], can significantly enhance the efficacy of primary prevention practices.

Climate change and its associated consequences, such as changing weather patterns and increased disaster occurrences [18], have shifted the epidemiological patterns of VBDs, as well as the volume and spread of the at-risk population, thus affecting the development policies and strategies for mitigating the VBD burden on health systems. Rising temperatures and unpredictable precipitation patterns, for example, lengthen peak-biting periods and further complicate the capacity for outdoor avoidance, especially in tropical areas which are sultry throughout the year. The increased incidence of hydro-meteorological hazards such as floods and cyclones brings about more extreme rainfall, as well as increased humidity and water accumulation [18], and impact stagnant water management, thus possibly facilitating further larval habitat development for disease vectors [18]. Insect vectors cannot regulate their internal temperatures and are very sensitive to changes, which has caused them to invade new areas in order to adapt [177]. This puts previously unexposed populations at risk, who may lack protective immunity or the experience, resources or services necessary to mitigate the prevalence of disease [6]. The WHO health-EDRM framework stresses the importance of strengthening health systems, with an increased emphasis on climate change adaptation [14], to reducing health risks associated with hazardous events, including VBD outbreaks. It is important for governing bodies to consider the associated challenges of climate change during policy formulation, with the inclusion of climate change scenarios in disaster risk assessments [18]. Considering the limitation of the predicted impact of climate change on VBD transmission, governing bodies should enhance individual capacities and community resilience in cases of sudden VBD surges [178]. For instance, early warning systems should be in place to communicate the health risks associated with seasonal VBD outbreaks to vulnerable populations in advance [18]. As such, primary prevention measures that emphasise the broader aspects of environmental management, resource distribution and public education must not be overlooked. Public education, to encourage early symptom identification and subsequent health-seeking behaviours, can serve as a steppingstone in propagating secondary and tertiary VBD intervention amongst vulnerable populations.

In light of the growing burden of VBDs and emerging public health threats, a progressive primary prevention model is key to disaster risk reduction, as encompassed in the four priorities set out in the Sendai Framework for Disaster Risk Reduction (risk understanding, governance, preparedness and resilience) [16]. In terms of disaster risk understanding, a thorough examination of the enabling and limiting circumstances is required in at-risk populations, including local disease prevention capacity, specific VBD characteristics, and risk drivers such as climate change [16,18]. Disaster governance should be strengthened through stakeholder involvement and multi-sectorial collaboration, as well as through adopting a well-coordinated top-down approach to empowering bottom-up community initiatives in a sustainable manner. Resilience enhancement should be driven by global investments in innovation and research, for instance the development of better prophylactic strategies and better vector-prevention commodity designs for utilisation against VBDs. Finally, disaster preparedness can be reinforced through raised awareness, secured healthcare accessibility and health-seeking behaviour encouragement, so as to better equip vulnerable populations facing future VBD outbreaks.

5. Conclusions

This narrative study identified 10 health-EDRM primary prevention measures against VBDs. Resource availability, risk awareness and systemic support were identified as the core enabling factors for the success of these measures. Resources, health and civil infrastructure, policy formulation, geographical climate and socioeconomic factors were the core sources of limitations, which necessitate the need to consider alternatives. Evidence supporting the effectiveness of alternative preventive measures is lacking, in particular with regards to prevention in resource-poor settings. Similarly, evidence related to preventive measures focusses heavily on mosquitoes, whereas research on effective prevention against diseases transmitted by other vectors such as sand flies and ticks is lacking. At a global level, the necessity of VBD prevention increases with the growing impact of climate change and globalisation.

Health risks associated with VBDs will remain an ongoing biological hazard to communities, and thus sustainability of practice is crucial. As recommended by the WHO health-EDRM framework, in addition to the health sector, the successful adoption of primary prevention measures against VBDs requires a multi-faceted, multi-sectoral and coordinated response, encompassing sectors such as meteorology for hazard prediction, education for health awareness and promotion, and the environmental and civil engineering sectors for waste collection and water management.

In conclusion, this review has shown that evidence of the effectiveness and management of primary prevention practices is focused on a narrow spectrum of VBDs and vector types. In order to fill research gaps, the scope of VBD research should be broadened, and standardised protocols should be adopted so as to better prepare communities for disaster risk mitigation and to build the capacities of populations that are vulnerable with regards to health-EDRM practices.

Supplementary Materials: The following is available online at http://www.mdpi.com/1660-4601/17/16/5981/s1, Table S1: Relevant Intervention(s), Study Design, Relevant Key Finding(s) and/or Conclusion of Each Reviewed Article Referenced ($n = 134$).

Author Contributions: Conceptualization, E.Y.Y.C. and C.D.; methodology, T.S.T.S. and T.S.S.; formal analysis, T.S.T.S; T.S.S.; writing—original draft preparation, E.Y.Y.C.; T.S.T.S.; T.S.S.; C.D.; writing—review and editing, Z.H.; S.L.; K.K.C.H.; S.L.A.T.; K.O.K.; P-H.C.; R.K.; R.S.; supervision, E.Y.Y.C.; funding acquisition, E.Y.Y.C. All authors have read and agreed to the published version of the manuscript.

Funding: This research was funded by the CCOUC-University of Oxford research fund (2019–2023).

Conflicts of Interest: The authors declare no conflict of interest. Professor Emily Ying Yang Chan serves as the Co-Chair of the Health-EDRM Global Research Network and Ryoma Kayano serves as the Secretary of the Health-EDRM Global Research Network.

Appendix A. Keywords Used for Literature Search

'bed nets', 'blue-light irradiation', 'bottom-up approach', 'breeding sites', 'carbon dioxide', 'cement', 'chemoprophylaxis', 'chikungunya', 'climate change', 'clothes moth larvae', 'clothes wear and tear', 'cockroaches', 'crack repair', 'dengue', 'diethyltoluamide (DEET) ', 'disease burden', 'door screening', 'doors and windows burglary', 'electricity access', 'fall injury water', 'floods', 'food decay', 'food fermentation', 'food mould and fungi', 'food-borne pathogens', 'forests', 'health hazards', 'health-EDRM', 'heat stroke', 'heat-seeking ability', 'heavy rain', 'household waste management', 'housing improvements', 'humidity', 'immunisation', 'infectious disease', 'insect repellents', 'insect traps', 'insecticide-treated nets', 'Japanese encephalitis', 'larval habitats', 'larvicides', 'lime', 'living environment', 'long clothing', 'long-lasting insecticide-treated nets', 'malaria', 'mosquito larvae', 'mosquito traps', 'mosquitoes', 'mould development water', 'mud', 'natural repellents', 'octenol', 'pesticide', 'primary prevention', 'protective behaviour', 'protective clothing', 'rodents', 'rubber plantations', 'sand flies', 'solid waste management', 'sticky traps', 'sunburns', 'temperature', 'tick-borne diseases', 'tick-borne encephalitis', 'ticks', 'top-down approach', 'tropical climates', 'ultraviolet irradiation', 'vaccination', 'vaccine complacency', 'vaccine hesitancy', 'VBDs', 'vector attraction', 'vector biting', 'vector contamination', 'vector exposure risk', 'vector human movement', 'vector landing preference', 'vector light clothing', 'vector net', 'vector traps', 'vectors', 'wall cracks', 'waste management', 'waste mismanagement', 'water storage', 'water supply', 'West Nile virus', 'window screening', 'yellow fever', 'Zika'.

References

1. Vector-Borne Diseases. Available online: https://www.who.int/news-room/fact-sheets/detail/vector-borne-diseases (accessed on 31 May 2020).
2. Lemon, S.M.; Sparling, P.F.; Hamburg, M.A.; Relman, D.A.; Choffnes, E.R.; Mack, A. *Vector-Borne Diseases: Understanding the Environmental, Human Health, and Ecological Connections*; The National Academies Press: Washington, DC, USA, 2008; pp. 1–27. ISBN 9780309108973.
3. WHO. *Global Vector Control Response 2017–2030*; World Health Organization: Geneva, Switzerland, 2017; ISBN 9789241564090.
4. Wu, X.; Lu, Y.; Zhou, S.; Chen, L.; Xu, B. Impact of climate change on human infectious diseases: Empirical evidence and human adaptation. *Environ. Int.* **2016**, *86*, 14–23. [CrossRef] [PubMed]
5. Hoshen, M.B.; Morse, A.P. A weather-driven model of malaria transmission. *Malar. J.* **2004**, *3*. [CrossRef]
6. Caminade, C.; McIntyre, K.M.; Jones, A.E. Impact of recent and future climate change on vector-borne diseases. *Ann. N. Y. Acad. Sci.* **2019**, *1436*, 157–173. [CrossRef] [PubMed]
7. Fouque, F.; Reeder, J.C. Impact of past and on-going changes on climate and weather on vector-borne diseases transmission: A look at the evidence. *Infect. Dis. Poverty* **2019**, *8*. [CrossRef] [PubMed]
8. Mathers, C. Global Burden of Disease. In *International Encyclopedia of Public Health*; Academic Press: Cambridge, MA, USA, 2016; ISBN 9780128037089.
9. James, S.L.; Abate, D.; Abate, K.H.; Abay, S.M.; Abbafati, C.; Abbasi, N.; Abbastabar, H.; Abd-Allah, F.; Abdela, J.; Abdelalim, A.; et al. Global, regional, and national incidence, prevalence, and years lived with

disability for 354 Diseases and Injuries for 195 countries and territories, 1990-2017: A systematic analysis for the Global Burden of Disease Study 2017. *Lancet* **2018**, *392*, 1859–1922. [CrossRef]

10. World Health Organization. *World Malaria Report 2019*; World Health Organization: Geneva, Switzerland, 2019; ISBN 9789241565721.
11. Mccarthy, D.; Wolf, H.; Wu, Y. *Malaria and Growth*; The World Bank: Washington, DC, USA, 2000; pp. 2–26. [CrossRef]
12. United Nations. *The Sustainable Development Goals Report 2019*; United Nations: New York, NY, USA, 2019.
13. The Global Fund: Malaria. Available online: https://www.theglobalfund.org/en/malaria/ (accessed on 31 May 2020).
14. WHO. *Health Emergency and Disaster Risk Management: Overview*; World Health Organization: Geneva, Switzerland, 2019; ISBN 9789241516181.
15. World Health Organisation. *Emergency Risk Management for Health—Overview*; World Health Organization: Geneva, Switzerland, 2013.
16. World Health Organization. *Sendai Framework for Disaster Risk Reduction 2015–2030*; World Health Organization: Geneva, Switzerland, 2015.
17. Wright, N.; Fagan, L.; Lapitan, J.M.; Kayano, R.; Abrahams, J.; Huda, Q.; Murray, V. Health Emergency and Disaster Risk Management: Five Years into Implementation of the Sendai Framework. *Int. J. Disaster Risk Sci.* **2020**, *11*, 206–217. [CrossRef]
18. Chan, E.Y.Y.; Shaw, R. *Public Health and Disasters: Health Emergency and Disaster Risk Management in Asia*; Springer: Berlin/Heidelberg, Germany, 2020.
19. Boslaugh, S. Prevention: Primary, Secondary, and Tertiary. In *Encyclopedia of Epidemiology*; SAGE Publications, Inc.: Thousand Oaks, CA, USA, 2008; pp. 839–840.
20. Alison, M. Global Health Impacts of Vector-Borne Diseases. In *Global Health Impacts of Vector-Borne Diseases*; The National Academies Press: Washington, DC, USA, 2016; pp. 1–59.
21. World Health Organization. *A Global Brief on Vector-Borne Diseases*; World Health Organization: Geneva, Switzerland, 2014; p. 9.
22. World Health Organisation. *International Clinical Trials Registry Platform*; World Health Organization: Geneva, Switzerland, 2006.
23. OCEBM Levels of Evidence Working Group. "The Oxford 2009 Levels of Evidence". Oxford Center for Evidence-Based Medicine. Available online: https://www.cebm.net/index.aspx?o=5653 (accessed on 10 August 2020).
24. Achee, N.L.; Youngblood, L.; Bangs, M.J.; Lavery, J.V.; James, S. Considerations for the use of human participants in vector biology research: A tool for investigators and regulators. *Vector-Borne Zoonotic Dis.* **2015**, *15*, 89–102. [CrossRef]
25. Saavedra, M.P.; Conn, J.E.; Alava, F.; Carrasco-Escobar, G.; Prussing, C.; Bickersmith, S.A.; Sangama, J.L.; Fernandez-Miñope, C.; Guzman, M.; Tong, C.; et al. Higher risk of malaria transmission outdoors than indoors by Nyssorhynchus darlingi in riverine communities in the Peruvian Amazon. *Parasites Vectors* **2019**, *12*. [CrossRef]
26. Nakkhara, P.; Chongsuvivatwong, V.; Thammapalo, S. Risk factors for symptomatic and asymptomatic chikungunya infection. *Trans. R. Soc. Trop. Med. Hyg.* **2013**, *107*, 789–796. [CrossRef]
27. Wallace, J.W.; Nicholson, W.L.; Perniciaro, J.L.; Vaughn, M.F.; Funkhouser, S.; Juliano, J.J.; Lee, S.; Kakumanu, M.L.; Ponnusamy, L.; Apperson, C.S.; et al. Incident Tick-Borne Infections in a Cohort of North Carolina Outdoor Workers. *Vector-Borne Zoonotic Dis.* **2016**, *16*, 302–308. [CrossRef]
28. Tangena, J.A.A.; Thammavong, P.; Lindsay, S.W.; Brey, P.T. Risk of exposure to potential vector mosquitoes for rural workers in Northern Lao PDR. *PLoS Negl. Trop. Dis.* **2017**, *11*. [CrossRef] [PubMed]
29. Ndoen, E.; Wild, C.; Dale, P.; Sipe, N.; Dale, M. Dusk to dawn activity patterns of anopheline mosquitoes in West Timor and Java, Indonesia. *Southeast Asian J. Trop. Med. Public Health* **2011**, *42*, 550–561. [PubMed]
30. Van Bortel, W.; Trung, H.D.; Hoi, L.X.; Van Ham, N.; Van Chut, N.; Luu, N.D.; Roelants, P.; Denis, L.; Speybroeck, N.; D'Alessandro, U.; et al. Malaria transmission and vector behaviour in a forested malaria focus in central Vietnam and the implications for vector control. *Malar. J.* **2010**, *9*. [CrossRef] [PubMed]
31. Loeb, M.; Elliott, S.J.; Gibson, B.; Fearon, M.; Nosal, R.; Drebot, M.; D'Cuhna, C.; Harrington, D.; Smith, S.; George, P.; et al. Protective behavior and West Nile virus risk. *Emerg. Infect. Dis.* **2005**, *11*, 1433–1436. [CrossRef] [PubMed]

32. Bhatt, S.; Gething, P.W.; Brady, O.J.; Messina, J.P.; Farlow, A.W.; Moyes, C.L.; Drake, J.M.; Brownstein, J.S.; Hoen, A.G.; Sankoh, O.; et al. The global distribution and burden of dengue. *Nature* **2013**. [CrossRef]
33. Tokarevich, N.; Tronin, A.; Gnativ, B.; Revich, B.; Blinova, O.; Evengard, B. Impact of air temperature variation on the ixodid ticks habitat and tick-borne encephalitis incidence in the Russian Arctic: The case of the Komi Republic. *Int. J. Circumpolar Health* **2017**, *76*. [CrossRef]
34. Chowdhury, F.R.; Ibrahim, Q.S.U.; Shafiqul Bari, M.; Jahangir Alam, M.M.; Dunachie, S.J.; Rodriguez-Morales, A.J.; Ismail Patwary, M. The association between temperature, rainfall and humidity with common climate-sensitive infectious diseases in Bangladesh. *PLoS ONE* **2018**, *15*, e0199579. [CrossRef]
35. Vázquez, M.; Muehlenbein, C.; Cartter, M.; Hayes, E.B.; Ertel, S.; Shapiro, E.D. Effectiveness of personal protective measures to prevent lyme disease. *Emerg. Infect. Dis.* **2008**, *14*, 210–216. [CrossRef]
36. Barnard, D.R. *Global Collaboration for Development of Pesticides for Public Health (GCDPP) Repellents and Toxicants for Personal Protection*; World Health Organization: Geneva, Switzerland, 2000; Volume 46, pp. 408–418.
37. Donohoe, H.; Pennington-Gray, L.; Omodior, O. Lyme disease: Current issues, implications, and recommendations for tourism management. *Tour. Manag.* **2015**, *46*, 408–418. [CrossRef]
38. Linos, E.; Keiser, E.; Fu, T.; Colditz, G.; Chen, S.; Tang, J.Y. Hat, shade, long sleeves, or sunscreen? Rethinking US sun protection messages based on their relative effectiveness. *Cancer Causes Control* **2011**. [CrossRef]
39. Szykitka, W. *Big Book of Self-Reliant Living: Advice and Information on just about Everything You Need to Know to Live on Planet Earth*; The Lyons Press: Guilford, CT, USA, 2010; p. 65.
40. Harahap, R. Sumatran Tigers Seen on Plantation in Riau. Available online: https://www.thejakartapost.com/news/2019/02/28/sumatran-tigers-seen-on-plantation-in-riau.html (accessed on 31 May 2020).
41. Takahata, C.; Nielsen, S.E.; Takii, A.; Izumiyama, S. Habitat selection of a large carnivore along human-wildlife boundaries in a highly modified landscape. *PLoS ONE* **2014**, *9*, e0086181. [CrossRef] [PubMed]
42. Gu, S.; Wang, A.; Bian, G.; He, T.; Yi, B.; Lu, B.; Li, X.; Xu, G. Relationship between weather factors and heat stroke in Ningbo city. *Chin. J. Endem.* **2016**, *37*, 1131–1136. [CrossRef]
43. Kenny, G.P.; Wilson, T.E.; Flouris, A.D.; Fujii, N. Heat exhaustion. In *Handbook of Clinical Neurology*; Elsevier: Amsterdam, The Netherlands, 2018; pp. 505–529.
44. Zeng, J.; Zhang, X.; Yang, J.; Bao, J.; Xiang, H.; Dear, K.; Liu, Q.; Lin, S.; Lawrence, W.R.; Lin, A.; et al. Humidity may modify the relationship between temperature and cardiovascular mortality in Zhejiang province, China. *Int. J. Environ. Res. Public Health* **2017**, *14*, 1383. [CrossRef] [PubMed]
45. Lin, L.W.; Lin, H.Y.; Hsu, C.Y.; Rau, H.H.; Chen, P.L. Effect of weather and time on trauma events determined using emergency medical service registry data. *Injury* **2015**, *46*, 1814–1820. [CrossRef]
46. Crawshaw, A.F.; Maung, T.M.; Shafique, M.; Sint, N.; Nicholas, S.; Li, M.S.; Roca-Feltrer, A.; Hii, J. Acceptability of insecticide-treated clothing for malaria prevention among migrant rubber tappers in Myanmar: A cluster-randomized non-inferiority crossover trial. *Malar. J.* **2017**, *16*. [CrossRef]
47. Ruiu, L.; Floris, I. Susceptibility of environmentally friendly sheep wool insulation panels to the common clothes moth tineola bisselliella in laboratory assays. *Insects* **2019**, *10*, 379. [CrossRef]
48. Gao, C.; Kuklane, K.; Östergren, P.O.; Kjellstrom, T. Occupational heat stress assessment and protective strategies in the context of climate change. *Int. J. Biometeorol.* **2018**, *62*, 359–371. [CrossRef]
49. Unger, A.; Riley, L.W. Slum health: From understanding to action. *PLoS Med.* **2007**, *4*, 1561–1566. [CrossRef]
50. Sobel, A.H. Tropical Weather. *Nat. Educ. Knowl.* **2012**, *3*, 2.
51. Stjernberg, L.; Berglund, J. Detecting ticks on light versus dark clothing. *Scand. J. Infect. Dis.* **2009**, *37*, 361–364. [CrossRef]
52. Dejenie, T.; Yohannes, M.; Assmelash, T. Characterization of Mosquito Breeding Sites in and in the Vicinity of Tigray Microdams. *Ethiop. J. Health Sci.* **2011**, *21*, 57–66. [CrossRef] [PubMed]
53. Sumodan, P.K. Species diversity of mosquito breeding in rubber plantations of Kerala, India. *J. Am. Mosq. Control Assoc.* **2012**, *28*, 114–115. [CrossRef] [PubMed]
54. Mackensie, J.S.; Lindsay, M.D.; Broom, A.K. Effect of climate and weather on the transmission of Ross River and Murray Valley encephalitis viruses. *Microbiol. Aust.* **2000**, *21*, 40.
55. Reinhold, J.M.; Lazzari, C.R.; Lahondère, C. Effects of the environmental temperature on Aedes aegypti and Aedes albopictus mosquitoes: A review. *Insects* **2018**, *9*, 158. [CrossRef]
56. Eldridge, B.F.; Edman, J.D.; Moncayo, A.C. Medical Entomology: A Textbook on Public Health and Veterinary Problems Caused by Arthropods. *J. Med. Entomol.* **2000**, *116*, 15086–15095. [CrossRef]

57. Sherrard-Smith, E.; Skarp, J.E.; Beale, A.D.; Fornadel, C.; Norris, L.C.; Moore, S.J.; Mihreteab, S.; Charlwood, J.D.; Bhatt, S.; Winskill, P.; et al. Mosquito feeding behavior and how it influences residual malaria transmission across Africa. *Proc. Natl. Acad. Sci. USA* **2019**. [CrossRef]
58. Sutherst, R.W. Global Change and Human Vulnerability to Vector-Borne Diseases. *Clin. Microbiol. Rev.* **2004**, *17*, 136–167. [CrossRef]
59. Leal, W.S. The enigmatic reception of DEET—The gold standard of insect repellents. *Curr. Opin. Insect Sci.* **2014**, *6*, 93–98. [CrossRef]
60. CDC, Centers for Disease Control and Prevention. *Fight the Bite for Protection from Malaria Guidelines for DEET Insect Repellent Use*; CDC: Atlanta, GA, USA, 2005; p. 1.
61. Staub, D.; Debrunner, M.; Amsler, L.; Steffen, R. Effectiveness of a repellent containing DEET and EBAAP for preventing tick bites. *Wilderness Environ. Med.* **2002**, *13*, 12–20. [CrossRef]
62. Onyett, H.; Bortolussi, R.; Bridger, N.A.; Finlay, J.C.; Martin, S.; McDonald, J.C.; Robinson, J.L.; Salvadori, M.I.; Vanderkooi, O.G.; Allen, U.D.; et al. Preventing mosquito and tick bites: A Canadian update. *Paediatr. Child Health* **2014**, *19*, 326–328. [CrossRef]
63. Tips for Using Insect Repellents. Available online: https://www.chp.gov.hk/en/features/38927.html (accessed on 31 May 2020).
64. Msellemu, D.; Shemdoe, A.; Makungu, C.; Mlacha, Y.; Kannady, K.; Dongus, S.; Killeen, G.F.; Dillip, A. The underlying reasons for very high levels of bed net use, and higher malaria infection prevalence among bed net users than non-users in the Tanzanian city of Dar es Salaam: A qualitative study. *Malar. J.* **2017**, *16*. [CrossRef] [PubMed]
65. Ochomo, E.O.; Bayoh, N.M.; Walker, E.D.; Abongo, B.O.; Ombok, M.O.; Ouma, C.; Githeko, A.K.; Vulule, J.; Yan, G.; Gimnig, J.E. The efficacy of long-lasting nets with declining physical integrity may be compromised in areas with high levels of pyrethroid resistance. *Malar. J.* **2013**, *12*. [CrossRef] [PubMed]
66. Shah, M.P.; Steinhardt, L.C.; Mwandama, D.; Mzilahowa, T.; Gimnig, J.E.; Bauleni, A.; Wong, J.; Wiegand, R.; Mathanga, D.P.; Lindblade, K.A. The effectiveness of older insecticide-treated bed nets (ITNs) to prevent malaria infection in an area of moderate pyrethroid resistance: Results from a cohort study in Malawi. *Malar. J.* **2020**, *19*. [CrossRef] [PubMed]
67. Insecticide-Treated Bed Nets. Available online: https://www.cdc.gov/malaria/malaria_worldwide/reduction/itn.html (accessed on 31 May 2020).
68. Jayanti, P.; Acharya, I.A. A Study on Efficacy of LLINS As Compared To In-Use ITNs Amongst Troops in a Malaria Endemic Area. *J. Trop. Dis.* **2015**, *3*. [CrossRef]
69. Clem, A.S. Fundamentals of vaccine immunology. *J. Glob. Infect. Dis.* **2011**, *3*, 73–78. [CrossRef]
70. McBride, W.J.H. Chemoprophylaxis of tropical infectious diseases. *Pharmaceuticals* **2010**, *3*, 1561–1575. [CrossRef] [PubMed]
71. Wilson, A.L.; Dhiman, R.C.; Kitron, U.; Scott, T.W.; van den Berg, H.; Lindsay, S.W. Benefit of Insecticide-Treated Nets, Curtains and Screening on Vector Borne Diseases, Excluding Malaria: A Systematic Review and Meta-analysis. *PLoS Negl. Trop. Dis.* **2014**, *8*. [CrossRef]
72. Xu, J.W.; Liao, Y.M.; Liu, H.; Nie, R.H.; Havumaki, J. Use of bed nets and factors that influence bed net use among jinuo ethnic minority in southern China. *PLoS ONE* **2014**, *9*, e0103780. [CrossRef]
73. Das, M.L.; Singh, S.P.; Vanlerberghe, V.; Rijai, S.; Rai, M.; Karki, P.; Sundar, S.; Boelaert, M. Population preference of net texture prior to bed net trial in Kala-Azar-endemic areas. *PLoS Negl. Trop. Dis.* **2007**, *1*. [CrossRef]
74. Maia, M.F.; Moore, S.J. Plant-based insect repellents: A review of their efficacy, development and testing. *Malar. J.* **2011**, *10*. [CrossRef]
75. Batish, D.R.; Singh, H.P.; Kohli, R.K.; Kaur, S. Eucalyptus essential oil as a natural pesticide. *For. Ecol. Manag.* **2008**, *256*, 2166–2174. [CrossRef]
76. McHenry, M.; Lacuesta, G. Severe allergic reaction to diethyltoluamide (DEET) containing insect repellent. *Allergy, Asthma Clin. Immunol.* **2014**, *10*. [CrossRef]
77. Nelson, K.E.; Williams, C.M. *Infectious Disease Epidemiology: Theory and Practice*; Jones & Bartlett Publishers: Burlington, MA, USA, 2008; pp. 1014–1015.
78. Von Seidlein, L.; Ikonomidis, K.; Bruun, R.; Jawara, M.; Pinder, M.; Knols, B.G.J.; Knudsen, J.B. Airflow attenuation and bed net utilization: Observations from Africa and Asia. *Malar. J.* **2012**, *11*. [CrossRef] [PubMed]

79. Ntonifor, N.H.; Veyufambom, S. Assessing the effective use of mosquito nets in the prevention of malaria in some parts of Mezam division, Northwest Region Cameroon. *Malar. J.* **2016**, *15*. [CrossRef] [PubMed]
80. Pulford, J.; Hetzel, M.W.; Bryant, M.; Siba, P.M.; Mueller, I. Reported reasons for not using a mosquito net when one is available: A review of the published literature. *Malar. J.* **2011**, *10*. [CrossRef]
81. Pugliese-Garcia, M.; Heyerdahl, L.W.; Mwamba, C.; Nkwemu, S.; Chilengi, R.; Demolis, R.; Guillermet, E.; Sharma, A. Factors influencing vaccine acceptance and hesitancy in three informal settlements in Lusaka, Zambia. *Vaccine* **2018**, *36*, 5617–5624. [CrossRef]
82. Muhsen, K.; Abed El-Hai, R.; Amit-Aharon, A.; Nehama, H.; Gondia, M.; Davidovitch, N.; Goren, S.; Cohen, D. Risk factors of underutilization of childhood immunizations in ultraorthodox Jewish communities in Israel despite high access to health care services. *Vaccine* **2012**, *30*, 2109–2115. [CrossRef]
83. The Lancet Infectious Diseases Malaria vaccination: A major milestone. *Lancet Infect. Dis.* **2019**, *19*, 559. [CrossRef]
84. Malande, O.O.; Munube, D.; Afaayo, R.N.; Annet, K.; Bodo, B.; Bakainaga, A.; Ayebare, E.; Njunwamukama, S.; Mworozi, E.A.; Musyoki, A.M. Barriers to effective uptake and provision of immunization in a rural district in Uganda. *PLoS ONE* **2019**, *14*, e0212270. [CrossRef]
85. Rodriguez, S.D.; Drake, L.L.; Price, D.P.; Hammond, J.I.; Hansen, I.A.; Liu, N. The efficacy of some commercially available insect repellents for Aedes aegypti (Diptera: Culicidae) and Aedes albopictus (Diptera: Culicidae). *J. Insect Sci.* **2015**, *15*. [CrossRef]
86. Legeay, S.; Clere, N.; Hilairet, G.; Do, Q.T.; Bernard, P.; Quignard, J.F.; Apaire-Marchais, V.; Lapied, B.; Faure, S. The insect repellent N,N-diethyl-m-Toluamide (DEET) induces angiogenesis via allosteric modulation of the M3 muscarinic receptor in endothelial cells. *Sci. Rep.* **2016**, *6*. [CrossRef] [PubMed]
87. Swale, D.R.; Bloomquist, J.R. Is DEET a dangerous neurotoxicant? *Pest Manag. Sci.* **2019**, *75*. [CrossRef] [PubMed]
88. Koren, G.; Matsui, D.; Bailey, B. DEET-based insect repellents: Safety implications for children and pregnant and lactating women. *Can. Med. Assoc. J.* **2003**, *169*, 209–212.
89. Lenhart, A.; Orelus, N.; Maskill, R.; Alexander, N.; Streit, T.; McCall, P.J. Insecticide-treated bednets to control dengue vectors: Preliminary evidence from a controlled trial in Haiti. *Trop. Med. Int. Heal.* **2008**, *13*, 56–57. [CrossRef] [PubMed]
90. Bhatt, S.; Weiss, D.J.; Cameron, E.; Bisanzio, D.; Mappin, B.; Dalrymple, U.; Battle, K.E.; Moyes, C.L.; Henry, A.; Eckhoff, P.A.; et al. The effect of malaria control on Plasmodium falciparum in Africa between 2000 and 2015. *Nature* **2015**, *526*, 207–211. [CrossRef] [PubMed]
91. Hawley, W.A.; Phillips-Howard, P.A.; Ter Kuile, F.O.; Terlouw, D.J.; Vulule, J.M.; Ombok, M.; Nahlen, B.L.; Gimnig, J.E.; Kariuki, S.K.; Kolczak, M.S.; et al. Community-wide effects of permethrin-treated bed nets on child mortality and malaria morbidity in western Kenya. *Am. J. Trop. Med. Hyg.* **2003**, *68*, 121–127. [CrossRef]
92. Killeen, G.F.; Smith, T.A.; Ferguson, H.M.; Mshinda, H.; Abdulla, S.; Lengeler, C.; Kachur, S.P. Preventing childhood malaria in Africa by protecting adults from mosquitoes with insecticide-treated nets. *PLoS Med.* **2007**, *4*, 1246–1258. [CrossRef]
93. Hauser, G.; Thiévent, K.; Koella, J.C. The ability of Anopheles gambiae mosquitoes to bite through a permethrin-treated net and the consequences for their fitness. *Sci. Rep.* **2019**, *9*. [CrossRef]
94. World Health Organization. Vaccines and vaccination against yellow fever WHO Position Paper—June Note de synthèse: Position de l' OMS sur les vaccins et la vaccination contre la fièvre jaune, juin 2013. *Relevé Épidémiologique Hebdomadaire* **2013**, *88*, 269–284.
95. Gotuzzo, E.; Yactayo, S.; Córdova, E. Review article: Efficacy and duration of immunity after yellow fever vaccination: Systematic review on the need for a booster every 10 years. *Am. J. Trop. Med. Hyg.* **2013**, *89*, 434–444. [CrossRef]
96. WHO Publication. Vaccines against tick-borne encephalitis: WHO position paper—Recommendations. *Vaccine* **2011**, *86*, 241–256. [CrossRef]
97. Bogovic, P. Tick-borne encephalitis: A review of epidemiology, clinical characteristics, and management. *World J. Clin. Cases* **2015**. [CrossRef] [PubMed]
98. World Health Organization. Japanese Encephalitis Vaccines: WHO position paper, February 2015—Recommendations. *Vaccine* **2016**, *90*, 69–88. [CrossRef]

99. Hegde, N.R.; Gore, M.M. Japanese encephalitis vaccines: Immunogenicity, protective efficacy, effectiveness, and impact on the burden of disease. *Hum. Vaccines Immunother.* **2017**, *13*, 1320–1337. [CrossRef] [PubMed]
100. Malaria Vaccine Pilot Launched in Malawi. Available online: https://www.who.int/news-room/detail/23-04-2019-malaria-vaccine-pilot-launched-in-malawi (accessed on 31 May 2020).
101. Jover, J.A.; Leon, L.; Pato, E.; Loza, E.; Rosales, Z.; Matias, M.A.; Mendez-Fernandez, R.; Díaz-Valle, D.; Benitez-del-Castillo, J.M.; Abasolo, L. Long-term use of antimalarial drugs in rheumatic diseases. *Clin. Exp. Rheumatol.* **2012**, *30*, 380–387.
102. Schwartz, E. Prophylaxis of Malaria. *Mediterr. J. Hematol. Infect. Dis.* **2012**, *4*. [CrossRef]
103. Chen, L.H.; Wilson, M.E.; Schlagenhauf, P. Prevention of malaria in long-term travelers. *J. Am. Med. Assoc.* **2006**, *296*, 2234–2244. [CrossRef]
104. First FDA-Approved Vaccine for the Prevention of Dengue Diseases in Endemic Regions. Available online: https://www.fda.gov/news-events/press-announcements/first-fda-approved-vaccine-prevention-dengue-disease-endemic-regions#:~{}:text=The_U.S._Food_and_Drug,who_live_in_endemic_areas (accessed on 31 May 2020).
105. Da Silveira, L.T.C.; Tura, B.; Santos, M. Systematic review of dengue vaccine efficacy. *BMC Infect. Dis.* **2019**, *19*. [CrossRef]
106. Du, S.; Liu, Y.; Liu, J.; Zhao, J.; Champagne, C.; Tong, L.; Zhang, R.; Zhang, F.; Qin, C.F.; Ma, P.; et al. Aedes mosquitoes acquire and transmit Zika virus by breeding in contaminated aquatic environments. *Nat. Commun.* **2019**, *10*. [CrossRef]
107. Monteiro, V.V.S.; Navegantes-Lima, K.C.; De Lemos, A.B.; Da Silva, G.L.; De Souza Gomes, R.; Reis, J.F.; Junior, L.C.R.; Da Silva, O.S.; Romão, P.R.T.; Monteiro, M.C. Aedes-chikungunya virus interaction: Key role of vector midguts microbiota and its saliva in the host infection. *Front. Microbiol.* **2019**, *10*. [CrossRef]
108. Soleimani-Ahmadi, M.; Vatandoost, H.; Zare, M. Characterization of larval habitats for anopheline mosquitoes in a malarious area under elimination program in the southeast of Iran. *Asian Pac. J. Trop. Biomed.* **2014**, *4*, 73–80. [CrossRef] [PubMed]
109. Ziraba, A.K.; Haregu, T.N.; Mberu, B. A review and framework for understanding the potential impact of poor solid waste management on health in developing countries. *Arch. Public Health* **2016**, *74*. [CrossRef] [PubMed]
110. Hori, M.; Shibuya, K.; Sato, M.; Saito, Y. Lethal effects of short-wavelength visible light on insects. *Sci. Rep.* **2014**, *4*. [CrossRef] [PubMed]
111. Puri, A.; Kumar, M.; Johal, E. Solid-waste management in Jalandhar city and its impact on community health. *Indian J. Occup. Environ. Med.* **2008**, *12*, 76–81. [CrossRef]
112. Achudume, A.C.; Olawale, J.T. Microbial pathogens of public health significance in waste dumps and common sites. *J. Environ. Biol.* **2007**, *28*, 151–154.
113. Bell, J.L.; Collins, J.W.; Wolf, L.; Gronqvist, R.; Chiou, S.; Chang, W.R.; Sorock, G.; Courtney, T.; Lombardi, D.; Evanoff, B. Evaluation of a comprehensive slip, trip and fall prevention programme for hospital employees. *Ergonomics* **2009**, *51*, 1905–1925. [CrossRef]
114. Weinhold, B. A spreading concern: Inhalational health effects of mold. *Environ. Health Perspect.* **2007**, *115*, 300–305. [CrossRef]
115. Mattiello, A.; Chiodini, P.; Bianco, E.; Forgione, N.; Flammia, I.; Gallo, C.; Pizzuti, R.; Panico, S. Health effects associated with the disposal of solid waste in landfills and incinerators in populations living in surrounding areas: A systematic review. *Int. J. Public Health* **2013**, *58*, 725–735. [CrossRef]
116. Ferronato, N.; Torretta, V. Waste mismanagement in developing countries: A review of global issues. *Int. J. Environ. Res. Public Health* **2019**, *16*, 1060. [CrossRef]
117. Abeyewickreme, W.; Wickremasinghe, A.R.; Karunatilake, K.; Sommerfeld, J.; Axel, K. Community mobilization and household level waste management for dengue vector control in Gampaha district of Sri Lanka; an intervention study. *Pathog. Glob. Health* **2012**, *106*, 479–487. [CrossRef]
118. SDG7: Data and Projections. Available online: https://www.iea.org/reports/sdg7-data-and-projections/access-to-electricity (accessed on 31 May 2020).
119. Ritchie, S.A.; Cortis, G.; Paton, C.; Townsend, M.; Shroyer, D.; Zborowski, P.; Hall-Mendelin, S.; Van Den Hurk, A.F. A Simple Non-Powered Passive Trap for the Collection of Mosquitoes for Arbovirus Surveillance. *J. Med. Entomol.* **2013**, *50*, 185–194. [CrossRef] [PubMed]

120. Lu, Y.; Bei, Y.; Zhang, J. Are Yellow Sticky Traps an Effective Method for Control of Sweetpotato Whitefly, Bemisia tabaci, in the Greenhouse or Field? *J. Insect Sci.* **2012**, *12*. [CrossRef]
121. García-Betancourt, T.; Higuera-Mendieta, D.R.; González-Uribe, C.; Cortés, S.; Quintero, J. Understanding water storage practices of urban residents of an endemic dengue area in Colombia: Perceptions, rationale and socio-demographic characteristics. *PLoS ONE* **2015**, *10*, e0129054. [CrossRef] [PubMed]
122. Dambach, P.; Jorge, M.M.; Traoré, I.; Phalkey, R.; Sawadogo, H.; Zabré, P.; Kagoné, M.; Sié, A.; Sauerborn, R.; Becker, N.; et al. A qualitative study of community perception and acceptance of biological larviciding for malaria mosquito control in rural Burkina Faso. *BMC Public Health* **2018**, *18*. [CrossRef] [PubMed]
123. Yukalang, N.; Clarke, B.; Ross, K. Barriers to effective municipal solid waste management in a rapidly urbanizing area in Thailand. *Int. J. Environ. Res. Public Health* **2017**, *14*, 1013. [CrossRef]
124. Shockley Cruz, M.; Lindner, R.; Cruz, M.S.; Lindner, R. Insect Vision: Ultraviolet, Color, and LED Light. Ph.D. Thesis, University of Georgia Department of Entomology, Athens, GA, USA, 2011.
125. Van Loon, J.J.A.; Smallegange, R.C.; Bukovinszkiné-Kiss, G.; Jacobs, F.; De Rijk, M.; Mukabana, W.R.; Verhulst, N.O.; Menger, D.J.; Takken, W. Mosquito Attraction: Crucial Role of Carbon Dioxide in Formulation of a Five-Component Blend of Human-Derived Volatiles. *J. Chem. Ecol.* **2015**, *41*, 567–573. [CrossRef] [PubMed]
126. O'Hara, J.E.; UsUpensky, I.; Bostanian, N.J.; Capinera, J.L.; Chapman, R.; Barfield, C.S.; Swisher, M.E.; Barfield, C.S.; Heppner, J.; Fitzgerald, T.D.; et al. Traps for Capturing Insects. In *Encyclopedia of Entomology*; Springer Science & Business Media: Berlin, Germany, 2008; pp. 3675–4007.
127. Zhou, Y.H.; Zhang, Z.W.; Fu, Y.F.; Zhang, G.C.; Yuan, S. Carbon dioxide, odorants, heat and visible cues affect wild mosquito landing in open spaces. *Front. Behav. Neurosci.* **2018**, *12*. [CrossRef] [PubMed]
128. Lorenzi, O.D.; Major, C.; Acevedo, V.; Perez-Padilla, J.; Rivera, A.; Biggerstaff, B.J.; Munoz-Jordan, J.; Waterman, S.; Barrera, R.; Sharp, T.M. Reduced incidence of Chikungunya virus infection in communities with ongoing aedes aegypti mosquito trap intervention studies—Salinas and Guayama, Puerto Rico, November 2015–february 2016. *Morb. Mortal. Wkly. Rep.* **2016**, *65*, 479–480. [CrossRef]
129. Junnila, A.; Kline, D.L.; Müller, G.C. Comparative efficacy of small commercial traps for the capture of adult Phlebotomus papatasi. *J. Vector Ecol.* **2011**, *36*, 172–178. [CrossRef]
130. Sliney, D.H.; Gilbert, D.W.; Lyon, T. Ultraviolet safety assessments of insect light traps. *J. Occup. Environ. Hyg.* **2016**, *13*, 413–424. [CrossRef]
131. Urban, J.E.; Broce, A. Killing of flies in electrocuting insect traps releases bacteria and viruses. *Curr. Microbiol.* **2000**, *41*, 267–270. [CrossRef] [PubMed]
132. Getachew, D.; Tekie, H.; Gebre-Michael, T.; Balkew, M.; Mesfin, A. Breeding sites of aedes aegypti: Potential dengue vectors in dire Dawa, east Ethiopia. *Interdiscip. Perspect. Infect. Dis.* **2015**, *2015*. [CrossRef] [PubMed]
133. UNICEF. *Djibouti Humanitarian Situation Report No. 2 Flood Response*; UNICEF: New York, NY, USA, 2019; pp. 1–5.
134. Krystosik, A.; Njoroge, G.; Odhiambo, L.; Forsyth, J.E.; Mutuku, F.; LaBeaud, A.D. Solid Wastes Provide Breeding Sites, Burrows, and Food for Biological Disease Vectors, and Urban Zoonotic Reservoirs: A Call to Action for Solutions-Based Research. *Front. Public Health* **2020**, *7*. [CrossRef] [PubMed]
135. Banerjee, S.; Aditya, G.; Saha, G.K. Household wastes as larval habitats of dengue vectors: Comparison between urban and rural areas of Kolkata, India. *PLoS ONE* **2015**, *10*, e0138082. [CrossRef]
136. Becher, P.G.; Hagman, A.; Verschut, V.; Chakraborty, A.; Rozpędowska, E.; Lebreton, S.; Bengtsson, M.; Flick, G.; Witzgall, P.; Piškur, J. Chemical signaling and insect attraction is a conserved trait in yeasts. *Ecol. Evol.* **2018**, *8*, 2962–2974. [CrossRef]
137. Billeter, J.C.; Wolfner, M.F. Chemical Cues that Guide Female Reproduction in Drosophila melanogaster. *J. Chem. Ecol.* **2018**, *44*, 750–769. [CrossRef]
138. Boadi, K.O.; Kuitunen, M. Environmental and health impacts of household solid waste handling and disposal practices in Third World cities: The case of the Accra Metropolitan Area, Ghana. *J. Environ. Health* **2005**, *68*, 32–36.
139. Barreiro, C.; Albano, H.; Silva, J.; Teixeira, P. Role of Flies as Vectors of Foodborne Pathogens in Rural Areas. *ISRN Microbiol.* **2013**, *2013*. [CrossRef]
140. Zamora, D.M.B.; Hernández, M.M.; Torres, N.; Zúñiga, C.; Sosa, W.; De Abrego, V.; Escobar, M.C.M. Information to act: Household characteristics are predictors of domestic infestation with the Chagas vector Triatoma dimidiata in central America. *Am. J. Trop. Med. Hyg.* **2015**, *93*. [CrossRef]

141. Jawara, M.; Jatta, E.; Bell, D.; Burkot, T.R.; Bradley, J.; Hunt, V.; Kandeh, B.; Jones, C.; Manjang, A.M.; Pinder, M.; et al. New prototype screened doors and windows for excluding mosquitoes from houses: A pilot study in rural Gambia. *Am. J. Trop. Med. Hyg.* **2018**, *99*, 1475–1484. [CrossRef]
142. Che-Mendoza, A.; Medina-Barreiro, A.; Koyoc-Cardeña, E.; Uc-Puc, V.; Contreras-Perera, Y.; Herrera-Bojórquez, J.; Dzul-Manzanilla, F.; Correa-Morales, F.; Ranson, H.; Lenhart, A.; et al. House screening with insecticide-treated netting provides sustained reductions in domestic populations of Aedes aegypti in Merida, Mexico. *PLoS Negl. Trop. Dis.* **2018**, *12*. [CrossRef] [PubMed]
143. Tusting, L.S.; Ippolito, M.M.; Willey, B.A.; Kleinschmidt, I.; Dorsey, G.; Gosling, R.D.; Lindsay, S.W. The evidence for improving housing to reduce malaria: A systematic review and meta-analysis. *Malar. J.* **2015**, *14*. [CrossRef] [PubMed]
144. Massebo, F.; Lindtjørn, B. The effect of screening doors and windows on indoor density of Anopheles arabiensis in south-west Ethiopia: A randomized trial. *Malar. J.* **2013**, *12*. [CrossRef] [PubMed]
145. Musoke, D.; Karani, G.; Ssempebwa, J.C.; Musoke, M.B. Integrated approach to malaria prevention at household level in rural communities in Uganda: Experiences from a pilot project. *Malar. J.* **2018**, *18*, 1144–1156. [CrossRef]
146. Matsui, E.C. Management of rodent exposure and allergy in the pediatric population. *Curr. Allergy Asthma Rep.* **2013**, *13*. [CrossRef]
147. Hopkins, A.S.; Whitetail-Eagle, J.; Corneli, A.L.; Person, B.; Ettestad, P.J.; DiMenna, M.; Norstog, J.; Creswell, J.; Khan, A.S.; Olson, J.G.; et al. Experimental evaluation of rodent exclusion methods to reduce hantavirus transmission to residents in a Native American community in New Mexico. *Vector Borne Zoonotic Dis.* **2002**, *2*, 61–68. [CrossRef]
148. Jones, C.H.; Benítez-Valladares, D.; Guillermo-May, G.; Dzul-Manzanilla, F.; Che-Mendoza, A.; Barrera-Pérez, M.; Selem-Salas, C.; Chablé-Santos, J.; Sommerfeld, J.; Kroeger, A.; et al. Use and acceptance of long lasting insecticidal net screens for dengue prevention in Acapulco, Guerrero, Mexico. *BMC Public Health* **2014**, *14*. [CrossRef]
149. Bonner, P.C.; Schmidt, W.P.; Belmain, S.R.; Oshin, B.; Baglole, D.; Borchert, M. Poor housing quality increases risk of rodent infestation and lassa fever in refugee camps of sierra leone. *Am. J. Trop. Med. Hyg.* **2007**, *77*, 169–175. [CrossRef]
150. Safan, M.A.; Etman, Z.A.; Konswa, A. Evaluation of polyurethane resin injection for concrete leak repair. *Case Stud. Constr. Mater.* **2019**, *11*. [CrossRef]
151. Tseloni, A.; Farrell, G.; Thompson, R.; Evans, E.; Tilley, N. Domestic burglary drop and the security hypothesis. *Crime Sci.* **2017**, *6*. [CrossRef]
152. Carter, A.D. Are Housing Improvements an Effective Supplemental Vector Control Strategy to Reduce Malaria Transmission? A Systematic Review. Ph.D. Thesis, Georgia State University, Atlanta, GA, USA, 2014.
153. Bublitz, D.A.C.; Poché, R.M.; Garlapati, R. Measures to control Phlebotomus argentipes and visceral leishmaniasis in India. *J. Arthropod. Borne. Dis.* **2016**, *10*, 113–126. [PubMed]
154. Kaindoa, E.W.; Finda, M.; Kiplagat, J.; Mkandawile, G.; Nyoni, A.; Coetzee, M.; Okumu, F.O. Housing gaps, mosquitoes and public viewpoints: A mixed methods assessment of relationships between house characteristics, malaria vector biting risk and community perspectives in rural Tanzania. *Malar. J.* **2018**, *17*. [CrossRef] [PubMed]
155. Ogoma, S.B.; Kannady, K.; Sikulu, M.; Chaki, P.P.; Govella, N.J.; Mukabana, W.R.; Killeen, G.F. Window screening, ceilings and closed eaves as sustainable ways to control malaria in Dar es Salaam, Tanzania. *Malar. J.* **2009**, *8*. [CrossRef] [PubMed]
156. Ranjan, A.; Sur, D.; Singh, V.P.; Siddique, N.A.; Manna, B.; Lal, C.S.; Sinha, P.K.; Kishore, K.; Bhattacharya, S.K. Risk factors for Indian kala-azar. *Am. J. Trop. Med. Hyg.* **2005**, *73*, 74–78. [CrossRef] [PubMed]
157. Chan, E.Y.Y.; Shaw, R. *Public Health Humanitarian Responses to Natural Disasters*; Springer: Berlin/Heidelberg, Germany, 2017; ISBN 9781317357445.
158. Ryan, J. Environmental Health in Emergencies and Disasters: A Practical Guide. *Emerg. Med. J.* **2002**, *22*, 610. [CrossRef]
159. Laaser, U.; Dorey, S.; Nurse, J. A plea for global health action bottom-up. *Front. Public Health* **2016**, *4*. [CrossRef] [PubMed]
160. Hou, S.I. *Health Education: Theoretical Concepts, Effective Strategies and Core Competencies*; World Health Organization: Geneva, Switzerland, 2012; Volume 15, ISBN 9789290218289.

161. Naranjo, D.P.; Qualls, W.A.; Jurado, H.; Perez, J.C.; De Xue, R.; Gomez, E.; Beier, J.C. Vector control programs in Saint Johns County, Florida and Guayas, Ecuador: Successes and barriers to integrated vector management. *BMC Public Health* **2014**, *14*. [CrossRef]
162. Demanou, M.; Pouillot, R.; Grandadam, M.; Boisier, P.; Kamgang, B.; Hervé, J.P.; Rogier, C.; Rousset, D.; Paupy, C. Evidence of Dengue Virus Transmission and Factors Associated with the Presence of Anti-Dengue Virus Antibodies in Humans in Three Major Towns in Cameroon. *PLoS Negl. Trop. Dis.* **2014**, *8*. [CrossRef]
163. Poinsignon, A.; Boulanger, D.; Binetruy, F.; Elguero, E.; Darriet, F.; Gallian, P.; De Lamballerie, X.; Charrel, R.N.; Remoue, F. Risk factors of exposure to Aedes albopictus bites in mainland France using an immunological biomarker. *Epidemiol. Infect.* **2019**, *147*. [CrossRef]
164. Reiter, P.; Lathrop, S.; Bunning, M.; Biggerstaff, B.; Singer, D.; Tiwari, T.; Baber, L.; Amador, M.; Thirion, J.; Hayes, J.; et al. Texas lifestyle limits transmission of dengue virus. *Emerg. Infect. Dis.* **2003**, *9*, 86–89. [CrossRef]
165. Bloch, D.; Roth, N.M.; Caraballo, E.V.; Muñoz-Jordan, J.; Hunsperger, E.; Rivera, A.; Pérez-Padilla, J.; Rivera Garcia, B.; Sharp, T.M. Use of Household Cluster Investigations to Identify Factors Associated with Chikungunya Virus Infection and Frequency of Case Reporting in Puerto Rico. *PLoS Negl. Trop. Dis.* **2016**, *10*. [CrossRef]
166. Mathanga, D.P.; Mwandama, D.A.; Bauleni, A.; Chisaka, J.; Shah, M.P.; Landman, K.Z.; Lindblade, K.A.; Steinhardt, L.C. The effectiveness of long-lasting, insecticide-treated nets in a setting of pyrethroid resistance: A case-control study among febrile children 6 to 59 months of age in Machinga District, Malawi. *Malar. J.* **2015**, *14*. [CrossRef] [PubMed]
167. Pryce, J.; Richardson, M.; Lengeler, C. Insecticide-treated nets for preventing malaria. *Cochrane Database Syst. Rev.* **2019**, *11*. [CrossRef] [PubMed]
168. Deletre, E.; Martin, T.; Duménil, C.; Chandre, F. Insecticide resistance modifies mosquito response to DEET and natural repellents. *Parasites Vectors* **2019**, *12*. [CrossRef] [PubMed]
169. WHO. *Handbook for Integrated Vector Management*; World Health Organization: Geneva, Switzerland, 2013; ISBN 9789241502801.
170. Wilson, A.L.; Boelaert, M.; Kleinschmidt, I.; Pinder, M.; Scott, T.W.; Tusting, L.S.; Lindsay, S.W. Evidence-based vector control? Improving the quality of vector control trials. *Trends Parasitol.* **2015**, *31*, 380–390. [CrossRef]
171. Corrin, T.; Waddell, L.; Greig, J.; Young, I.; Hierlihy, C.; Mascarenhas, M. Risk perceptions, attitudes, and knowledge of chikungunya among the public and health professionals: A systematic review. *Trop. Med. Health* **2017**, *45*. [CrossRef]
172. Degroote, S.; Zinszer, K.; Ridde, V. Interventions for vector-borne diseases focused on housing and hygiene in urban areas: A scoping review. *Infect. Dis. Poverty* **2018**, *7*. [CrossRef]
173. Giantsis, I.A.; Chaskopoulou, A. Broadening the tools for studying sand fly breeding habitats: A novel molecular approach for the detection of phlebotomine larval DNA in soil substrates. *Acta Trop.* **2019**, *190*, 123–128. [CrossRef]
174. Moncaz, A.; Faiman, R.; Kirstein, O.; Warburg, A. Breeding sites of Phlebotomus sergenti, the sand fly vector of cutaneous leishmaniasis in the Judean desert. *PLoS Negl. Trop. Dis.* **2012**, *6*. [CrossRef]
175. Vivero, R.J.; Torres-Gutierrez, C.; Bejarano, E.E.; Peña, H.C.; Estrada, L.G.; Florez, F.; Ortega, E.; Aparicio, Y.; Muskus, C.E. Study on natural breeding sites of sand flies (Diptera: Phlebotominae) in areas of Leishmania transmission in Colombia. *Parasites Vectors* **2015**, *8*. [CrossRef]
176. World Health Organization. *Dengue Guidelines for Diagnosis, Treatment, Prevention and Control*; World Health Organization: Geneva, Switzerland, 2009.
177. Iwamura, T.; Guzman-Holst, A.; Murray, K.A. Accelerating invasion potential of disease vector Aedes aegypti under climate change. *Nat. Commun.* **2020**, *1*. [CrossRef] [PubMed]
178. Campbell-Lendrum, D.; Manga, L.; Bagayoko, M.; Sommerfeld, J. Climate change and vector-borne diseases: What are the implications for public health research and policy? *Philos. Trans. R. Soc. B Biol. Sci.* **2015**, *370*. [CrossRef] [PubMed]

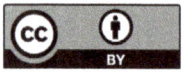

© 2020 by the authors. Licensee MDPI, Basel, Switzerland. This article is an open access article distributed under the terms and conditions of the Creative Commons Attribution (CC BY) license (http://creativecommons.org/licenses/by/4.0/).

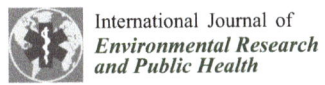 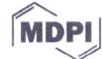

Commentary

The Asia Pacific Disaster Mental Health Network: Setting a Mental Health Agenda for the Region

Elizabeth A. Newnham [1,2,*], Peta L. Dzidic [1], Enrique L.P. Mergelsberg [1], Bhushan Guragain [3], Emily Ying Yang Chan [2,4,5], Yoshiharu Kim [6], Jennifer Leaning [2], Ryoma Kayano [7], Michael Wright [8], Lalindra Kaththiriarachchi [9], Hiroshi Kato [10], Tomoko Osawa [10] and Lisa Gibbs [11]

1. School of Psychology, Curtin University, Perth 6845, Australia; peta.dzidic@curtin.edu.au (P.L.D.); enrique.mergelsberg1@curtin.edu.au (E.L.P.M.)
2. François-Xavier Bagnoud Center for Health & Human Rights, Harvard University, Boston, MA 02115, USA; emily.chan@cuhk.edu.hk (E.Y.Y.C.); jleaning@hsph.harvard.edu (J.L.)
3. Centre for Victims of Torture, Kathmandu 44600, Nepal; bhushan@cvict.org.np
4. Division of Global Health and Humanitarian Medicine, CUHK, Hong Kong 999077, China
5. Nuffield Department of Medicine, University of Oxford, Oxford OX3-7LF, UK
6. National Institute of Mental Health, Tokyo 187-0031, Japan; joice21@yc4.so-net.ne.jp
7. World Health Organization Kobe Centre, Kobe 651-0073, Japan; kayanor@who.int
8. School of Occupational Therapy, Social Work and Speech Pathology, Curtin University, Perth 6845, Australia; m.wright@curtin.edu.au
9. Department of Physiology, Faculty of Medicine, General Sir John Kotelawala Defense University, Rathmalana 10390, Sri Lanka; lasakamd@ymail.com
10. Hyogo Institute for Traumatic Stress, Kobe 651-0073, Japan; kato@j-hits.org (H.K.); osawa@j-hits.org (T.O.)
11. Child and Community Wellbeing Unit, Melbourne School of Population and Global Health, University of Melbourne, Melbourne 3010, Australia; lgibbs@unimelb.edu.au
* Correspondence: Elizabeth.Newnham@curtin.edu.au; Tel.: +61-8-9266-3376

Received: 30 July 2020; Accepted: 21 August 2020; Published: 24 August 2020

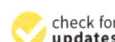

Abstract: Addressing the psychological mechanisms and structural inequalities that underpin mental health issues is critical to recovery following disasters and pandemics. The Asia Pacific Disaster Mental Health Network was established in June 2020 in response to the current disaster climate and to foster advancements in disaster-oriented mental health research, practice and policy across the region. Supported by the World Health Organization (WHO) Thematic Platform for Health Emergency and Disaster Risk Management (Health EDRM), the network brings together leading disaster psychiatry, psychology and public health experts. Our aim is to advance policy, research and targeted translation of the evidence so that communities are better informed in preparation and response to disasters, pandemics and mass trauma. The first meetings of the network resulted in the development of a regional disaster mental health agenda focused on the current context, with five priority areas: (1) Strengthening community engagement and the integration of diverse perspectives in planning, implementing and evaluating mental health and psychosocial response in disasters; (2) Supporting and assessing the capacity of mental health systems to respond to disasters; (3) Optimising emerging technologies in mental healthcare; (4) Understanding and responding appropriately to addressing the mental health impacts of climate change; (5) Prioritising mental health and psychosocial support for high-risk groups. Consideration of these priority areas in future research, practice and policy will support nuanced and effective psychosocial initiatives for disaster-affected populations within the Asia Pacific region.

Keywords: disaster; mental health; psychosocial; Asia Pacific; COVID-19; Health EDRM

1. Introduction

Disasters create an environment of disruption, trauma and grief, with potential for sustained mental health impacts. Heightened stress during pandemics and disasters can impair individual wellbeing (with effects on psychological health and sleep), cognitive function (memory, concentration and executive function), high-risk behaviours (alcohol and substance use, increased rates of domestic violence) and behavioural outcomes (such as compliance or disregard for public health orders) [1,2]. The mental health effects of disasters result not only from trauma exposure but may also arise from the implementation of public health response strategies such as quarantine, physical and social distancing or evacuation [3,4]. Economic insecurity, unemployment or underemployment, school closures and the shutdown of regional infrastructure can have devastating effects for population mental health. In addition, concerns regarding safety measures and sufficient supply of personal protective equipment can contribute to psychological distress [4,5]. Moreover, while many people demonstrate tremendous resilience during emergencies and in the immediate aftermath [6], the long-term psychological effects of disasters and pandemics are often debilitating [7,8].

The Asia Pacific region records the highest frequency of hazards and greatest number of people affected by disasters annually [9,10]. The immense psychological consequences are particularly concerning in nations with developing mental health systems and services [11]. A significant proportion of mental health need is unmet, and this has substantial effects on the social ecology and economic stability of affected communities. As climate change, growing urbanization, population density and animal–human viral transmission generate increasingly severe impacts of hazards and health emergencies, attention to mental health will be critical.

In response, the Asia Pacific Disaster Mental Health Network was established in June 2020 to create a collaborative platform for rigorous research, evidence-based practice and tailored policy designed to support improvements in mental health among disaster-affected communities. The network is supported by the World Health Organization (WHO) Thematic Platform for Health Emergency and Disaster Risk Management (Health EDRM) and its research network [12]. At its formation, the network represented seven Asian-Pacific nations, and it is growing. The network's membership represents practitioners and scholars with broad interdisciplinary expertise in the fields of humanitarian response, psychiatry, psychology, public health, disaster risk reduction, human rights and security, indigenous mental health, emergency and mental health services and climate change action. In its first meetings, the network sought to determine an agenda for the advancement of disaster mental health evidence and practice within the region that would inform the design of future collaborative research, policy development and delivery of services.

2. Materials and Methods

The Asia Pacific Disaster Mental Health Network comprises fifteen representatives (57% female), selected for their expertise in responding to health emergencies and natural disasters, and work with trauma-affected communities within the region. The network is open to all Asia Pacific nations and currently includes representatives from Australia, Japan, China, Nepal, Sri Lanka, India and the USA. The purpose of the network's early meetings was to establish a collaborative platform for future research and policy development and set overarching priorities in line with the goals of the WHO Thematic Platform for Health EDRM and its research network. Monthly meetings are conducted via videoconference. The selection of research priorities was conducted through open consultation within the network. An iterative-generative reflective method was adopted, whereby experiential knowledge of network members gleaned through their immersion with affected communities allowed for iterative debate [13]. As reflective-generative practitioners, each network member provided community-relevant insights as to potential priority areas. An iterative and deliberative discussion occurred across two meetings, held in June and July 2020. A list of key priorities identified by the group as central to mental health practice, research and policy within the region was generated. Thirteen representatives attended the first meeting and ten representatives attended the second. Impromptu responses on the priority list were systematically collated; the list was adapted following a second round of discussion and then circulated among the representatives for feedback. An additional round of input from representatives on the priorities and supporting evidence was incorporated into the write-up. All network members contributed to and provided feedback on the final priority list.

3. Results

3.1. Key Priorities for Disaster Mental Health

Large-scale climate disasters, severe wildfires and the COVID-19 pandemic have drawn renewed global attention to disaster response this year. The COVID-19 pandemic has amplified the structural injustices of race, faith, gender, age, migration and economic inequality within and across societies, with significant implications for mental health (e.g., [14–18]). Addressing structural disadvantage and inequality is vital, and without attention to these issues, many mental health difficulties during and after disasters may not be amenable to psychological treatment. Mental health practitioners and researchers play a vital role in highlighting injustice, community needs and the role of economic empowerment in supporting mental health. It is critical that psychological first aid and evidence-based interventions suitable for response to mass trauma events are implemented to support individual, family and community level improvements in mental health, recognizing that psychological distress occurs on a continuum and multi-level strategies are required [19,20]. First, broad public health strategies such as psychological first aid, mental health education, family reunification and child-friendly spaces, should be implemented at the community level to address general distress following an event; second, delivery of low-intensity programs to assist those dealing with sustained distress and psychological difficulties; third, clinical treatment provided for those with diagnosable conditions [19,21,22]. However, the effectiveness of treatments will vary due to the sociocultural context in which they are delivered [23]. A nuanced, solution-based approach will support significant advancements in this field. In line with this point, we identified the following priorities for a regional disaster mental health agenda.

3.2. Strengthening Community Engagement and the Integration of Diverse Perspectives in Planning, Implementing and Evaluating Mental Health Response

Reinforcing local social networks, social solidarity and engagement with community groups in responding to disasters and other mass trauma events will enhance psychosocial outcomes [24–26]. Community-driven responses are led by the community and may invite external agency partnership, whereas community-supported responses are facilitated by an external agency with the endorsement of the community [27]. Central to both approaches is that the community be recognised as valued authorities on their own lived experience. Listening to and incorporating diverse knowledges and multiple perspectives are essential to ensure that mental health services and psychosocial initiatives designed for any community are accessible, acceptable, culturally secure and developmentally appropriate [28] and that intervention models, disaster risk reduction strategies and mental health policy are designed and delivered in ways that are meaningful and relevant [29]. Furthermore, emerging evidence suggests that mutual reinforcement of public health messages and actions among community members has positive implications for health-related behaviors and compliance with public health directives during pandemics [30]. Restoring connections to the natural environment will have additional mental health benefits [31]. Working within existing community social structures and across a broad cross section of the community—with Elders, youth, local faith leaders and community groups—helps to establish respectful and collaborative relationships. Measures to access broad input and community guidance will result in treatment models, services and strategies that meet the diversity of mental health needs [32–34].

3.3. Supporting the Capacity of Mental Health Systems to Respond to Disasters

Disasters create multiple waves of healthcare need. Early response requires a focus on physical injuries, bereavement and re-establishing critical infrastructure for survival [35]. Establishing conditions for safe recovery will lessen distress for a vast majority of the population [19,36]. Mental illness tends to emerge in a second surge of health need, often months and years following the initial emergency [37]. However, the COVID-19 pandemic highlighted mental health needs that required immediate support during this crisis [2,5]. Health systems need to be prepared to address the short- and long-term mental health needs that arise within disaster-affected settings. Disaster response must begin with a diverse and well-supported workforce and include ensuring that workers are trained and supported with ongoing supervision and further training in psychological care for traumatized people—including how to cope with the added overlay of mass trauma impacts. Where disasters are more likely to affect remote areas, infrastructure to support regional health workers and digital health platforms will be important [38]. Lessons learned from the COVID-19 pandemic have already sparked significant expansion of mental health systems in many nations, including in China, where an increased workforce was engaged in order to address the psychological distress and grief arising from the pandemic in Wuhan [39,40]. Similar initiatives have been developed in other parts of the Asia Pacific region, including increased mental health budget funding in Australia [41], improved and expanded mental health helpline services in Nepal [42] and increased in-person and remote counselling services in Japan [43]. The challenge will be an ongoing commitment to the long-term sustainability of services to address the growing incidence of disaster-related trauma and grief within our region and ensuring that first responders, medical, nursing and allied health staff are well supported [44,45]. Mental health services research is both urgent and critical to evaluate the efficacy of models for rapid upskilling and ongoing support of the healthcare workforce, and to design and implement the appropriate expansion of access; acceptability and cultural security of services; effectiveness of trauma-informed treatments in low resource settings and community-based strategies to prevent the escalation of psychological distress.

3.4. Optimising the Integration of Digital Platforms in Mental Healthcare to Support Access and Acceptability of Care

The COVID-19 pandemic has fast-tracked the development and widespread adoption of technology in mental healthcare in many settings. Digital mental health services include treatment sessions conducted via video call, telephone helplines, clinical text messaging services, digital health applications and platforms, online streaming and therapy services and mass dissemination of mental health resources on social media [39,46]. Enabling the safe continuation of mental health services during lockdown or physical distancing, tele-mental health services have been widely implemented in many nations including China, Japan, Australia and New Zealand and have received additional funding for development and dissemination globally [39,47,48]. New and adapted technologies have the potential to transform the delivery of mental healthcare, as care can be tailored on a personal level, provided anywhere, be perceived as less stigmatizing and can empower people to take a more active role in their own healthcare decisions [49–51]. Although many settings within the Asia Pacific region still lack reliable access to electricity, internet and phone coverage, all limiting the use of digital mental healthcare [52]; the growing ubiquity of smartphone use has enabled rapid communication of disaster and mental health messaging, reaching populations less likely to be engaged with mainstream health services, such as international migrant workers [53]. Technology may also enable people to maintain the social connections that are critical to mental health and wellbeing outcomes. However, the digitalization of mental healthcare has possible negative implications. Reliance on technology can lead to social disengagement, and there are increasing concerns about the potential for misinformation with unregulated online information, as well as technical issues, unreliable internet access, low digital competences of health providers and clients, safety of data handling and perceived loss of therapeutic relationships [49,54]. It is thus essential to now identify which services and strategies have proven to be protective and efficient in improving mental health outcomes in the context of COVID-19 so as to design approaches that will have relevance beyond this pandemic.

3.5. Addressing the Mental Health Impacts of Climate Change

Climate change has increased the frequency and severity of natural disasters in the Asia Pacific region, with resulting risks for mental health problems [55–57]. The relationship between climate change and mental health impacts can be direct, by experiencing trauma caused by climate hazards, or indirect, through resulting physical health consequences, increased economic vulnerability and detrimental effects on community cohesion [55,56]. Further indirect effects from climate change may arise through a reduced sense of hope and self- and community-efficacy, identified as essential elements in recovery from mass trauma events such as natural disasters [58]. Within the Asia Pacific region, Indigenous communities and those dependent on agricultural production or coastal fishing experience disproportionate adverse impacts of climate change [55,56,59]. However, the effects are broadening—the Australian 2020 wildfires demonstrated widespread ecological and economic damage—with substantial psychological effects [38,60]. Similarly, climate change has had significant effects on mental health in the Pacific Island of Tuvalu [59], where the changing climate threatens irreversible changes to the way of life [61]. Climate-related hazards (i.e., tropical cyclones and increasing ocean temperatures) combined with urbanization, land shortages, overcrowding, limitations in infrastructure, services and poor governance have resulted in high levels of stress, anxiety and depressive symptoms among the Tuvaluan population [59]. Similar issues accompanied the impact of 2013 super typhoon Haiyan in the Philippines [62]. Direct and indirect mental health consequences from climate change are current and understudied [57]. This gap in our knowledge requires our immediate and collective attention in order to bring about an efficient, effective and holistic approach to mitigating the inequity of climate change impacts on mental health, led by local experts. This effort must become a central focus of disaster risk reduction in the coming decades.

3.6. Prioritising Mental Health and Psychosocial Support for High-Risk Groups

High-risk groups, including those disadvantaged or discriminated against due to the characteristics and intersection of age, gender, sexuality, ethnicity, faith, ability, migration and economic status, may be at greater risk of mental health difficulties during and after disasters [63,64]. In addition, those affected by domestic violence, chronic mental illness, forced displacement, job loss or homelessness will require tailored solutions [65]. The damage to the natural environment from climatic hazards may also generate an additional level of pain and loss for First Nations people with historical and cultural connections to the land [66], as well as for many others who find solace and peace in the persistence of nature. Failure to recognize historical circumstances and cultural values can result in interventions reinforcing existing patterns of disadvantage and prejudice [67]. Risk factors are dynamic, and an individual's level of vulnerability during disasters is dependent on a range of contextual factors, resulting in resilience at times and vulnerability at others [63]. For example, there is a complex relationship between disaster exposure and suicide risk, with increased risk associated with large-scale disaster impacts and length of time following exposure [68]. Specific groups, such as working-age men and older women, and factors including limited social connections, economic insecurity, living in temporary housing and pre-existing or new mental health conditions may increase suicide risk following disasters [68,69]. COVID-19 has demonstrated the potential for mental health risks to emerge as a result of both disaster-related trauma and the public health safety measures implemented to reduce transmission. This has been highlighted in Nepal, where widespread job loss and economic insecurity arising from government lockdown measures during the pandemic has resulted in a tragic spike in suicides, with 1200 deaths reported due to suicide during the 74 day lockdown [70,71]. Established mental health services in Nepal are working to provide helpline services through telephone and social media and further improve the capacity of community psychosocial workers to respond to individuals experiencing psychological distress [42]. Thus, effective services working within high-risk communities must be supported to continue and, where needed, expand their services during and after disasters. As we see an increasingly sophisticated global response to disaster risk reduction, inclusion and support for high-risk groups will be vital for effective mental healthcare.

4. Conclusions

The Asia Pacific Disaster Mental Health Network was established to foster advancements and coordination of psychosocial supports and mental health service delivery, policy development and collaborative research in the region. In line with the priorities of the WHO Thematic Platform for Health EDRM and its research network [12,72], the Asia Pacific Network aims to contribute to improvements in mental healthcare and psychosocial support through rigorous research and policy. Within the context of the COVID-19 pandemic and recent climatic hazards, the network set an agenda that prioritises strengthened community engagement, improved capacity for mental health and community services to respond to the needs of disaster-affected populations, integrating emerging technologies, addressing the impacts of climate change and supporting high-risk groups. Through multidisciplinary regional partnerships, the network will contribute to effective and culturally secure intervention design and delivery, translation of evidence to support community preparedness and response, and the collection of high-quality data to inform knowledge, policy and practice specific to the Asia Pacific region and relevant across the globe.

Author Contributions: Conceptualization, E.A.N., E.Y.Y.C., P.L.D., L.G.; B.G., Y.K., J.L., L.K., H.K., writing—original draft preparation, E.A.N., E.L.P.M., P.L.D.; writing—review and editing, E.A.N., P.L.D., E.L.P.M., B.G., E.Y.Y.C., Y.K., J.L., R.K., M.W., L.K., H.K., T.O., L.G., funding acquisition, E.A.N., Y.K., H.K., L.G., P.L.D., J.L. All authors have read and agreed to the published version of the manuscript.

Funding: This research was supported by the World Health Organization Centre for Health Development (WHO Kobe Centre—WKC: K19007).

Conflicts of Interest: The funders had no role in the design of the study; in the collection, analyses, or interpretation of data; or in the decision to publish the results.

References

1. Holmes, E.A.; O'Connor, R.C.; Perry, V.H.; Tracey, I.; Wessely, S.; Arseneault, L.; Ballard, C.; Christensen, H.; Silver, R.C.; Everall, I. Multidisciplinary research priorities for the COVID-19 pandemic: A call for action for mental health science. *Lancet Psychiatry* **2020**, *7*, 547–560. [CrossRef]
2. Pfefferbaum, B.; North, C.S. Mental health and the Covid-19 pandemic. *N. Engl. J. Med.* **2020**, *383*, 510–512. [CrossRef] [PubMed]
3. Brooks, S.K.; Webster, R.K.; Smith, L.E.; Woodland, L.; Wessely, S.; Greenberg, N.; Rubin, G.J. The psychological impact of quarantine and how to reduce it: Rapid review of the evidence. *Lancet* **2020**, *395*, 912–920. [CrossRef]
4. Li, H.Y.; Cao, H.; Leung, D.Y.; Mak, Y.W. The psychological impacts of a COVID-19 outbreak on college students in China: A longitudinal study. *Int. J. Environ. Res. Public Health* **2020**, *17*, 3933. [CrossRef] [PubMed]
5. Choi, E.P.H.; Hui, B.P.H.; Wan, E.Y.F. Depression and anxiety in Hong Kong during COVID-19. *Int. J. Environ. Res. Public Health* **2020**, *17*, 3740. [CrossRef] [PubMed]
6. Bonanno, G.A.; Brewin, C.R.; Kaniasty, K.; Greca, A.M.L. Weighing the costs of disaster: Consequences, risks, and resilience in individuals, families, and communities. *Psychol. Sci. Public Interest* **2010**, *11*, 1–49. [CrossRef] [PubMed]
7. Beaglehole, B.; Mulder, R.T.; Frampton, C.M.; Boden, J.M.; Newton-Howes, G.; Bell, C.J. Psychological distress and psychiatric disorder after natural disasters: Systematic review and meta-analysis. *Br. J. Psychiatry* **2018**, *213*, 716–722. [CrossRef] [PubMed]
8. Bryant, R.A.; Gibbs, L.; Gallagher, H.C.; Pattison, P.; Lusher, D.; MacDougall, C.; Harms, L.; Block, K.; Sinnott, V.; Ireton, G. Longitudinal study of changing psychological outcomes following the Victorian black Saturday bushfires. *Aust. N. Z. J. Psychiatry* **2018**, *52*, 542–551. [CrossRef] [PubMed]
9. CRED; UNISDR. *2018 Review of Disaster Events*; Centre for Research on the Epidemiology of Disasters: Brussels, Belgium, 2019.

10. Below, R.; Wallemacq, P. *Annual Disaster Statistical Review 2017*; Centre for Research on the Epidemiology of Disasters: Brussels, Belgium, 2018.
11. Henderson, L.J. Emergency and disaster: Pervasive risk and public bureaucracy in developing nations. *Public Organ. Rev.* **2004**, *4*, 103–119. [CrossRef]
12. Kayano, R.; Chan, E.Y.; Murray, V.; Abrahams, J.; Barber, S.L. WHO Thematic Platform for Health Emergency and Disaster Risk Management Research Network (TPRN): Report of the Kobe Expert Meeting. *Int. J. Environ. Res. Public Health* **2019**, *16*, 1232. [CrossRef]
13. Dokecki, P.R. On knowing the community of caring persons: A methodological basis for the reflective-generative practice of community psychology. *J. Community Psychol.* **1992**, *20*, 26–35. [CrossRef]
14. Matache, M.; Bhabha, J. Anti-Roma Racism is Spiraling during COVID-19 Pandemic. *Health Hum. Rights* **2020**, *22*, 379. [PubMed]
15. Tai, D.B.G.; Shah, A.; Doubeni, C.A.; Sia, I.G.; Wieland, M.L. The Disproportionate Impact of COVID-19 on Racial and Ethnic Minorities in the United States. *Clin. Infect. Dis.* **2020**. [CrossRef] [PubMed]
16. Kihato, C.W.; Landau, L.B. Coercion or the social contract? COVID 19 and spatial (in) justice in African cities. *City Soc.* **2020**, *32*. [CrossRef] [PubMed]
17. Xafis, V. 'What is Inconvenient for You is Life-saving for Me': How Health Inequities are playing out during the COVID-19 Pandemic. *Asian Bioeth. Rev.* **2020**, 1. [CrossRef] [PubMed]
18. Pirtle, W.N.L. Racial capitalism: A fundamental cause of novel coronavirus (COVID-19) pandemic inequities in the United States. *Health Educ. Behav.* **2020**. [CrossRef]
19. Tol, W.A.; Barbui, C.; Galappatti, A.; Silove, D.; Betancourt, T.S.; Souza, R.; Golaz, A.; Van Ommeren, M. Mental health and psychosocial support in humanitarian settings: Linking practice and research. *Lancet* **2011**, *378*, 1581–1591. [CrossRef]
20. Zhang, Y.; Ma, Z.F. Impact of the COVID-19 pandemic on mental health and quality of life among local residents in Liaoning Province, China: A cross-sectional study. *Int. J. Environ. Res. Public Health* **2020**, *17*, 2381. [CrossRef]
21. Forbes, D.; O'Donnell, M.; Bryant, R. Psychosocial recovery following community disasters: An international collaboration. *Aust. N. Z. J. Psychiatry* **2017**, *51*, 660–662. [CrossRef]
22. Kim, Y.; Akiyama, T. Post-disaster mental health care in Japan. *Lancet* **2011**, *378*, 317–318. [CrossRef]
23. Newnham, E.A.; McBain, R.K.; Hann, K.; Akinsulure-Smith, A.M.; Weisz, J.; Lilienthal, G.M.; Hansen, N.; Betancourt, T.S. The Youth Readiness Intervention for war-affected youth. *J. Adolesc. Health* **2015**, *56*, 606–611. [CrossRef] [PubMed]
24. Bryant, R.; Gallagher, H.; Waters, E.; Gibbs, L.; Pattison, P.; MacDougall, C.; Harms, L.; Block, K.; Baker, E.; Sinnott, V. Mental health and social networks after disaster. *Am. J. Psychiatry* **2017**, *173*, 277–285. [CrossRef] [PubMed]
25. Gallagher, H.C.; Block, K.; Gibbs, L.; Forbes, D.; Lusher, D.; Molyneaux, R.; Richardson, J.; Pattison, P.; MacDougall, C.; Bryant, R.A. The effect of group involvement on post-disaster mental health: A longitudinal multilevel analysis. *Soc. Sci. Med.* **2019**, *220*, 167–175. [CrossRef] [PubMed]
26. Hawdon, J.; Räsänen, P.; Oksanen, A.; Ryan, J. Social solidarity and wellbing after critical incidents: Three cases of mass shootings. *J. Crit. Incid. Anal.* **2012**, *3*, 2–25.
27. Rodriguez-García, R.; Bonnel, R.; N'Jie, N.D.; Olivier, J.; Pascual, F.B.; Wodon, Q. *Analyzing Community Responses to HIV and AIDS: Operational Framework and Typology*; The World Bank: Washington, DC, USA, 2011.
28. Wright, M.; Lin, A.; O'Connell, M. Humility, inquisitiveness, and openness: Key attributes for meaningful engagement with Nyoongar people. *Adv. Ment. Health* **2016**, *14*, 82–95. [CrossRef]
29. Tol, W.A.; Song, S.; Jordans, M.J. Annual research review: Resilience and mental health in children and adolescents living in areas of armed conflict–a systematic review of findings in low-and middle-income countries. *J. Child Psychol. Psychiatry* **2013**, *54*, 445–460. [CrossRef]
30. Lim, S.; Nakazato, H. The emergence of risk communication networks and the development of citizen health-related behaviors during the COVID-19 pandemic: Social selection and contagion processes. *Int. J. Environ. Res. Public Health* **2020**, *17*, 4148. [CrossRef]
31. Block, K.; Molyneaux, R.; Gibbs, L.; Alkemade, N.; Baker, E.; MacDougall, C.; Ireton, G.; Forbes, D. The role of the natural environment in disaster recovery: "We live here because we love the bush". *Health Place* **2019**, *57*, 61–69. [CrossRef]

32. Harr, C.R.; Yancey, G.I. Social work collaboration with faith leaders and faith groups serving families in rural areas. *J. Relig. Spiritual. Soc. Work Soc. Thought* **2014**, *33*, 148–162. [CrossRef]
33. Israel, B.A.; Schulz, A.J.; Parker, E.A.; Becker, A.B. Review of community-based research: Assessing partnership approaches to improve public health. *Annu. Rev. Public Health* **1998**, *19*, 173–202. [CrossRef]
34. Wright, M.; Crisp, N.; Newnham, E.A.; Flavell, H.; Lin, A. Addressing mental health in Aboriginal young people in Australia. *Lancet Psychiatry* **2020**. [CrossRef]
35. Bar-On, E.; Abargel, A.; Peleg, K.; Kreiss, Y. Coping with the challenges of early disaster response: 24 years of field hospital experience after earthquakes. *Disaster Med. Public Health Prep.* **2013**, *7*, 491–498. [CrossRef] [PubMed]
36. North, C.S.; Pfefferbaum, B. Mental health response to community disasters: A systematic review. *JAMA* **2013**, *310*, 507–518. [CrossRef] [PubMed]
37. Gibbs, L.; Waters, E.; Bryant, R.A.; Pattison, P.; Lusher, D.; Harms, L.; Richardson, J.; MacDougall, C.; Block, K.; Snowdon, E. Beyond Bushfires: Community, Resilience and Recovery-a longitudinal mixed method study of the medium to long term impacts of bushfires on mental health and social connectedness. *BMC Public Health* **2013**, *13*, 1036. [CrossRef]
38. Newnham, E.A.; Titov, N.; McEvoy, P. Preparing mental health systems for climate crisis. *Lancet Planet. Health* **2020**, *4*, e89–e90. [CrossRef]
39. Liu, S.; Yang, L.; Zhang, C.; Xiang, Y.T.; Liu, Z.; Hu, S.; Zhang, B. Online mental health services in China during the COVID-19 outbreak. *Lancet Psychiatry* **2020**, *7*, e17–e18. [CrossRef]
40. Li, W.; Yang, Y.; Liu, Z.H.; Zhao, Y.J.; Zhang, Q.; Zhang, L.; Cheung, T.; Xiang, Y.T. Progression of mental health services during the COVID-19 outbreak in China. *Int. J. Biol. Sci.* **2020**, *16*, 1732. [CrossRef]
41. Australian Government, Department of Health. *Supporting the Mental Health of Australians through the Coronavirus Pandemic*; Australian Government: Canberra, Australia, 2020.
42. MHIN. A global Community of Mental Health Innovators, and Department of Mental Health and Substance Use WHO. Resources for Mental Health and Psychosocial Support during the COVID-19 Pandemic. Available online: https://www.mhinnovation.net/collaborations/resources-mental-health-and-psychosocial-support-during-covid-19-pandemic (accessed on 23 July 2020).
43. Health, Centre for Japanese Mental. In-Person and Remote Counseling. Available online: https://cjmh.org/counseling/ (accessed on 23 July 2020).
44. Matsuishi, K.; Kawazoe, A.; Imai, H.; Ito, A.; Mouri, K.; Kitamura, N.; Miyake, K.; Mino, K.; Isobe, M.; Takamiya, S. Psychological impact of the pandemic (H1N1) 2009 on general hospital workers in Kobe. *Psychiatry Clin. Neurosci.* **2012**, *66*, 353–360. [CrossRef]
45. Krystal, J.H.; McNeil, R.L. Responding to the hidden pandemic for healthcare workers: Stress. *Nat. Med.* **2020**, *26*, 639. [CrossRef]
46. Ben-Zeev, D. The digital mental health genie is out of the bottle. *Psychiatr. Serv.* **2020**. [CrossRef]
47. Zhou, X.; Snoswell, C.L.; Harding, L.E.; Bambling, M.; Edirippulige, S.; Bai, X.; Smith, A.C. The role of telehealth in reducing the mental health burden from COVID-19. *Telemed. E-Health* **2020**, *26*, 377–379. [CrossRef] [PubMed]
48. Marshall, J.M.; Dunstan, D.A.; Bartik, W. The role of digital mental health resources to treat trauma symptoms in australia during COVID-19. *Psychol. Trauma Theory Res. Pract. Policy* **2020**, *12*, S269–S271. [CrossRef] [PubMed]
49. Bucci, S.; Schwannauer, M.; Berry, N. The digital revolution and its impact on mental health care. *Psychol. Psychother. Theory Res. Pract.* **2019**, *92*, 277–297. [CrossRef] [PubMed]
50. Hollis, C.; Sampson, S.; Simons, L.; Davies, E.B.; Churchill, R.; Betton, V.; Butler, D.; Chapman, K.; Easton, K.; Gronlund, T.A. Identifying research priorities for digital technology in mental health care: Results of the James Lind Alliance Priority Setting Partnership. *Lancet Psychiatry* **2018**, *5*, 845–854. [CrossRef]
51. World Economic Forum. *Empowering 8 Billion Minds: Enabling Better Mental Health for All Via the Ethical Adoption of Technologies*; World Economic Forum: Geneva, Switzerland, 2019.
52. Statica. Internet Penetration Rate in Asia Compared to the Global Penetration Rate from 2009 to 2020. Available online: https://www.statista.com/statistics/265156/internet-penetration-rate-in-asia/ (accessed on 23 July 2020).
53. Liem, A.; Wang, C.; Wariyanti, Y.; Latkin, C.A.; Hall, B.J. The neglected health of international migrant workers in the COVID-19 epidemic. *Lancet Psychiatry* **2020**, *7*, e20. [CrossRef]

54. Christensen, H.; Griffiths, K.M.; Farrer, L. Adherence in internet interventions for anxiety and depression: Systematic review. *J. Med. Internet Res.* **2009**, *11*, e13. [CrossRef]
55. Berry, H.L.; Bowen, K.; Kjellstrom, T. Climate change and mental health: A causal pathways framework. *Int. J. Public Health* **2010**, *55*, 123–132. [CrossRef]
56. Fritze, J.G.; Blashki, G.A.; Burke, S.; Wiseman, J. Hope, despair and transformation: Climate change and the promotion of mental health and wellbeing. *Int. J. Ment. Health Syst.* **2008**, *2*, 13. [CrossRef]
57. Hayes, K.; Blashki, G.; Wiseman, J.; Burke, S.; Reifels, L. Climate change and mental health: Risks, impacts and priority actions. *Int. J. Ment. Health Syst.* **2018**, *12*, 28. [CrossRef]
58. Hobfoll, S.E.; Watson, P.; Bell, C.C.; Bryant, R.A.; Brymer, M.J.; Friedman, M.J.; Friedman, M.; Gersons, B.P.; De Jong, J.T.; Layne, C.M. Five essential elements of immediate and mid–term mass trauma intervention: Empirical evidence. *Psychiatrynterpers. Biol. Process.* **2007**, *70*, 283–315. [CrossRef]
59. Gibson, K.; Haslam, N.; Kaplan, I. Distressing encounters in the context of climate change: Idioms of distress, determinants, and responses to distress in Tuvalu. *Transcult. Psychiatry* **2019**, *56*, 667–696. [CrossRef] [PubMed]
60. Miller, V.M.; Davies, M.J.; Etherton-Beer, C.; McGough, S.; Schofield, D.; Jensen, J.F.; Watson, N. Increasing patient activation through diabetes self-management education: Outcomes of DESMOND in regional Western Australia. *Patient Educ. Couns.* **2020**, *103*, 848–853. [CrossRef]
61. Nunn, P.D. The end of the P acific? Effects of sea level rise on P acific I sland livelihoods. *Singap. J. Trop. Geogr.* **2013**, *34*, 143–171. [CrossRef]
62. Chan, C.; Tang, K.; Hall, B.; Yip, S.; Maggay, M. Psychological sequelae of the 2013 Super Typhoon Haiyan among survivor-responders. *Psychiatry Interpers. Biol. Process.* **2016**, *79*, 282–296. [CrossRef]
63. Newnham, E.A.; Ho, J.Y.; Chan, E.Y.Y. Identifying and engaging high-risk groups in disaster research. In *World Health Organization Guidance on Research Methods for Health Emergency and Disaster Risk Management*; Clarke, M., Murray, V., Chan, E.Y.Y., Kayano, R., Abrahams, J., O'Sullivan, T., Eds.; World Health Organization: Geneva, Switzerland, 2020, in press.
64. Collins, P.H.; Bilge, S. *Intersectionality*; Polity Press: Cambridge, UK, 2016.
65. Chan, E.Y.Y.; Gobat, N.; Kim, J.H.; Newnham, E.A.; Huang, Z.; Hung, H.; Dubois, C.; Hung, K.K.C.; Wong, E.L.Y.; Wong, S.Y.S. Informal home care providers: The forgotten health-care workers during the COVID-19 pandemic. *Lancet* **2020**, *395*, 1957–1959. [CrossRef]
66. Williamson, B.; Markham, F.; Weir, J. *Aboriginal Peoples and the Response to the 2019–2020 Bushfires*; Centre for Aboriginal Economic Policy Research, Australian National University: Canberra, Australia, 2020.
67. Hsu, M.; Howitt, R.; Miller, F. Procedural Vulnerability and Institutional Capacity Deficits in Post-Disaster Recovery and Reconstruction: Insights from Wutai Rukai Experiences of Typhoon Morakot. *Hum. Organ.* **2015**, *74*, 308–318. [CrossRef]
68. Matsubayashi, T.; Sawada, Y.; Ueda, M. Natural disasters and suicide: Evidence from Japan. *Soc. Sci. Med.* **2013**, *82*, 126–133. [CrossRef]
69. Safarpour, H.; Sohrabizadeh, S.; Malekyan, L.; Safi-Keykaleh, M.; Pirani, D.; Daliri, S.; Bazyar, J. Suicide death rate after disasters: A meta-analysis study. *Arch. Suicide Res.* **2020**. [CrossRef]
70. Singh, R.; Baral, K.P.; Mahato, S. An urgent call for measures to fight against increasing suicides during COVID-19 pandemic in Nepal. *Asian J. Psychiatry* **2020**, *54*, 102259. [CrossRef]
71. Poudel, A. Over 1,200 people killed themselves during 74 days of lockdown in Nepal. *The Kathmandu Post*, 21 August 2020.
72. Newnham, E.A.; Reifels, L.; Gibbs, L. Disaster mental health research. In *World Health Organization Guidance on Research Methods for Health Emergency and Disaster Risk Management*; larke, M., Murray, V., Chan, E.Y.Y., Kayano, R., Abrahams, J., O' Sullivan, T., Eds.; World Health Organization: Geneva, Switzerland, 2020, in press.

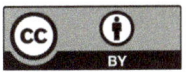

© 2020 by the authors. Licensee MDPI, Basel, Switzerland. This article is an open access article distributed under the terms and conditions of the Creative Commons Attribution (CC BY) license (http://creativecommons.org/licenses/by/4.0/).

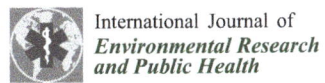 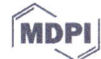

Article

Long-Term Impact of Disasters on the Public Health System: A Multi-Case Analysis

Nina Lorenzoni [1,*], Verena Stühlinger [1], Harald Stummer [1,2] and Margit Raich [1]

1 Department for Public Health, Health Services Research and Health Technology Assessment, UMIT TIROL—Private University for Health Sciences, Medical Informatics and Technology, 6060 Hall in Tirol, Austria; verena.stuehlinger@umit.at (V.S.); harald.stummer@umit.at (H.S.); margit.raich@umit.at (M.R.)
2 Department of Business, University Seeburg Castle, 5201 Seekirchen am Wallersee, Austria
* Correspondence: nina.lorenzoni@umit.at

Received: 31 July 2020; Accepted: 25 August 2020; Published: 27 August 2020

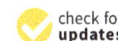

Abstract: As past events have shown, disasters can have a tremendous impact on the affected population's health. However, research regarding the long-term impact on a systems level perspective is still scarce. In this multi-case study, we analyzed and compared the long-term impacts on the public health system of five disasters which took place in Europe: avalanche (Austria), terror attack (Spain), airplane crash (Luxembourg), cable-car tunnel fire (Austria), and a flood in Central Europe. We used a mixed-methods approach consisting of a document analysis and interviews with key stakeholders, to examine the various long-term impacts each of the disasters had on health-system performance, as well as on security and health protection. The results show manifold changes undertaken in the fields of psychosocial support, infrastructure, and contingency and preparedness planning. The holistic approach of this study shows the importance of analyzing long-term impacts from the perspective of the type (e.g., disasters associated with natural hazards) and characteristic (e.g., duration and extent) of a disaster, as well as the regional context where a disaster took place. However, the identified recurring themes demonstrate the opportunity of learning from case studies in order to customize the lessons and apply them to the own-disaster-management setting.

Keywords: long-term impact; disaster; public health; case study; disaster management; multi-case analysis; Europe

1. Introduction

The impact of disasters on the health of the people affected and on the public health system can be far-reaching and long lasting. However, studies examining these long-term influences months or even years (mid- to long-term periods) after the event are rare, although their importance is repeatedly underlined [1–3]. Nomura et al. (2016) emphasize the need for a better understanding of long-term health impacts of disasters, in order to be able to set measures and guide actions (before, during, and after the event) to reduce health risks [4]. Moreover, the Sendai Framework for Disaster Risk Reduction points out, in Priority 4 ("Enhancing disaster preparedness for effective response and to 'Build Back Better' in recovery, rehabilitation and reconstruction"), that the importance of post-disaster reviews as they offer a valuable source for learning lessons for the public health system and consequently raise disaster preparedness [5]. Such a systematic review of challenges, dysfunctions, and, consequently, changes, as well as impacts, would be essential to improve preparedness for future events [6]. A better understanding of the impacts of disasters on the public health system and which determinants influence these impacts would be an important contribution to reduce disaster risk. The Sendai Framework advocates for the collection and analysis of the impacts of disasters and consequently the dissemination of the resulting lessons learned across all relevant stakeholders. Researchers are asked for their contributions, sharing their evaluations with practitioners, government officials, and policy makers, to support decision-making and the implementation of good practices on local, regional, and national level [5]. Especially studies on mid- to long-term periods, i.e., months to years after the event, would be needed. A long-term study is difficult, since data are hardly available in a consistent form, and the quality of these data also varies greatly depending on jurisdiction and time frame [7]. Furthermore, the literature review provided no recommendations for the definition of "long-term". The studies differed in the use of time spans, but no discussion was found as to why the authors used specific time spans.

Investigations on the long-term impact of disasters on the health of people affected cover a wide field of research topics (e.g., disaster impacts such as economic losses of the affected population or effects on mental and/or physical health; or focus on specific target groups such as children or the elderly [8–13]). Research on economic and human loss or damage tends to focus on short-term effects, while longer-term effects are difficult to track, and public attention often shifts on the next disaster event [4,14]. Murthy et al. [15] analyzed the progress made in public health preparedness within the US after 9/11, until 2016, by using self-reports from "Centers for Disease Control and Prevention" and reports of congress funding. Fitter et al. [16] examined the recovery of the public health system of Haiti following the 2010 earthquake and cholera outbreak. By using a framework consisting of 10 essential public health services, their research demonstrated progress and improvement made regarding the public health system seven years after the disaster. Our literature review revealed that the research on long-term impact mainly focuses on individual or population health, but less on the systems perspective.

The purpose of this study was to investigate the various long-term impacts on the public health system of five different disasters occurring in Europe, from 1999 to 2013. The chosen holistic research approach allowed the representation of the complexity, specific circumstances, and undertaken measures for each disaster in detail. This process allowed us to identify undertaken adaptions and changes that result in longer-term impacts.

2. Materials and Methods

2.1. Design

We decided to use a case study approach, as it allowed for us to capture both the diversity in disaster management and the complexity of specific circumstances. An extensive collection of rich data makes an embedded multiple-case analysis and presentation possible. The selection of multiple cases resulted from replication logic [17]. We built upon contrasting cases [18], since a variety of contexts, circumstantial factors, and their impact on each case could offer a more complete picture of the longer-term impact of disasters on public health. Since the study was conducted within the EU project PsyCris (PSYchosocial support in CRISis Management), the selected case studies all took place in the European Union. The project consortium decided to use disasters, which are relevant for many EU countries. In addition to the high probability, further criteria for the decision of which cases to use were the scale of the disaster, complexity and number of institutions involved, long-term consequences, and data availability. Moreover, the analysis should include disasters caused by natural hazards, as well as human-caused disasters (e.g., technological or mass-violence).

We decided to use a mixed-method approach consisting of document analysis and expert interviews. As we could not identify a standardized assessment tool to investigate the long-term impact of disasters to the public health system in the literature, we decided to focus on impact models [19–22] that serve as a foundation for the development of the interview guide and the category grid used for the document analysis.

The main categories in the grid were as follows:

- Information about the chosen disaster (what happened, number of people affected, which organizations were involved in disaster management and response, and reaction of the healthcare system);
- General coping strategies and direct effects on health;
- Direct costs and follow-up costs;
- Long-term effects on the public healthcare system;
- Long-term effects on culture and the community.

For our analysis, we reviewed key documents relevant to the disaster-management process and the long-term impact of chosen disasters. The reviewed documents included governmental and organizational reports, legislative documents, journal articles, books, letters, TV documentaries, brochures, and newspaper articles.

As a reconstruction of the complex disaster management process is not possible with existing public documents only, we also conducted expert interviews.

The interview partners all played key roles in the management of the respective disaster. When selecting the interview partners, care was taken to obtain a picture as broad and holistic as possible of the most diverse organizations and units. The professional fields of the interview partners included fire department, emergency psychologists, politicians, armed forces, police, physicians, red cross, forensic, and priests. The average interview duration was 60 min. Table 1 shows the number of interviewees per case study.

Table 1. Overview of number of interviewees per case study.

Case Study	Number of Interviewees
Avalanche, 1999 (Austria)	7
Cable-Car Accident, 2000 (Austria)	7
Airplane Crash, 2002 (Luxembourg)	7
Terror Attack, 2004 (Spain)	7
Flood, 2013 (Austria/Germany)	8

The main themes of the interviews were as follows:

- Job description and responsibilities of the interviewed person;
- Description of the event and the disaster-management process;
- Organization and cooperation of rescue organizations and teams;
- Psychosocial support and challenges for the disaster managers;
- Community resilience;
- Security/protection of population.

For the interview analysis, we used GABEK® (Holistic Processing of Complexity) (Josef Zelger, Innsbruck, Austria), a qualitative method of knowledge organization developed by Josef Zelger, supporting analysis of unstructured texts on the basis of the theory of "linguistic gestalten". The method helps to handle individual thoughts and attitudes and present them in a structured and systematic way. GABEK allows for the transparent organization of knowledge and captures the holistic representation of complex social situations, like disasters, from the perspective of those affected [23]. The analysis was conducted with the corresponding software application GABEK–WinRelan, which combines qualitative content analysis (e.g., coding of keywords, evaluations, or causal relationships) and quantitative measures (e.g., frequencies of keywords and relations) and therefore offers a profound understanding of data, their interlinkages, and their weight [24].

2.2. The Case Studies

2.2.1. Avalanche, Austria, 1999

On 23 February 1999, shortly after 4:00 p.m., an avalanche buried around 100 people in the village of Galtuer (Austria). Ongoing snowfall in the previous days triggered high avalanche risk in the entire federal state of Tyrol. The Paznaun valley, in which Galtuer is located, was already cut off from the outside world before the avalanche, due to the snow conditions. The avalanche hit areas in the village center, which had previously been considered safe from avalanches. Due to the bad weather conditions, no rescue teams were able to reach Galtuer for assistance. The people affected were left to their own devices to rescue the buried victims. Only on the 24 February did the first helicopters could take off and bring the injured from the village to the surrounding hospitals. The Austrian government asked NATO (North Atlantic Treaty Organisation) and neighboring countries for support with additional helicopters. On 25 February, aerial evacuation of the whole valley began with 37 helicopters from Austria, Germany, Switzerland, France, and the US. Thirty-one people died in the avalanche, and 35 were injured (11 of them severely).

2.2.2. Cable-Car Accident, Austria, 2000

In Kaprun (Salzburg), on 11 November 2000, in the tunnel of the cable-car, a fire occurred in the ascending train. The glacier around the Kitzsteinhorn is a popular all-the-year skiing region. On 11 November, the train started at 8:57 in the morning, with 161 passengers aboard. At 9:02 a.m., the first smoke formed. At 9:05 a.m., the train stopped after 600 m in the tunnel; the total distance from the entrance to the exit was 3.8 km. Passengers broke the windows. Smoke rose from the train at the back. The operator saw the fire and gave alarm. Twelve passengers walked with their ski boots downstairs and survived. The other 149 passengers and the operator were in the tunnel. At 9:35 a.m., because of the danger of explosion, the outfall of electricity, and the formation of toxic smoke, the fire brigade had to stop the rescue mission. The mountain station had to be evacuated. At 10:16 a.m., a rescue team started to enter the tunnel. Three people died at the mountain station because of exhaust-gas poisoning. One person survived. At 12:00 p.m., a second team of the fire brigade entered the tunnel. In total, 155 passengers died on 11th of November.

2.2.3. Airplane Crash, Luxembourg, 2002

On Wednesday, 6 November 2002, an airplane of the national air company crashed during the approach to Luxembourg airport. At 10:05 a.m., the airplane reported difficulties during the landing procedure, and 42 s later, the plane disappeared from the radar. The reasons for the airplane crash are based on a mix of technical problems, human errors, and bad weather conditions. At 10:06 a.m., the plane ploughed into a field, and one side of the plane was ripped open. Six passengers were catapulted out. After the crash, the aviation fuel caught fire, and the plane began to burn. Both pilots were trapped in the wreckage. After fire brigades had extinguished the fire, the rescue of the trapped passengers began. The only survivors had been sitting in the front of the aircraft, which had been torn off during the crash, leaving the nose cone embedded in the ground. Twenty people died and two survived severely injured.

2.2.4. Terror Attack, Spain, 2004

On 11 March 2004, ten explosions occurred aboard four commuter trains in the city of Madrid. It was later reported that thirteen improvised explosive devices had been hidden on the trains. The explosions happened during rush hour, on a normal workday, between 7:37 a.m. and 7:39 a.m. At 7:37 a.m., three bombs exploded on train number 21,431, on track two, inside Atocha station, the main capital railway station. At 7:38 a.m., two bombs exploded in train number 21,435, at El Pozo del Tío Raimundo Station. One bomb exploded on train number 21,713, at Santa Eugenia Station, at 7:38 a.m. Then, at 7:39 a.m., four bombs exploded on train number 17,305, on Calle Téllez, approximately 500 m from Atocha station. The bombing was the deadliest terror attack in the history of Spain: 191 people died, and more than 2000 were injured.

2.2.5. Flood, Austria/Germany, 2013

Due to exceptionally heavy rainfalls in early June 2013, extreme flooding of the major river systems occurred throughout Central Europe (particularly Switzerland, Germany, Austria, Czech Republic, Slovakia Hungary, and Serbia). Thousands of people needed to be evacuated from their houses. Twice as much rainfall as average during the month in Austria resulted in the soil becoming saturated. Although forecasts predicted a high rise of water levels, the prognoses have been too low. The water level exceeded the levels seen during the disastrous "once in a century" Central European floods of 2002 in many areas. In Austria, six people died in the flood, and thousands of people had to be evacuated. The infrastructural damages were extensive; railway lines, roads, bridges, and houses were damaged severely.

3. Results

The following section describes the long-term effects of the disasters on the public health system. Figure 1 gives an overview of the framework of analysis. We decided to categorize the identified impact factors into the categories health system performance, and security and health protection. The increased demand during and after a disaster has a direct effect on the health system performance, i.e., the delivering of services, the creation of resources, the stewardship, and, finally, the related financing [25]. Security and health protection refers to post-disaster efforts aiming at optimizing leadership and governance, contingency and preparedness planning, infrastructure, and training, or may lead to an increase in security research funding activities, as well as information and communication activities. The information stated in this section was extracted from the stated sources, as well as from the expert interviews.

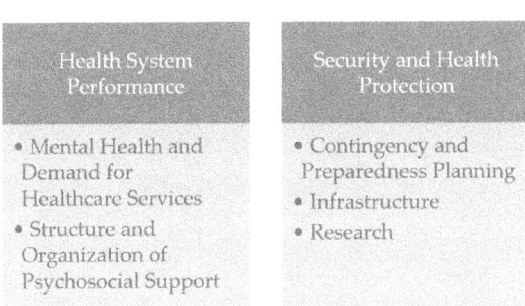

Figure 1. Overview of the aggregated long-term impacts of the analyzed disasters on the public health system (source: the authors).

3.1. Long-Term Impact on Health System Performance

3.1.1. Mental Health and Demand for Healthcare Services

For an adequate public health policy, different dimensions have to be taken into account to optimize the offer for healthcare services, including mental health. The identification and evaluation of how many people are affected by a disaster and develop adjustment disorders because of distress seems to be a challenge for health service providers. For the chosen disasters, statistics about the health status of people affected and derived demand for healthcare services are rare.

Distinction of Target Groups

For an analysis of the demand for healthcare services, a distinction of target groups has to be undertaken. Standardized programs for psychosocial and psychological support are not sufficient, as one crisis manager from Luxembourg stated. The demand for psychosocial and psychological support, but also for medical and physical treatments, mainly differs depending on who is affected. The target groups have to be defined carefully, to guarantee adequate support. A study conducted by the Complutense University of Madrid, with 526 victims of the bombings in Madrid, shows that, ten years later, almost 30% of them presented symptoms of anxiety, depression, and PTSD (posttraumatic stress disorder). Ten years later, nearly 200 victims still received psychological treatment [26]. Moreover, a care program has been launched for people with hearing disabilities after the terror attack in Madrid. The explosions and the effects of the blast caused hearing impairments resulting in total deafness in many victims of these attacks. The General Directorate of Support for Victims of Terrorism taught sign language to victims of these attacks and to their families to help them recover communication within their families [27].

Psychosocial Support for Specific Target Groups

An important lesson that has been identified in all cases is the demand for performance-linked psychosocial support. Target-oriented healthcare delivery has to consider the different needs of people affected (e.g., survivors, families, witnesses, and volunteers). Standardization in the provision of services is seen critically by most of the interview partners. One interview partner from Luxembourg explained: "The pilot survived, there was certainly a different need, with the family, than with those where people died; I also think that people had different approaches to dealing with the accident ... To accommodate these different "points of view", that's extremely difficult. It is often the case that you think you have a solution to a problem, but actually you have to realize in retrospect that you need many solutions for many types of people ... and you also have to give people the freedom to deal with the problem in their own way which is enormously difficult". Because of the fact that nearly all people in the airplane died, the psychosocial support for families played the most important role. The challenge for the disaster management team was the information management to the relatives of the victims, the organization of their arrivals and accommodation, and how to offer psychosocial support.

Compared to our analyzed disasters associated with natural hazards (avalanche and flood), only a small number of passengers survived in the case of the airplane crash or cable-car accident. The main target group for psychosocial support was the relatives who had to arrive from longer distance or respectively from abroad. Locals and tourists have been identified as important relevant target groups for psychosocial and psychological support after the avalanche. Results have shown that the cohesiveness of the community in Galtuer (=locals) had an essential impact on the demand for psychosocial and psychological support.

The terror attack in Spain, with its destructive power for humans and infrastructure, caused a large number of deaths and people injured. Because of the characteristic of the disaster that occurred in this urban area, more walk-in volunteers entered the scene during the acute phase of the disaster, for help. This has an effect on the demand of psychosocial and psychological support in order to consider a large number of walk-in volunteers.

People Affected Who Originate from Abroad

Additionally, in some of the analyzed disasters, no information about psychosocial and psychological support, as well as medical or physical treatment of people who originate from other countries, was given. Especially in the case of the airplane crash, the avalanche and the cable-car accident many victims came from abroad. They were tourists or traveling persons. Survivors and relatives stayed for a certain period time in the country of the event. This leads to the inability to diagnose disorders and reactions, especially of those who were not directly affected by the disaster since some diagnoses cannot be identified immediately after the event, but occur later on (e.g., flashbacks and posttraumatic stress reaction). About 100 of the evacuated tourists in Galtuer were traumatized seriously, and some eventually were confronted with posttraumatic stress disorders later on [28,29].

Refusal of Psychosocial or Psychological Support

Individuals or a community may refuse psychosocial or psychological support. An interview partner involved in psychosocial support after the terror attack in Spain explained the following: "I've learned not to take it personally but as a normal reaction to emotional trauma. Sometimes we had to work with volunteers who were affected by the comments of relatives, like "if you're not going to return my son to me I don't know what you're doing here ... Emotional trauma can cause aggressive reactions and that's normal". Some families who lost relatives during the airplane crash in Luxembourg refused psychosocial support. One survivor of the avalanche was buried for several hours. He preferred to talk with his family to cope with the disaster. It was reported that only one woman with adjustment disorders consulted a psychologist after the avalanche disaster in Galtuer [30].

A community may also refuse psycho0social and psychological support. In Galtuer, locals dealt intensively with the event and experienced common grief. In the first year, they talked among themselves about the disaster and about their experiences, until they felt some relief from their burden. From the cultural point of view, the locals preferred to talk with family, relatives, or friends, but not with outsiders. Locals also had negative associations with psychologists because of two reasons. First, they experienced an insufficient management of psychosocial support directly after the event. Second, a big distance from and distrust of mental healthcare services were observed. The trust into the community was more helpful for the locals to recreate a meaningful life, as compared to professional organized support.

Risk Perceptions

Results gave interesting insights in the awareness of possible causes of risks. People living in endangered zones may perceive possible causes of risks induced by predictable disasters (e.g., risk of a flood or avalanche) as neutral compared to events that arise abruptly without any advanced warning (e.g., airplane crash or terror attack). The resistance of people living in an endangered zone can be influenced of their motivation and individual risk perception living in such an area. This conscious decision has an impact on the mental and physical health in the context of a disaster. The persons may dispose of a higher acceptance of the forces of nature, given the fact that the inhabitants of Galtuer do not evaluate the avalanches negatively [30]. Moreover, in the investigated flood case, in an area that is prone to flood, people are used to dealing with the flood. One interview partner explained the following: "The people down there, they can handle the water... they have their own strategies, they can handle it. And the humility and the acceptance with which they take the flood there, that's fascinating for me. I couldn't imagine that every 10 years I clean out my house, clear out the silt, pump out the water. For them, it's just the water, it's as simple as that". Moreover, most people had family or friends close by with whom they could stay during evacuation, when needed. These two factors are assumed to be a huge reduction of stress for the effected people.

Legal Proceedings

A relevant aspect in dealing with disasters is the way of legal response, especially in the case of organizational failures. One important impact on health was identified in the context of legal proceedings after the cable-car accident. Many family members of the victims complained about the lack of empathy during the legal proceedings. The trial was experienced as unfair by many families, leading to a lot of anger and disappointment. The need for clarity and mental processing was not fulfilled [31,32]. During the trial, a self-help initiative was founded which fought for years for resumption of the legal process [33]. Moreover, after the airplane crash, the legal proceedings lasted over years. One interview partner said the following: "[These] court proceedings have simply taken far too long, and that is disastrous for the people who are affected, who simply want decisions and that they can finish their mourning at some point. It has simply taken far too long".

3.1.2. Structure and Organization of Psychosocial Support

Different longer-term impacts in the structure and organization of psychosocial support have been identified. In one case, the formation of a new organization was induced; in other cases, major or smaller organizational improvements were undertaken. After the avalanche, the disorganization of psychosocial support caused enormous costs for the life assurances, public authorities, and governments. Good management of psychosocial and psychological support, distinct functional attributions, structures, and responsibilities lead to the reduction of conflicts between organizations and institutions involved in the management of a disaster. After the disaster, a discussion was started with regard to financial responsibilities of long-term mental treatments. In the context of psychosocial support, the responsibilities and financing structures for further events were revised.

Formation of New Organizations and Units

A completely new organization for psychosocial support was formed after the Galtuer avalanche. The management of psychosocial support was not organized by one central responsible body. Competition between psychologists and psychotherapists was the source of many conflicts. Additionally, journalists disguised themselves as psychologists and psychotherapists to access the disaster scene. In the years following the disaster, the Austrian Red Cross established the crisis intervention team (KIT—Kriseninterventionsteam). Moreover, it was decided to provide uniforms for the emergency psychologists as they were not associated as professionals by the surviving dependents. An interview partner who was in Galtuer after the avalanche explained the following: "Today it is taken for granted that already the emergency doctor asks if you want a crisis intervention team. But it was different in the past. We didn't wear a uniform, that was a big problem. And nobody knew the service. The care of uninjured survivors simply didn't exist". Although Kaprun, where the cable-car accident happened, is located in Salzburg, in the neighboring province of Tyrol, no structure for psychosocial support existed there at the time of the disaster. However, the tunnel fire was seen as trigger event to also establish a crisis intervention team in Salzburg. In the context of psychosocial support, the extent of the event has led to the formation of a special psychological care unit which takes over the organization and management of psychosocial support. Because of the huge dimension of the terror attack, a systemized supply of psychosocial support for rescue workers in their organizations was established. The awareness for the necessity of psychosocial support for people affected (victims, relatives, and also rescue teams) has grown after all of the analyzed disasters.

3.2. Long-Term Impact on Security and Health Protection

3.2.1. Contingency and Preparedness Planning

Plans and Checklists

An important long-term impact that was identified in all analyzed disasters is the update of existing emergency, civil protection, and national rescue plans and the development or adaption of checklists. Protocols for different contexts have been developed (e.g., intervention protocols for psychological intervention), as well protocols for recruiting people to participate in emergency volunteer management and psychological interventions. The emergency plans and the interfaces between the participating organizations were modified to improve the cooperation and coordination between security teams, armed forces, medical teams (doctors and nurses) in hospitals, social workers, and psychologists. After the airplane crash, psychosocial support was officially integrated as a necessary component into the national rescue plan of Luxembourg.

Establishment of Working Groups and New Units

As a central long-term impact, many different units and working groups were created after the disasters. The established working groups with experts and persons concerned analyzed past events, with the objective of developing recommendations for further improvements. The National Counter-Terrorism Coordination Centre has also been created, aiming to improve coordination between the National Police and the Guardia Civil, and terrorism experts have been sent from the Ministry of Interior to key embassies, to improve exchanges of information. After the airplane crash, an airline emergency committee was rebuilt, and a crisis-support center for Luxair accidents abroad was established. After the avalanche, the local government established a center to link research institutions, non-profit organizations, and businesses in the field of environmental hazards, to improve security measures, create databases, and develop efficient and up-to-date scenario plans.

Legal Changes

Several changes in laws (fire safety regulations and railway act, which also includes funiculars) have occurred after the Kaprun tunnel fire [34]. As a response to the disaster in Galtuer, the federal minister decided to update the guidelines of the danger areas. Basics of the administration procedures are the danger-zone plans, state-specific land-use planning laws, and the forest law of 1975. As a consequence of the flood, the land registry plans have been re-evaluated, and danger zones have been updated. However, various interview partners pointed out the difficulty of keeping danger zones up in the long-term: "The danger is simply that the pressure on the administrative employees comes when nothing has happened for a long time, that one says the yellow zone is no longer necessary. Or people demand the red zone to become a yellow zone in which building, under certain conditions, is possible. The pressure is certainly there, because we are in need of soil that can be built on". Moreover, concepts for resettlement from the endangered areas have been developed. However, it is unclear if and how many people have agreed to resettlement. A decision of the airline management after the crash in Luxembourg led to the implementation of all recommendations from aircraft designers concerning technical details in a compulsory way.

3.2.2. Infrastructure

For all investigated disasters, measures concerning infrastructure were initiated. These measures are referred to as items that improve security, in general, or specific measures to optimize processes, to be better prepared for future disasters. The costs of these infrastructure measures differ substantially.

Large-Scale Investments

After the avalanche, the avalanche barriers around Galtuer were improved and extended. In order to protect the houses of Galtuer in the future, an avalanche barrier was built in the middle of the village center. This special construction, called "Alpinarium", combines avalanche protection and an integrated museum, which deals with the history of Galtuer and the avalanche risk in the area. Further infrastructural measures were the improvement of the meteorological station, a reforestation project, and the extension of the security tunnels at the access road to Galtuer.

High investments were also undertaken in the case of the Austrian flood. Improvements and extended flood protection measures with 34 new building projects were realized. The building process had to be sped up after the flood because 17 projects had not been realized until then. Compared to the building projects, public authorities weighed the importance of the security of the public and decided not to invest in a dam, because of the complex construction project, the enormous monetary investment, and low benefit [35]. For affected public buildings like kindergartens and community buildings, the high possibility of future floods was considered, and a flood-proof way of construction and the addition of flood-resistant materials were implemented. For better forecasts and accurate prognosis, automated water-level measurement stations have been installed. However, improved technical equipment does not automatically lead to better flood protection, as one interview partner explains: "The most difficult thing is the final interpretation of the measured values. A river is a living organism, constantly changing". The damage of the transport medium—as what took place in Kaprun—catalyzed the building of a new ropeway instead of a new funicular due to security reasons. Due to the legal adaptions, many existing funiculars in Austria had to be adapted to guarantee a high level of security for the passengers. Finally, new helicopters with a higher load capacity were purchased for the Austrian Armed Forces, to ensure access to the valleys in the event of natural hazards restricting access to the population.

Small- and Medium-Scale Investments

Small- and medium-sized investments were undertaken in the case of Luxembourg, to improve transport by using more containers for meeting places or restrooms for rescue teams for future operations. These decisions were based on low costs and high flexibility. Additionally, a new operation control car was acquired. In Spain, public infrastructures were controlled more intensively after the terror attack, and constructional adaptions were undertaken. Security measures, like video surveillance, emergency exits, controls of specific infrastructure, and future usage of flak vests, were implemented.

3.2.3. Research

After the Galtuer avalanche, the local government invested in research projects which should reduce future disaster risks. One project was the "Alpine Safety and Information Centre (ASI)". The mission of this non-profit organization was to promote safety mountain environment and to act as a communication bridge between all participating institutions and local organizations. One product of these research investments that is now being used in practice is the "ESIS Tirol" mission information system, an internet platform that facilitates communication and coordination in the event of a disaster. Moreover, new calculations for avalanche simulation models have been developed.

3.3. Others

Because there were some problems in the flow of information between the response organizations, the communication processes have been updated in all investigated disasters. Moreover, technological improvements like the implementation of a uniform radio system in Tyrol and special software have been undertaken. The high media interest after the avalanche and the tunnel fire had a negative impact on the well-being and health of people affected. Therefore, improvements in media management were undertaken. Changes regarding the trainings and exercises (e.g., special topics such as media or psychosocial support, more joint trainings, and cross-border cooperation) could also be observed in all cases. Measures for improvements in the coordination of processes between the organizations and of the handling of professionals and volunteers have been initialized in all cases. Formal and informal networking was identified as a valuable basis for future cooperation. An interview partner pointed out the following: "I would add that in order to improve our response in emergencies, all the teams intervening in an emergency should have more meetings and we should learn to coordinate ourselves better, defining new plans on coordination, structure and control to make sure we all know who's in charge, where we have to go and what we have to do".

Tables 2 and 3 summarize the various impacts each disaster had on the public health system.

Table 2. Overview of long-term impacts on health-system performance.

	Avalanche	Cable Car Accident	Airplane Crash	Terror Attack	Flood
Mental health and demand for health care services	• Significance of different needs of target groups • Refusal of external psychosocial support	• Influence of legal proceedings on mental health and coping	• Significance of different needs of target groups	• Special long-term care for people with hearing impairment due to explosions needed • Sign language courses for families	
Structure and organisation of psychosocial support	• Establishment of KIT by Austrian Red Cross • Financing structure for psychological treatment • Uniforms for emergency psychologists	• Establishment of KIT by Austrian Red Cross		• Formation of special psychological care units	

Table 3. Overview of long-term impacts on security and health protection.

	Avalanche	Cable Car Accident	Airplane Crash	Terror Attack	Flood
Contingency and Preparedness Planning	• Adaption of danger areas • Creation of new working groups and units • Update emergency plans	• Update emergency plans • Changes in fire safety regulations and railway act	• Psychosocial support officially integrated in national rescue plan • Creation of new working groups and units • Update emergency plans	• Creation of new working groups and units • Update emergency plans • Creation of new psychological protocols and plans	• Re-evaluation of land registry pans
Infrastructure	• Avalanche barriers • Reforestation> • Extension security tunnel • Higher load capacity helicopters	• Ropeway instead of funicular	• Extended use of containers • Acquisition of operation control car	• More video surveillance • Adaptions of emergency exits • Flak vests	• Flood protection building measures • Flood-proof way of construction for public buildings • Automated water level measurement
Research	• ASI Centre • ESIS mission information system • Avalanche simulation models		-	-	-

211

Many of the identified impacts overlap with the recommendations in the Sendai Framework [5]: update of preparedness and contingency plans (Paragraph 33a), forecasting and early warning system (Paragraph 33b), trainings and exercises (Paragraphs 33f, 33h, 34f, and 34h), land-use planning (Paragraph 33j), provision of psychosocial support (Paragraph 33o), and revision of laws (Paragraph 33p). It can be concluded from this that the opportunity to "Build Back Better" and consequently enhance disaster preparedness has been taken.

4. Discussion

Based on the results of the literature review, we identified highly fragmented studies without any standardized approach to investigating the long-term impacts of disasters on public healthcare. We did not find any standard definition of long-term impact on the healthcare system. In the context of long-term impacts, the literature mainly focuses on long-term psychological impact effects on affected populations. A broader approach is missing. The studies have also chosen different time frames that do not allow any comparative conclusions.

The investigation of the case studies has shown that each disaster causes aftermaths in various fields. Learning circles [36] play a substantial role in the context of disaster management, as many of the identified long-term impacts on the public health system are the result of a learning process because of inadequate outputs in the past.

The changes observed all seem to have been sustained over the years. One exception is the ASI center, which, according to one interviewee, was closed for political reasons. The necessity of the acquired helicopters is regularly discussed in politics and media. However, landslides and roadblocks due to avalanche risk repeatedly demonstrate their importance for the protection of the affected population.

The study showed us that federalism and organizational boundaries can be a hindrance to improvements: After the 1999 avalanche in Galtuer, the Red Cross created a crisis intervention team in the province of Tyrol. In the neighboring province of Salzburg, however, there was no such infrastructure for psychosocial support yet established when the tunnel fire happened in November 2000. Christensen, Lægreid, and Rykkja (2013) describe something similar in their study: A major obstacle after the terrorist attack in Oslo was the fragmentation of responsibility within government departments. This might have hindered information-sharing and, consequently, taking measures which could have reduced the impact of the Oslo terror attack in 2011, as plans for improving the security of the building had already been established prior the attacks, but not implemented yet [37].

There is the need to analyze the individual and social circumstances of people affected. Results show the importance of analyzing long-term impacts from the perspective of the type (e.g., disaster associated with natural hazards or human-made disaster) and characteristic (e.g., duration and extent) of a disaster, as well as the regional context where a disaster took place. The effectiveness of disaster management procedures is dependent on a number of contingencies (e.g., not only how accurately one system is implemented, but also how well aligned a system is with cultural subsystems) [5,38,39]. As became apparent in Galtuer, the inhabitants applied coping strategies that are rooted in local traditions (e.g., importance of spiritual support). Nevertheless, the consequences of the avalanche led the local population to increasingly open up and cope with this specifically challenging situation by augmented communication. The ex post facto identification of local practices could be highly valuable as basis for discussion within a broader audience of special interest groups (e.g., experts for avalanche risk areas in Austria, Italy, and France).

The chosen cases include disasters caused by natural hazards, as well as human-made disasters. Both types of disasters have been demonstrated to have a potentially high impact on the public health system. However, they might have different consequences concerning preparedness planning. As avalanches and floods are often foreseeable, proactive actions like early warning and evacuation are possible in many cases. On the other hand, avalanches and floods result in relatively large impact areas, which makes response more difficult and requires thorough preparedness regarding mobilization and equipment. Differences between disasters caused by natural hazards and human-caused disasters are also observed with regards to mental health.

Dynes and Quarantelli [40] describe disasters caused by natural hazards as "consensus crises", leading to an increase of community cohesiveness and moral, whereas human-made disasters are characterized by human blame [41]. This has consequences for the coping process and the need for psychological support. Although the disasters analyzed in the case studies may have different characteristics, they share many similarities in their impact. Recurring themes in all the case studies were infrastructural measures, update of emergency plans, changes in communication procedures, and a raised awareness for the importance of mental health and providing psychosocial support. It might prove difficult to compare different individual disaster-management cases in order to elect one best practice example. However, the use of historical lessons can be a valuable source for improvements regarding disaster preparedness [38]. Gaining insights from out-of-sector lessons is often overlooked or considered as not relevant [42]. The recurring themes we identified across the various disasters analyzed in this study, however, demonstrate the learning opportunities from other fields or kinds of disasters. Crichton et al. [42] recommend broadening the perspective and trying to apply lessons beneficially to the own environment. Therefore, the learnings from these European cases can also be of use for countries with other structures and regulations regarding their public health system and disaster management structure. Even though political, socioeconomic, cultural, environmental, and hazard circumstances vary in every state, good practices might be transferable. This learning can be achieved when using a customized approach by "making use of others' experience, for instance by reviewing the contexts of particular measures and the nature of good practices and lessons learned, and then tailoring these to implement policies and activities that are appropriate for the local contexts" [43] (p. 5). Moreover, the Sendai Framework [5] points out the need for adaptions to the respective jurisdictions, capacities, and capabilities of each country.

Although each disaster is unique in its progress and coping, we ask for the design of a standardized assessment system for long-term disaster impacts. This would help to increase comparability of disasters. We share the recommendation expressed in the WHO Health-EDRM framework [1] regarding future research needs: a holistic all-hazard perspective across all disaster-management phases which includes physical, mental, and psychosocial needs. In order to achieve this, multidisciplinary and multi-sectoral collaboration between science, policy makers and practitioners is needed [39,44,45]. Such an exchange and dialogue between stakeholders is important in order to identify knowledge gaps, jointly develop knowledge, and, finally, to put scientific findings into practice [5].

5. Limitations

The chosen case-study methodology can be criticized because of its limited generalizability. The results of our case studies are a preliminary investigation with the intention of generating a first understanding of long-term impact and its underlying determinants. Although it is hardly possible to derive a holistic model covering all cumulative effects of disasters, such case studies can serve as a guide for researchers, policy makers, and disaster managers [3].

The case studies refer to disasters that have occurred in the European Union. Analyzing cases from other countries, which have different disaster management structures and health system regulations, might be an interesting task for future research offering further insights.

6. Conclusions

In this study, we investigated the long-term impacts of disasters on the public health system. We used a mixed-method approach consisting of document analysis and expert interviews. For our analysis, we chose the following cases: an avalanche, a cable-car accident, an airplane crash, a terror attack, and a flood. The analysis of the case studies revealed the variety of direct and indirect impacts on population health and health systems major incidents can have. We grouped the identified impacts into the categories of health-system performance, and security and health protection. Subcategories in health-system performance were mental health and demand for healthcare services, as well as structure and organization of psychosocial support. The subcategories for security and health protection were contingency and preparedness planning, infrastructure, and research. Although we chose contrasting cases, we identified recurring themes in all the cases investigated. A change in communication processes, updates of emergency plans, infrastructural measures, and a higher awareness for psychosocial support was observed in each case study. Our chosen holistic strategy gave us deep insights into each case study and helped us to better understand the undertaken or missing reactions concerning public health. By analyzing past events and their consequences on the public health system, one can develop strategies for better dealing with similar events in the future.

Author Contributions: Conceptualization, M.R., V.S., N.L., and H.S.; methodology, M.R. and V.S.; formal analysis, M.R. and N.L.; investigation, M.R., N.L., and V.S.; writing—original draft preparation, N.L.; writing—review and editing, N.L., M.R., V.S., and H.S.; supervision, M.R. and H.S.; project administration, M.R., N.L., and H.S.; funding acquisition, M.R. All authors have read and agreed to the published version of the manuscript.

Funding: This research was funded by the European Union's Seventh Framework Programme for research, technological development, and demonstration, under grant agreement No. 312395.

Acknowledgments: We thank all disaster managers and other stakeholders who shared their experiences with us, gave us feedback during these initial steps, and helped us develop the current concept. We would also like to thank all our project partners for their tireless support during the past months, to finally reach this point, where we can start to discuss our current research.

Conflicts of Interest: The authors declare no conflict of interest. The funders had no role in the design of the study; in the collection, analyses, or interpretation of data; in the writing of the manuscript; or in the decision to publish the results.

References

1. WHO. *Health Emergency and Disaster Risk Management Framework*; World Health Organization: Geneva, Switzerland, 2019; Available online: https://www.who.int/hac/techguidance/preparedness/health-emergency-and-disaster-risk-management-framework-eng.pdf?ua=1 (accessed on 30 July 2020).
2. Lucchini, R.G.; Hashim, D.; Acquilla, S.; Basanets, A.; Bertazzi, P.A.; Bushmanov, A.; Crane, M.; Harrison, D.J.; Holden, W.; Landrigan, P.J. A comparative assessment of major international disasters: The need for exposure assessment, systematic emergency preparedness, and lifetime health care. *BMC Public Health* **2017**, *17*, 46. [CrossRef] [PubMed]
3. Oloruntoba, R.; Sridharan, R.; Davison, G. A proposed framework of key activities and processes in the preparedness and recovery phases of disaster management. *Disasters* **2018**, *42*, 541–570. [CrossRef] [PubMed]
4. Nomura, S.; Parsons, A.J.; Hirabayashi, M.; Kinoshita, R.; Liao, Y.; Hodgson, S. Social determinants of mid- to long-term disaster impacts on health: A systematic review. *Int. J. Disaster Risk Reduct.* **2016**, *16*, 53–67. [CrossRef]
5. UNISDR. *Sendai Framework for Disaster Risk Reduction 2015–2030*; UNISDR: Geneva, Switzerland, 2015.
6. Sundnes, K.O. 18. Preparedness process. *Scand. J. Public Health* **2014**, *42*, 151–172. [CrossRef]
7. Hettige, S.; Haigh, R. An integrated social response to disasters: The case of the Indian Ocean tsunami in Sri Lanka. *Disaster Prev. Manag.* **2016**, *25*, 595–610. [CrossRef]
8. Dell'Osso, L.; Carmassi, C.; Massimetti, G.; Daneluzzo, E.; Di Tommaso, S.; Rossi, R. Full and partial PTSD among young adult survivors 10 months after the L'Aquila 2009 earthquake: Gender differences. *J. Affect. Disord.* **2011**, *131*, 79–83. [CrossRef]
9. Hussain, Y.; Bagguley, P. Funny Looks: British Pakistanis' experiences after 7 July 2005. *Ethn. Racial Stud.* **2013**, *36*, 28–46. [CrossRef]
10. Dorn, T.; Yzermans, J.C.; Spreeuwenberg, P.M.M.; Schilder, A.; Van Der Zee, J. A cohort study of the long-term impact of a fire disaster on the physical and mental health of adolescents. *J. Trauma. Stress* **2008**, *21*, 239–242. [CrossRef]
11. Rafiey, H.; Momtaz, Y.A.; Alipour, F.; Khankeh, H.; Ahmadi, S.; Khoshnami, M.S.; Haron, S.A. Are older people more vulnerable to long-term impacts of disasters? *Clin. Interv. Aging* **2016**, *11*, 1791–1795. [CrossRef]

12. Goenjian, A.K.; Roussos, A.; Steinberg, A.M.; Sotiropoulou, C.; Walling, D.; Kakaki, M.; Karagianni, S. Longitudinal study of PTSD, depression, and quality of life among adolescents after the Parnitha earthquake. *J. Affect. Disord.* **2011**, *133*, 509–515. [CrossRef]
13. Annang, L.; Wilson, S.; Tinago, C.; Sanders, L.W.; Bevington, T.; Carlos, B.; Cornelius, E.; Svendsen, E. Photovoice: Assessing the Long-Term Impact of a Disaster on a Communitys Quality of Life. *Qual. Health Res.* **2016**, *26*, 241–251. [CrossRef] [PubMed]
14. Coffman, M.; Noy, I. Hurricane Iniki: Measuring the long-term economic impact of a natural disaster using synthetic control. *Environ. Dev. Econ.* **2011**, *17*, 187–205. [CrossRef]
15. Murthy, B.P.; Molinari, N.-A.M.; Leblanc, T.T.; Vagi, S.J.; Avchen, R.N. Progress in Public Health Emergency Preparedness-United States, 20012016–. *Am. J. Public Health* **2017**, *107*, S180–S185. [CrossRef] [PubMed]
16. Fitter, D.L.; Delson, D.B.; Guillaume, F.D.; Schaad, A.W.; Moffett, D.B.; Poncelet, J.-L.; Lowrance, D.; Gelting, R.J. Applying a New Framework for Public Health Systems Recovery following Emergencies and Disasters: The Example of Haiti following a Major Earthquake and Cholera Outbreak. *Am. J. Trop. Med. Hyg.* **2017**, *97*, 4–11. [CrossRef] [PubMed]
17. Yin, R.K. *Case Study Research Design*; SAGE Publications: Thousand Oaks, CA, USA, 2009.
18. Mabry, L. Case study in social research. In *The Sage Handbook of Social Research Methods*; SAGE Publications Inc.: London, UK, 2008.
19. Shoaf, K.I.; Rottman, S.J. The role of public health in disaster preparedness, mitigation, response, and recovery. *Prehosp. Disaster Med.* **2000**, *15*, 18–20. [CrossRef]
20. A Scoping Study of Emergency Planning and Management in Health Care: What Further Research is Needed? Available online: http://www.netscc.ac.uk/netscc/hsdr/files/project/SDO_FR_09-1005-01_V01.pdf (accessed on 17 July 2020).
21. Lindell, M.K.; Prater, C.; Perry, R.W. *Introduction to Emergency Management*; John Wiley & Sons: Hoboken, NJ, USA, 2006.
22. Lindell, M.K. Disaster studies. *Curr. Sociol.* **2013**, *61*, 797–825. [CrossRef]
23. Zelger, J. Twelve Steps of GABEKWinRelan A Procedure for Qualitative Opinion Research, Knowledge Organization and Systems Development. In *GABEK II. Zur Qualitativen Forschung. On Qualitative Research*; Buber, R., Zelger, J., Eds.; Studienverlag: Innsbruck, Austria, 2000; pp. 205–220.
24. Raich, M.; Mueller, J.; Abfalter, D. Hybrid analysis of textual data. *Manag. Decis.* **2014**, *52*, 737–754. [CrossRef]
25. Evans, D.B.; Murray, C.; WHO. *Health Systems Performance Assessment: Debates, Methods and Empiricism*; World Health Organization: Geneva, Switzerland, 2003.
26. Seguimiento y Tratamiento Psicológico de las Víctimas de los Atentados. Available online: https://www.youtube.com/watch?v=_AdXnr_oWEA (accessed on 17 July 2020).
27. Ministerio de Interior Gobierno de España. *El Ministerio del Interior ha Indemnizado y Ayudado a las Víctimas de los Atentados del 11-M con 318,2 Millones de Euros en Diez Años*; Ministerio de Interior Gobierno de España: Madrid, Spain, 2014.
28. Brauchle, G.; Juen, B.; Hötzendorfer, C.; Bänninger-Huber, E. Notfallpsycho logie oder Psychotherapie. Aufgaben und Einsatzkriterien psychologischen Handelns in Großschadensereignissen. *Psychol. Österreich* **2000**, *20*, 260–264.
29. Brauchle, G.; Juen, B.; Hötzendorfer, C.; Bänninger-Huber, E. *Die "Entdeckung" der Katastrophe als Betätigungsfeld—Kritische Betrachtungen über Helfer als "Helden" am Beispiel der Lawinenkatastrophe von Galtür Brauchle Gernot, Juen Barbara, Hötzendorfer Christian, Bänninger-Huber Eva*; Texte der Fachhochschule Villingen-Schwenningen, Hochschule für Polizei: Villingen-Schwenningen, Germany, 2000; pp. 1–14.
30. Rieken, B. *Schatten über Galtür? Gespräche mit Einheimischen über die Lawine von 1999*; Waxmann: Münster, Germany, 2010.
31. Kaprun: Zurück ins Leben. Available online: https://tvthek.orf.at/history/Die-Katastrophe-von-Kaprun/9840723/Kaprun-Zurueck-ins-Leben/9485772 (accessed on 30 July 2020).
32. Kaprun Disaster Protokoll einer Katastrophe Teil 4. 2014. Available online: https://www.youtube.com/watch?v=s5jSnY4vKRE (accessed on 30 July 2020).
33. Godeysen, H. *Gerechtigkeit für Kaprun*; Die Zeit: Hamburg, Germany, 2009.
34. Meyer, H.J. The Kaprun cable car fire disaster—Aspects of forensic organisation following a mass fatality with 155 victims. *Forensic Sci. Int.* **2003**, *138*, 1–7. [CrossRef]
35. *Bures will Hochwasserschutz beschleunigen*; Die Presse: Vienna, Austria, 2013.

36. Hedberg, B. How organizations learn and unlearn. In *Handbook of Organziational Design*; Nyström, P.C., Starbuck, W.H., Eds.; Oxford University Press: New York, NY, USA, 1981; pp. 3–26.
37. Christensen, T.; Lægreid, P.; Rykkja, L.H. After a terrorist attack: Challenges for political and administrative leadership in Norway. *J. Contingencies Cris. Manag.* **2013**, *21*, 167–177. [CrossRef]
38. Roth, F.; Prior, T. Learning from Disaster Events and Exercises in Civil Protection Organizations. *Risk Resil. Rep.* **2016**, *5*, 1–27.
39. Généreux, M.; Lafontaine, M.; Eykelbosh, A. From science to policy and practice: A critical assessment of knowledge management before, during, and after environmental public health disasters. *Int. J. Environ. Res. Public Health* **2019**, *16*, 587. [CrossRef] [PubMed]
40. Dynes, R.R.; Quarantelli, E.L. *Organization Communications and Decision Making in Crises*; Disaster Research Center: Columbus, OH, USA, 1976.
41. Tierney, K.; Lindell, M.; Perry, R.W. *Facing the Unexpected: Disaster Preparedness and Response in the United States*; Natural Hazards and Disasters; Joseph Henry Press: Washington, DC, USA, 2001; Volume 2001, p. 281.
42. Crichton, M.T.; Ramsay, C.G.; Kelly, T. Enhancing Organizational Resilience Through Emergency Planning: Learnings from Cross-Sectoral Lessons. *J. Contingencies Cris. Manag.* **2009**, *17*, 24–37. [CrossRef]
43. UNISDR & UNOCHA. *Disaster Preparedness for Effective Response Guidance and Indicator Package for Implementing Priority Five of the Hyogo Framework, Hyogo Framework for Action: 2005–2015 Building the Resilience of Nations and Communities to Disasters*; United Nations: New York, NY, USA, 2008; p. 60.
44. Lo, S.T.T.; Chan, E.Y.Y.; Chan, G.K.W.; Murray, V.; Abrahams, J.; Ardalan, A.; Kayano, R.; Yau, J.C.W. Health Emergency and Disaster Risk Management (Health-EDRM): Developing the Research Field within the Sendai Framework Paradigm. *Int. J. Disaster Risk Sci.* **2017**, *8*, 145–149. [CrossRef]
45. Kayano, R.; Chan, E.Y.Y.; Murray, V.; Abrahams, J.; Barber, S.L. WHO thematic platform for health emergency and disaster risk management research network (TPRN): Report of the kobe expert meeting. *Int. J. Environ. Res. Public Health* **2019**, *16*, 1232. [CrossRef] [PubMed]

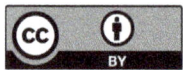

© 2020 by the authors. Licensee MDPI, Basel, Switzerland. This article is an open access article distributed under the terms and conditions of the Creative Commons Attribution (CC BY) license (http://creativecommons.org/licenses/by/4.0/).

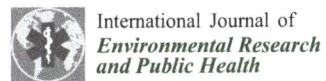

Article

Increased Medical Visits and Mortality among Adults with Cardiovascular Diseases in Severely Affected Areas after Typhoon Morakot

Hsin-I Shih [1,2,3], Tzu-Yuan Chao [4], Yi-Ting Huang [2], Yi-Fang Tu [2,5], Tzu-Ching Sung [6], Jung-Der Wang [3] and Chia-Ming Chang [2,7,*]

1. Department of Emergency Medicine, National Cheng Kung University Hospital, College of Medicine, National Cheng Kung University, Tainan 70403, Taiwan; hshihnckutw@gmail.com
2. School of Medicine, College of Medicine, National Cheng Kung University, Tainan 70101, Taiwan; alage@gs.ncku.edu.tw (Y.-T.H.); nckutu@gmail.com (Y.-F.T.)
3. Department of Public Health, College of Medicine, National Cheng Kung University, Tainan 70101, Taiwan; jdwang121@gmail.com
4. Department of Urban Planning, National Cheng Kung University, Tainan 70101, Taiwan; tychao@mail.ncku.edu.tw
5. Department of Paediatrics, National Cheng Kung University Hospital, College of Medicine, National Cheng Kung University, Tainan 70403, Taiwan
6. School of Medicine for International Students, I-Shou University, Kaohsiung 82445, Taiwan; vivian1223@isu.edu.tw
7. Division of Geriatrics & Gerontology, Department of Internal Medicine, National Cheng Kung University Hospital, Tainan 70403, Taiwan
* Correspondence: 10108040@gs.ncku.edu.tw

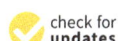

Received: 19 June 2020; Accepted: 2 September 2020; Published: 8 September 2020

Abstract: Natural disasters have negative health impacts on chronic diseases in affected populations. Severely affected areas are usually rural areas with limited basic infrastructure and a population have that has limited access to optimal healthcare after a disaster. Patients with cardiovascular diseases are required to maintain quality care, especially after disasters. A population-based case-control study enrolled adults from the National Health Insurance Registry who had ischemic heart disease and cerebrovascular disease histories and lived in the area affected by Typhoon Morakot in 2009. Monthly medical visits for acute cerebrovascular and ischemic heart diseases markedly increased at approximately 1–2 months after the typhoon. Survival analysis during the two years following the typhoon indicated a significant increase in mortality in adults with an acute ischemic heart disease history who lived in the severely affected area. Mortality hazard analysis showed that among affected adults with previous cerebrovascular diseases and acute ischemic heart diseases, patients with diabetes (adjusted hazard ratio [HR]: 1.3–1.7), Chronic Kidney Disease (CKD) (adjusted HR: 2.0–2.7), chronic obstructive pulmonary diseases (COPD) and asthma (adjusted HR: 1.7–2.1), liver cirrhosis (adjusted HR: 2.3–3.3) and neoplasms (adjusted HR: 1.1–2.1) had significantly increased mortality rates. Consequently, high-quality and accessible primary healthcare plans should be made available to maintain and support affected populations after disasters.

Keywords: disaster; typhoon; flood; elderly; cardiovascular diseases; cerebrovascular diseases

---

1. Introduction

The number of reported weather-related natural disasters has been increasing since the 1960s. These disasters result in over 60,000 deaths each year worldwide [1,2]. Increasingly variable rainfall patterns have increased the frequency and intensity of flooding, which has had great impacts on human health. People may be forced to move, which heightens the risk of health effects on mental disorders, communicable diseases, and chronic comorbidities. Heavy floods cause substantial infrastructure damage and lead to massive economic and personal losses for communities [3,4]. These disasters require large-scale, multinational coordination to provide urgent humanitarian aid and continuous relief [5] to the affected areas.

Severely affected areas are usually rural and coastal areas with limited basic infrastructure and a small population. Rural and coastal areas are more likely than urban areas to have an inequitably high burden due to healthcare disparities. These disparities contribute to the inadequate provision of basic healthcare services that arise from few medical facilities, a minimal number of providers, few specialty practices, and a lack of accompanying technical innovations and health promotion programs [6–8]. In medically underserved rural settings, people experiencing barriers to primary healthcare tend to have a low income, low education level and high rate of unemployment [9]. Patients with chronic comorbidities need to maintain a delicate balance of care to decrease complications during and after disasters. A previous study found that 24.3% of visits to emergency treatment facilities after Hurricane Katrina were for chronic diseases or related conditions [10]. Following the March 2011 earthquake and tsunami in Japan, increased mortality was observed in some patients with chronic comorbidities [11]. Increased numbers of visits for acute ischemic heart disease and stroke following natural disasters have been identified after natural disasters. Survivors also have to cope with stressors such as searching for food and shelter, relocating, crowding, financial hardship, and navigating social services [12]. Stressors from hurricanes and other natural disasters can cause chronic and acute mental stress, which can trigger cardiovascular events. Affected communities, especially those who are severely affected and in a rural area, are faced with a myriad of disparities, each posing a barrier to timely response and complete recovery from a disaster.

The Asia-Pacific region has been recognized as the region with the highest risk of major disasters [13]. Moreover, Taiwan may be the location most vulnerable to natural hazards, with 73% of its land and population exposed to three or more hazards [14]. Typhoon Morakot affected the West Pacific Region from August 6 to 11 August 2009. On August 7, it caused copious amounts of rainfall in Taiwan, peaking at 2777 mm (109.3 in). This extreme amount of rain triggered massive mudflows and severe flooding throughout southern Taiwan, causing 702 deaths and roughly US$6.76 billion in financial losses [15,16]. Almost all southern Taiwan experienced record-breaking heavy rain, and the associated flood damage required people to relocate to temporary shelters for approximately six months to one year. After Typhoon Morakot, multidisciplinary, large-scale reconstruction and relief actions were initiated. Residents who lived in the affected areas before the disaster were identified by the Ministry of Health and Welfare and received partial medical expense reimbursement for 3 months. Medical teams and clinics were established in the temporary shelters to provide primary basic healthcare in the severely affected areas for at least 6 months. A series of recovery and relief measures were implemented and initiated in the following years. To evaluate the parameters affecting health outcomes of cardiovascular and cerebrovascular diseases among different levels of affected areas (Appendix A Table A1), we conducted a longitudinal follow-up study to assess health parameters among adult residents in different areas affected by Typhoon Morakot, a major disaster.

2. Materials and Methods

2.1. Data Source

Data from the Taiwan National Health Insurance (NHI) Database from the National Health Research Institute (NHRI) was analyzed. All claims submitted by physicians to the National Health Insurance Registry must include a diagnostic code based on the International Classification of Diseases, Ninth Revision, Clinical Modification (ICD-9-CM) developed by the World Health Organization which allows the NHI Registry to verify claims and generate statistics about causes of illness and death [17].

The NHRI recorded data included residents' demographic data, medications, treatments (including operations), and disease diagnoses at four different levels of healthcare facilities. After Typhoon Morakot, the NHI Bureau identified residents who had lived in the affected areas before the disaster and provided partial reimbursement of their medical expenses based on the Regulation "National Health Insurance Reimbursement for Medical Expenses after Typhoon Morakot". Adult residents living in the affected area were enrolled for further analysis.

2.2. Study Design

A population-based longitudinal case-control study was conducted. In total, historical data of 715,244 adults who had lived in the affected areas were obtained for this study. Adult patients with healthcare facility visit records were analyzed. The index date was 8 August 2009, the date that Typhoon Morakot struck Taiwan. The adults were separated into non-elderly and elderly groups (18–64 years and 65 years and older, respectively). Patients with chronic medical conditions requiring long-term follow-up, such as diabetes mellitus (DM), hypertension, chronic kidney disease (CKD), heart disease, hyperlipidemia, chronic obstructive pulmonary disease (COPD), liver cirrhosis and neoplasms, were identified from long-term medical records, and records of their most recent follow-up visit for their chronic medical conditions were reviewed to assess their comorbidities after the disaster. The observation period of the study was from January 2008 to December 2011.

Patients with underlying medical comorbidities, including hypertension (ICD-9-CM: 401–405), DM (ICD-9-CM: 250), asthma (ICD-9-CM: 493), chronic heart failure (ICD-9-CM: 428, 410–414), COPD (ICD-9-CM: 491–496, excluding 493, 495), liver cirrhosis (ICD-9-CM: 571.5), neoplasms (ICD-9-CM: 140–239) and CKD (ICD-9-CM: 585, 582, 583.9), that were recorded before the index date were selected and noted. All medical service utilization records after the index date were reviewed. The calculated Charlson Comorbidity Index (CCI) values indicated the severity of these patients' comorbidities. The patients' socioeconomic statuses were based on their income records, as reported to the NHI bureau.

The rates of acute ischemic heart diseases and cerebrovascular diseases in adults who lived in the affected areas were analyzed. The study analyzed patients with acute ischemic heart disease (ICD-9-CM: 410–414), intracranial hemorrhage (ICH) (ICD-9-CM: 430–432) and ischemic stroke (ICD-9-CM: 433–437) before and after Typhoon Morakot. The above diseases that occurred after the index date were evaluated to determine patients' health outcomes before and after Typhoon Morakot. The monthly visits of acute illnesses were measured from the patients' medical records. For each person, the occurrence of the same event within the same one-month period was counted only once. Hospitalization records after Typhoon Morakot were also analyzed to evaluate the health hazards, heart failure (ICD-9-CM: 428); common infections such as lower respiratory tract infection (ICD-9-CM: 480–488), urinary tract infection (ICD-9-CM: 590, 595, 597, 599), and skin and soft tissue infections (ICD-9-CM: 680–686); and trauma and injury (ICD-9-CM: 850–959).

The validated definition of mortality was adapted from the NHI database and was based on the insurance status among those affected adults enrolled in our study. Mortality cases were defined as enrolled adults withdrawn due to death or critical discharge with the diagnosis of one of the most common twenty causes of death (ICD-9-CM) of National Statistics in Taiwan, and without any medical records after withdrawal date, missing for more than six months, and were disqualified as an insurance applicant of the NHI program such as immigration and the expiration of the duration of stay of aliens [18]. All causes of death for the affected adults enrolled in this study between August 2009 and December 2011 were enrolled for further survival and hazard ratio analysis.

2.3. Spatial-Temporal Analysis

The classification of township and metropolitan areas in Taiwan was adapted from the 2005 Taiwan Social Change Survey, which tracks and provides insights into long-term societal trends and developments in each town or metropolitan area in six prospective areas through nationally representative survey data obtained through cluster sampling; data obtained included the proportion of the working population employed in the service sector, the proportion of the industrial population, the proportion of the population 15–64 years old, the proportion of the elderly population, the proportion of the population that attained at least a bachelor's degree, and the population density of the area. In total, three different town or metropolitan areas (urban, suburban, and rural) were included [19].

2.4. Covariates

In addition to age and sex, area of residence was incorporated into the study design as a demographic variable. Comorbidities considered in this study included hypertension, DM, hypertension, COPD and asthma, liver cirrhosis, and neoplasms, which were defined by major diagnosis codes with at least three months' long-term prescriptions before the index date with relevant ICD-9-CM codes mentioned above.

2.5. Statistical Analysis

The distribution of the study population, which was based on demographic and disease history data such as sex, age, diabetes, chronic kidney, pulmonary, and liver diseases, living place, social economic status, cardiovascular, cerebrovascular diseases, and mortality was analyzed. Besides A case control study to evaluate time-to-event outcomes was applied. To evaluate differences among different study groups, the chi-square test was used for categorical variables, and the Student's *t* test was used for continuous variables. The control group was matched for age and sex using propensity scoring methods. Major underlying diseases and living locations were selected from the univariate and multi-variate Cox proportional hazard regression models with backward eliminations to estimate hazard ratios of mortality among affected adults with a history of cardiovascular and cerebrovascular events. All tests of significance were 2-tailed, and a *p* value of 0.05 or less was considered statistically significant. Robust Cox models using robust sandwich variance estimators were applied considering clustering within matched sets. Moreover, stratified Cox models using stratification of the propensity scores were also adopted to treat the matched sets. The former approach resulted in an unbiased estimation of marginal hazard ratios that were compared with a biased estimation of marginal hazard ratios resulting from the latter approach. Each comparison value and its 95% confidence interval (95% CI) were also analyzed. All data management and statistical analyses were performed with SAS 9.4 software (SAS Institute, Cary, NC, USA). All statistical tests were 2-sided, and *p* values less than 0.05 were considered statistically significant.

2.6. Ethical Issues

All provisions of the study were performed in accordance with the principles of the Declaration of Helsinki and the Declaration of Taipei [20]. Patients' personal information was encrypted to protect their privacy, and the electronic databases were decoded for research; therefore, the requirement for informed consent was waived by the institutional review board (IRB). This study was approved by the IRB of the study hospital (IRB No: A-ER-103-176).

3. Results

A total of 715,244 adult patient files were identified; 199,991 patients (28%) were in the elderly group. Female patients were predominant (398,819, 56%). The study diagram is shown in the Appendix A Figure A1. The demographic characteristics of the study population between different severity of affected areas are presented in Table 1. Compared to the adults living in the moderately affected area, those in the severely affected area before Typhoon Morakot were older, lived more in rural areas, had a higher rate of multiple underlying diseases (CCI ≥ 1: 45% vs. 41%) and cardiovascular disease history (18% vs. 15%). Besides, the adults living in the severely affected area also had higher rates of underlying chronic diseases, such as DM (16% vs. 14%), hypertension (33% vs. 26%), heart disease (12% vs. 10%), COPD and asthma (6% vs. 4%).

Table 1. Demographic and clinical characteristics of adults living between different severity of affected areas before Typhoon Morakot.

Characteristics	Adults Living in the Affected Area			Chi²-Test p Value
	Moderately Affected (n = 574,089) No. (%)	Severely Affected (n = 141,155) No. (%)	Total (n = 715,244) No. (%)	
Sex				
Female	321,697 (56)	77,122 (55)	398,819 (56)	<0.0001
Age (years)				
Mean ± SD *	51.69 ± 17.87	55.29 ± 17.64	52.40 ± 17.88	
Age Group				
Elderly	151,801 (26)	48,190 (34)	199,991 (28)	<0.0001
Related Cardiovascular History (January 2008–July 2009)				
Either of the following	86,198 (15)	24,969 (18)	111,167 (16)	<0.0001
Ischemic heart diseases	59,226 (10)	17,093 (12)	76,319 (11)	<0.0001
Acute cerebrovascular diseases	36,559 (6)	11,003 (8)	47,562 (7)	<0.0001
Socioeconomic Status (USD/month)				
Low < $750 USD	301,416 (53)	93,431 (66)	394,847 (55)	
Location				
Urban	150,232 (26)	0 (0)	150,232 (21)	<0.0001
Suburban	276,951 (48)	47,890 (34)	324,841 (45)	
Rural	146,906 (26)	93,265 (66)	240,171 (34)	
CCI †				
0	338,653 (59)	77,717 (55)	416,370 (58)	<0.0001
1–2	183,175 (32)	49,034 (35)	232,209 (32)	
>2	52,261 (9)	14,404 (10)	66,665 (9)	
Underlying diseases				
DM	79,653 (14)	21,886 (16)	101,539 (14)	<0.0001
Hypertension	143,332 (26)	45,940 (33)	189,272 (26)	<0.0001
CKD	12,959 (2)	3058 (2)	16,017 (2)	0.04
Heart disease	57,835 (10)	17,171 (12)	75,006 (10)	<0.0001
COPD & asthma	25,612 (4)	8116 (6)	33,728 (6)	<0.0001
Liver cirrhosis	9570 (2)	2007 (1)	11,577 (1)	0.02
Neoplasms	32,304 (6)	7341 (5)	39,645 (6)	0.01

* Standard deviation; † Charlson Comorbidity Index. DM: Diabetes mellitus; CKD: Chronic kidney disease; COPD: Chronic obstructive pulmonary diseases.

Figure 1 shows the number of monthly visits for acute ischemic heart disease and cerebrovascular events by affected adults before and after Typhoon Morakot, i.e., from 2008 to 2010. There was a markedly increased peak in visits in the same month Typhoon Morakot occurred in both the severely and moderately affected areas and in both elderly and non-elderly adults. Compared to that for acute ischemic heart disease, the difference in the number of monthly visits for acute cerebrovascular diseases was more prominent in the moderately affected areas, particularly in the elderly group.

The demographic data before and after matching are summarized in Table 2. After matching for age and sex, the proportions of adults living in the severely affected area with a history of cerebrovascular diseases (44% vs. 42%, $p < 0.001$), hypertension (62% vs. 58%, $p < 0.0001$), hypertension (62% vs. 58%, $p < 0.0001$), COPD and asthma (12% vs. 11%, $p = 0.0001$) was higher than those in the moderately affected area. Adults living in the severely affected area had a higher proportion of living in rural area (71% vs. 32%, $p < 0.0001$) and low-income status than those living in the moderately affected area (monthly income < 750 USD: 73% vs. 60%, $p < 0.0001$). However, there was no significant difference in the CCI score between adults living in the moderately and severely affected areas.

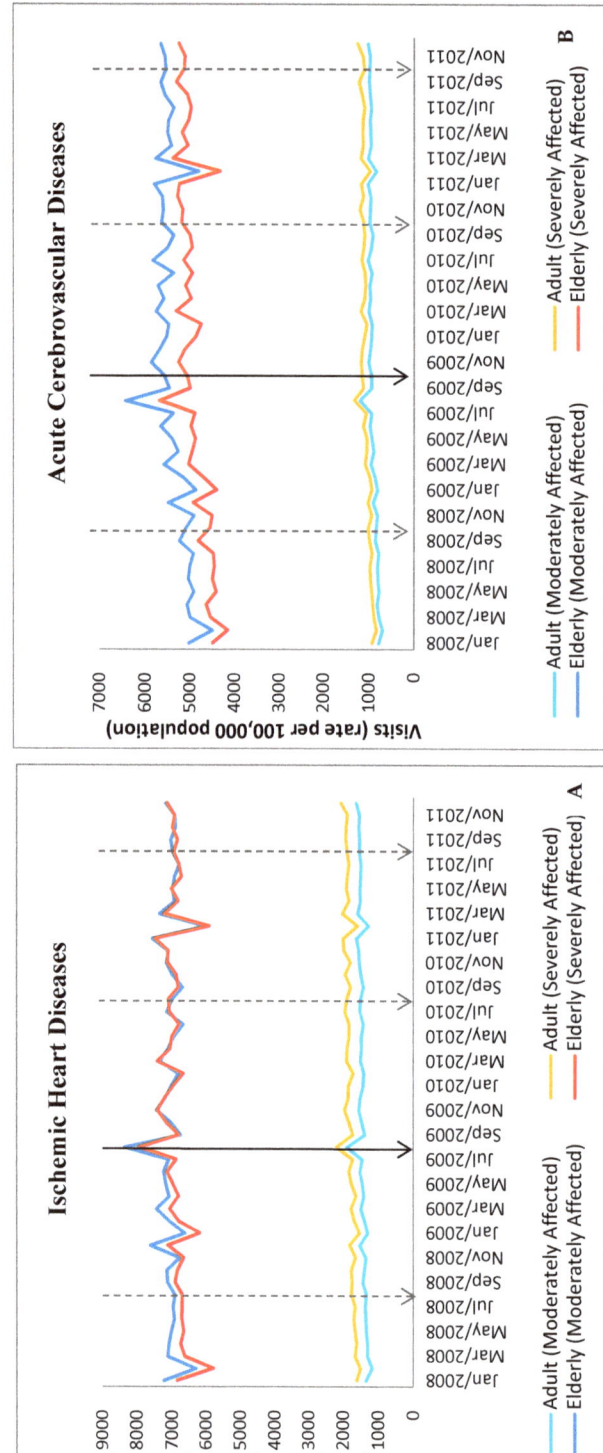

Figure 1. Monthly visits for acute cardiovascular and cerebrovascular events by affected adults before and after Typhoon Morakot. (**A**): Ischemic Heart Diseases; (**B**): Acute Cerebrovascular Diseases. Vertical solid lines: Index Month (August/2009); vertical dotted lines: August/2008, August/2010 and August/2011.

Table 2. Demographics of affected adults before and after matching.

Characteristics	Adult Patients with a Related Cardiovascular History (January 2008–July 2009)					
	Pre-Match			Post-Match		
	Moderately Affected ($n = 86{,}198$) No. (%)	Severely Affected ($n = 24{,}969$) No. (%)	Chi^2 Test p Value	Moderately Affected ($n = 24{,}969$) No. (%)	Severely Affected ($n = 24{,}969$) No. (%)	Chi^2 Test p Value
Sex						
Female	45,030 (52)	13,257 (53)	0.02	13,257 (53)	13,257 (53)	1.00
Age (years)						
Mean ± SD *	66.84 ± 12.76	67.72 ± 12.37		67.52 ± 12.63	67.72 ± 12.37	
Age Group						
Elderly	51,724 (60)	15,814 (63)	<0.0001	15,814 (63)	15,814 (63)	1.00
Related Cardiovascular History (January 2008–July 2009)						
Ischemic heart disease	59,226 (69)	17,093 (68)	0.45	17,158 (69)	17,093 (68)	0.53
Acute cerebrovascular diseases	36,559 (42)	11,003 (44)	<0.0001	10,568 (42)	11,003 (44)	<0.0001
Socioeconomic Status (USD/month)						
Low < $750 USD	51,230 (59)	18,169 (73)	<0.0001	14,985 (60)	18,169 (73)	<0.0001
Location						
Urban	21,279 (25)	0 (0)		6213 (25)	0 (0)	<0.0001
Suburban	36,826 (42)	7267 (29)	<0.0001	10,650 (43)	7267 (29)	
Rural	28,093 (33)	17,702 (71)		8106 (32)	17,702 (71)	
CCI †						
0	17,928 (21)	4918 (20)	0.0007	5102 (20)	4918 (20)	0.11
1–2	44,003 (51)	12,911 (52)		12,744 (51)	12,911 (52)	
> 2	24,267 (28)	7140 (29)		7123 (29)	7140 (29)	
Underlying diseases						
DM	24,863 (29)	7063 (28)	0.09	7225 (29)	7063 (28)	0.11
Hypertension	49,642 (58)	15,468 (62)	<0.0001	14,430 (58)	15,468 (62)	<0.0001
CKD	4613 (5.4)	1195 (4.8)	0.0004	1372 (5.5)	1195 (4.8)	0.0003
Heart disease	41,546 (48)	12,326 (49)	0.0012	12,111 (48)	12326 (49)	0.05
COPD & asthma	8891 (10)	2933 (12)	<0.0001	2662 (11)	2933 (12)	0.0001
Liver cirrhosis	1946 (2.3)	424 (1.6)	<0.0001	553 (2.2)	424 (1.7)	<0.0001
Neoplasms	6520 (7.6)	1748 (7.0)	0.0028	1933 (7.7)	1748 (7.0)	0.0015

* Standard deviation; † Charlson Comorbidity Index. DM: Diabetes mellitus; CKD: Chronic kidney disease; COPD: Chronic obstructive pulmonary diseases.

A mortality analysis of adults with cardiovascular and cerebrovascular disease histories was performed. Robust Cox models using robust sandwich variance estimators for clustering within matched sets were used to analyze survival after Typhoon Morakot in affected adults with cardiovascular and cerebrovascular disease histories in the moderately and severely affected areas. Before Typhoon Morakot, the robust sandwich estimation for three-year survival between moderately and severely affected areas revealed a significant difference in the survival rate of affected adults with a cardiovascular events history ($p = 0.0047$) but did not reveal a significant difference in the survival rate of affected adults with a cerebrovascular event history.

Hospitalizations after Typhoon Morakot in affected adults with cardiovascular and cerebrovascular histories before Typhoon Morakot were analyzed (Table 3). Compared to the hospitalization rate in affected adults in the moderately affected area, a slightly increased hospitalization rate was noted among affected adults living in the severely affected area after Typhoon Morakot in terms of acute ischemic heart diseases, acute cerebrovascular diseases, heart failure, infection-related diseases, trauma- and injury-related diseases ($p < 0.0001$).

Table 3. Hospitalizations after Typhoon Morakot in affected adults with preexisting histories of cardiovascular and cerebrovascular diseases before Typhoon Morakot.

Characteristics	Adult Patients with a Related Cardiovascular History (January 2008–July 2009/)			
	Post-Match			
	Moderately Affected ($n = 24{,}969$) No. (%)	Severely Affected ($n = 24{,}969$) No. (%)	OR 95% CI	Chi^2-Test p Value
Acute ischemic heart diseases	2607 (10)	2896 (12)	1.096 * (1.037–1.16)	<0.0001
Acute cerebrovascular diseases	1852 (7.4)	2118 (8.4)	1.129 * (1.058–1.205)	<0.0001
Heart failure	1399 (5.6)	1633 (6.5)	1.152 * (1.07–1.24)	<0.0001
Infection	4661 (19)	5301 (21)	1.123 * (1.075–1.173)	<0.0001
Trauma and injury	1238 (4.9)	1456 (5.8)	1.161 * (1.074–1.255)	<0.0001

* $p < 0.05$.

To determine the important risk factors for mortality among affected adults with cardiovascular and cerebrovascular disease histories and to eliminate confounding factors, a multivariate stratified Cox proportional hazards regression model was estimated (Table 4). Among affected adults with a cerebrovascular disease history, patients with diabetes (adjusted HR: 1.40, 95% CI: 1.29–1.52, $p < 0.0001$), CKD (adjusted HR: 2.05, 95% CI: 1.81–2.33), COPD and asthma (adjusted HR: 1.89, 95% CI: 1.72–2.08, $p < 0.0001$), liver cirrhosis (adjusted HR: 2.25 95% CI: 1.79–2.79, $p < 0.0001$) and neoplasms (adjusted HR: 1.51, 95% CI: 1.33–1.71, $p < 0.0001$) had significantly increased mortality rates. Additionally, among affected adults with acute ischemic heart disease histories, patients with diabetes (adjusted HR: 1.55, 95% CI: 1.43–1.68, $p < 0.0001$), CKD (adjusted HR: 2.40, 95% CI: 2.15–2.69), COPD and asthma (adjusted HR: 1.69, 95% CI: 1.54–1.86, $p < 0.0001$), liver cirrhosis (adjusted HR: 2.76, 95% CI: 2.29–3.32, $p < 0.0001$) and neoplasms (adjusted HR: 1.87, 95% CI: 1.67–2.09, $p < 0.0001$) had higher mortality.

Table 4. Hazard ratio of all-cause mortality in affected adults with previous histories of cerebrovascular and ischemic heart diseases before Typhoon Morakot.

	Cerebrovascular Disease History [†] ($n = 21{,}571$)				Ischemic Heart Disease History [†] ($n = 34{,}251$)			
	Univariate Analysis		Multivariate Analysis		Univariate Analysis		Multivariate Analysis	
	HR	95% CI	aHR	95% CI	HR	95% CI	aHR	95% CI
Location (Ref = Nonrural)								
Rural	0.93	0.86–1.00			1.01	0.93–1.09		
DM (Ref = No)								
Yes	1.43 *	1.32–1.56	1.40 *	1.29–1.52	1.58 *	1.46–1.71	1.55 *	1.43–1.68
Hypertension (Ref = No)								
Yes	0.96	0.88–1.04			0.85 *	0.79–0.92	0.84 *	0.77–0.91
CKD (Ref = No)								
Yes	2.24 *	1.97–2.54	2.05 *	1.81–2.33	2.60 *	2.32–2.91	2.40 *	2.15–2.69
COPD & asthma (Ref = No)								
Yes	1.88 *	1.71–2.07	1.89 *	1.72–2.08	1.69 *	1.54–1.86	1.69 *	1.54–1.85
Liver cirrhosis (Ref = No)								
	2.35 *	1.88–2.93	2.23 *	1.79–2.79	3.18 *	2.64–3.82	2.76 *	2.29–3.32
Neoplasms (Ref = No)								
	1.61 *	1.42–1.82	1.51 *	1.33–1.71	2.07 *	1.85–2.31	1.87 *	1.67–2.09

[†] Enrolled variables in Cox model for cerebrovascular disease history and cerebrovascular disease history: Location, DM, Hypertension, CKD, COPD and asthma, liver cirrhosis, Neoplasm. DM: Diabetes mellitus; CKD: Chronic kidney disease, COPD: Chronic obstructive pulmonary diseases. * $p < 0.05$.

4. Discussion

This study suggested that affected adults with acute ischemic heart diseases and acute cerebrovascular disease histories before Typhoon Morakot had an increased numbers of visits healthcare facilities for acute ischemic heart disease and acute cerebrovascular diseases two months after Typhoon Morakot in both the moderately and severely affected areas. The survival analysis suggested that affected adults with acute ischemic heart disease history before Typhoon Morakot living in the severely affected area had significantly higher mortality than those living in the moderately affected area. Compared with those of affected adults in the moderately affected area, slightly more hospitalizations were noted among affected adults living in the severely affected area after Typhoon Morakot. Increased mortality rates were observed in affected adults with cerebrovascular disease and ischemic heart disease histories who had comorbidities such as diabetes, CKD, COPD and asthma, liver cirrhosis, and neoplasms.

Increases in the numbers of hospital visits for acute ischemic heart disease and stroke following natural disasters have been reported. A medical records analysis after the Great Hanshin-Awaji Earthquake in 1995 found that acute coronary syndrome and stroke rates rapidly increased and then decreased within 7 weeks, similar to rates after the Great East Japan Earthquake in 2011 [21,22]. After Hurricane Sandy in 2012, researchers detected increases in hospitalizations and deaths due to myocardial infarction and stroke during the 2 weeks following the hurricane compared to the same 2 weeks from 5 years previously [23]. In Taiwan, the rate of hospitalization due to acute myocardial infarction increased during the 6 weeks after the Ji-Ji Earthquake in 1999, and a significantly higher number of patients were hospitalized with acute myocardial infarction during that period than during the same 6-week period in the previous year [24]. Our study revealed similar results. Increased numbers of visits for acute cardiovascular and cerebrovascular events were observed in the first two months after Typhoon Morakot. The survival analysis also indicated a significant increase in mortality in the two years following the typhoon in those with previous acute ischemic heart disease who had lived in the severely affected area. Typhoon Morakot has had significantly short- and long-term health impacts on affected adults with acute ischemic heart diseases and cerebrovascular disease histories, especially those with chronic comorbidities such as DM, CKD or end-stage renal disease (ESRD), COPD, liver cirrhosis and neoplasms.

The abrupt increase in cardiovascular diseases (CVDs) in the acute phase was likely due to psychosocial and posttraumatic stress caused by the disaster and inadequate response after the disaster, especially in the severely affected areas [25–27]. Early morbidity from some cardiovascular events was likely predominantly attributable to the psychological stress of the event2 and corresponding physiologic derangements; psychosocial factors such as missed medications, changed diet, poor living conditions, and the stress of disorders following a disaster have been noted as well [26,28,29]. Psychosocial stressors and lack of medication and a proper support system likely play a key role. After Hurricane Katrina, multiple reports indicated high rates of psychosocial stress and posttraumatic stress [30]. Survivors had to cope with stressors such as searching for food and shelter, relocating, crowding, financial hardship, and navigating social services. Events such as hurricanes and other natural disasters can cause chronic and acute mental stress, which can trigger cardiovascular events [31]. Traditional cardiac risk factors account for only half of the incidence of CVDs, with most of the remaining risk explained by psychosocial factors [31]. Our study revealed similar results and indicated a short-term increase in the numbers of visits for acute ischemic heart and cerebrovascular diseases by affected adults with cardiovascular and cerebrovascular disease histories after Typhoon Morakot. After matching, increased two-year mortality was observed in severely affected adults with an acute ischemic heart disease history, highlighting the importance of the care of high-risk populations with cardiovascular diseases, especially those residing in severely affected rural areas. However, our study also suggested that affected populations with more co-morbidities (i.e., liver cirrhosis, CKD, COPD, asthma and neoplasms other than cardiovascular disease) have higher all-cause mortality hazards. The increased all-cause mortality occurred when patients with multimorbidity and pre-existing cardiovascular diseases such as stroke and ischemic heart diseases had increased risk of complications from either underlying diseases or comorbidities [32–37].

Health disparities are differences in the health statuses of specific populations and the general population. Health disparities are usually defined as "a particular type of health difference that is closely linked with social, economic, and/or environmental disadvantages" [8,38]. Although medical teams and acute social and financial relief programs are provided to affected populations in affected areas, affected populations with chronic comorbidities in severely affected areas still have an increased risk of mortality. Specialty and subspecialty healthcare services are usually less likely to be available in rural areas, and rural areas are less likely to offer specialized and highly sophisticated or high-intensity care than suburban or urban areas. Reliable transportation to healthcare facilities might also be a barrier for rural residents due to long distances, poor road conditions, and the limited availability of public transportation options in rural areas. These exacerbate problems for rural patients seeking specialized care who are required to travel significant distances for treatment [39]. Following a disaster, medical infrastructure usually becomes overwhelmed with acute injury and illness patients [40,41]. If chronic diseases controlled, preexisting chronic health problems can quickly become acute in nature, and these diseases have been linked to increased mortality in vulnerable populations in the wake of a disaster [40]. Chronic disease within the context of a disaster might have a bidirectional effect, whereby initial acute disorders may advance to long-term illnesses if insufficiently treated. This effect creates a "secondary surge" in required medical treatment long after the event and amplifies health disparities among medically underserved populations. The secondary surge of chronic diseases after a disaster coupled with inherent healthcare disparities, such as those commonly found in medically deprived rural areas, makes access to routine healthcare very difficult during the recovery phase [7]. Our data revealed similar results. Severely affected areas were more likely to comprise households with low socioeconomic levels. Patients with underlying comorbidities had higher mortality rates and morbidities after Typhoon Morakot that those without underlying comorbidities. Affected adults with an acute ischemic heart disease history before Typhoon Morakot living in severely affected areas had substantially increased hospitalization and mortality rates, highlighting the importance of medical accessibility. Most of the acute medical teams departed the severely affected areas approximately 6 months after Typhoon Morakot. Although relocation villages with permanent houses and healthcare centers were established within one year after Typhoon Morakot in the severely affected area, the accessibility of public transportation from these relocation villages to advanced cardiovascular care centers was limited. Accessibility limitations have great negative impacts on affected adults with cardiovascular risks, resulting in negative health outcomes.

The effects of spatial disparities after a disaster could be improved by the adoption of an improved universal healthcare system. Previous studies have suggested that universal healthcare systems substantially reduce socioeconomic inequalities in primary care access and quality but lead to only modest reductions in disparities in healthcare outcomes [42–44]. The Sendai framework for disaster risk reduction 2015–2030 aims to achieve substantial reductions in disaster risks and losses by enhancing the resilience of national health systems; corresponding efforts include strengthening the development and implementation of inclusive policies and social safety-net mechanisms and ensuring access to basic healthcare services, with the ultimate aim of eradicating poverty [45]. High-quality and accessible universal healthcare systems could maintain and support affected populations after disasters and are regarded as an important aspect of community resilience [46]. In order to be well-prepared for the foreseeable catastrophic natural events caused by the climate change, after Typhoon Morakot, a series of laws have been enacted including the most important "Spatial Planning Act 2016" [47] (state of the new climate-adaptive and environmental-oriented land use policy). In 2018, the Ministry of the Interior announced the implementation of the National Spatial Plan in accordance with the law and further emphasized on prioritizing the conservation of environmentally sensitive areas as well as important public facilities including medical services in rural and coastal areas. In addition, the United Nations Sustainable Development Goals (SDGs) [48] (United Nations, 2015) form the basis of spatial plans at all levels to ensure the health inequality and urban-rural gaps are taken into account in future land use policies. At the same time, more comprehensive affected area response plans including early evacuation of vulnerable groups and more medical and mental resources deployments before and after the heavy rainfall in susceptible areas were implemented to decrease the vulnerabilities and increase the resilience of the communities [49].

This study has several strengths. First, the large sample of population-based data covering almost the entire population affected by this disaster provided a large enough sample size for matching. Second, in addition to the use of traditional analyses, stratified Cox models and robust Cox models using robust sandwich variance estimators considering clustering within matched sets were employed. The latter approach resulted in unbiased estimations of marginal hazard ratios that could be compared with biased estimations of marginal hazard ratios resulting from the former approach.

Some limitations also need to be mentioned. The limitations of this study include the fact that the clinical data were collected from a registry; thus, completely verifying the data was impossible. Additionally, the registry does not include non-affected adults as reference group and provide detailed cardiovascular risk information regarding smoking habits, alcohol consumption, body mass index, physical activity, and family history, which are potential confounding factors in the analysis of chronic diseases and populations affected by disasters. The estimates of mortality among patients in this study were not verified with death certificates; however, the missing for more than 6 months is closely related to death and the proportion of disqualifications as an insurance applicant is negligible given the fact that foreigners only constitute around 2% of all insured individuals of Taiwan's NHI from the insurance service database. The misclassification rate of the estimated mortality method was <2.37%, and the method we used has been adapted from some previous studies [50,51]. Sex and age were chosen to match in these two groups to minimize the effects of comorbidities in the elderly. Although the underlying diseases between the two groups were still different, the CCI between the two groups after matching was similar and revealed similar comorbidities between groups. Hypertension is known as an important risk factor for cardiovascular death during the acute phase of a disaster. In most patients, the increases in clinic blood pressure and self-measured blood pressure are transient, and the blood pressure levels return to the pre-disaster baseline levels within 4 weeks. The blood pressure levels should be monitored and the dose of antihypertensive medication should be reconsidered every 2 weeks during the disaster situation [52]. An inverse relationship between diastolic pressure and adverse cardiac ischemic events (i.e., the lower the diastolic pressure the greater the risk of coronary heart disease and adverse outcomes) has been observed in numerous studies. This effect is even more pronounced in patients with underlying coronary artery disease (CAD) [53]. Previous studies also indicated uncontrolled hypertension increased risk of all-cause and cardiovascular disease mortality but no significant differences were identified between normotensives, and treated and controlled hypertensives [54]. Non-adherence to antihypertensive medication increased the risk of all adverse health outcomes, including all-cause mortality and hospitalization for cardiovascular diseases such as myocardial infarction, heart failure and stroke [55,56]. The hypertension-mortality risk would be significant reduced if good adherence to anti-hypertension agents is achieved [57,58]. Our study suggested that hypertension did not increase all-cause mortality within two years among affected adults with an ischemic heart disease history after Typhoon Morakot; patients with hypertension have lower mortality hazard might be because patients marked as hypertension received regular anti-hypertensive agent treatment with relative good adherence and blood pressure levels. Further longer follow-up studies should be considered to observe the effects. The monthly visits and mortality rates after this disaster might be underestimated if affected adults were not enrolled in the national healthcare system or did not have medical records during the study period. Furthermore, the areas covered in the spatial-temporal analysis were based on the primary medical facilities that were most commonly used by the residents of the affected areas after the disaster. It was difficult to locate all the affected individuals because some patients visiting these medical facilities might not have been residing in the same area they did before the disaster. The database did not include the unaffected population as the reference group in evaluating the baseline status of mental health before and after Typhoon Morakot. The effects of Typhoon Morakot are difficult to evaluate precisely. Moreover, classifications of township development and the proportions of elderly individuals in the populations were based on the 2005 Taiwan Social Change Survey (Round 5), which primarily considered socioeconomic change and township development in Taiwan; thus, these results may not apply to other spatiotemporal analyses of the relationships between socioeconomic factors and diseases. However, data from the national census, such as the proportion of elderly individuals in the population and household income, were acquired to achieve optimal validity. Finally, nondifferential misclassification of diseases in the registry at baseline might lead to bias toward the null.

In conclusion, the health status of patients with histories of acute cerebrovascular and cardiovascular diseases before Typhoon Morakot was negative effected in both the short term and long term after Typhoon Morakot. The increase in mortality was predominant among the elderly population and was associated with comorbidities and living in the severely affected area. High-quality and accessible universal healthcare systems are important to maintain and support affected populations after disasters. Further long-term spatial and socioeconomic analyses of the health of affected populations with chronic diseases are warranted to build community resilience with optimal deployment, beneficial healthcare strategies and a collaborative framework.

Author Contributions: Conceived and designed the study: H.-I.S., C.-M.C. Provided study materials and assembled the data: H.-I.S., T.-Y.C., C.-M.C., Y.-F.T. Analysed and interpreted the data: H.-I.S., C.-M.C., Y.-T.H., T.-C.S. and J.-D.W. Wrote the paper: H.-I.S., C.-M.C., T.-C.S. and Y.-T.H. Final approval of the manuscript: H.-I.S. and C.-M.C. All authors have read and agreed to the published version of the manuscript.

Funding: The funders played no role in the study design, data collection and analysis, decision to publish, or preparation of the manuscript. No additional external funding was received for this study.

Conflicts of Interest: The authors declare no conflict of interest.

Appendix A

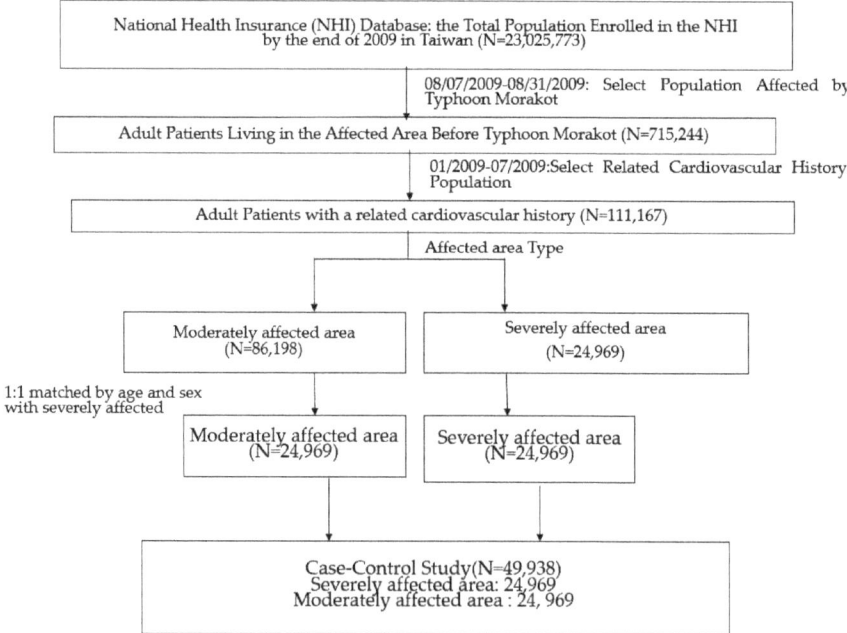

Figure A1. Flow diagram for patients enrolled in this study.

Table A1. Affected Townships of Typhoon Morakot.

County	Severely Affected Townships
Kaohsiung County *	Jiaxian, Taoyuan, Namaxia, Maolin, Neimen, Liugui, Qishan, Dashu, Shanlin, Meinong
Pingtung County *	Jiadong, Linbian, Neipu, Sandimen, Gaoshu, Taiwu, Shizi, Chunri, Wutai, Laiyi, Mudan, Donggang Majia
Chiayi County *	Dongshi, Alishan, Meishan, Zhuqi, Fanlu, Dapu
Taitung County	Taimali, Jinfeng, Dawu, Daren, Haiduan
Tainan County *	Nanhua, Danei, Yujing, Madou, Xuejia
Nantou County	Xinyi, Ren'ai, Shuili, Guoxing
Yulin County	Gukeng, Kouhu, Yuanchang

* All townships were severely affected.

References

1. Costello, A.; Abbas, M.; Allen, A.; Ball, S.; Bellamy, R.; Friel, S.; Groce, N.; Johnson, A.; Kett, M.; Lee, M.; et al. Managing the health effects of climate change. *Lancet* **2009**, *373*, 1693–1733. [CrossRef]
2. Smith, K.R.; Woodward, A.; Campbell-Lendrum, D.; Chadee, D.D.; Honda, Y.; Liu, Q.; Olwoch, J.M.; Revich, B.; Sauerborn, R. Human health: Impacts, adaptation, and co-benefits. In *Climate Change 2014: Impacts, Adaptation, and Vulnerability*; Field, C.B., Barros, V.R., Dokken, D.J., Mach, K.J., Mastrandrea, M.D., Bilir, T.E., Chatterjee, M., Ebi, K.L., Estrada, Y.O., Genova, R.C., et al., Eds.; Cambridge University Press: Cambridge, UK, 2014; pp. 709–754.
3. World Health Organization. Climate Change and Health. Available online: https://www.who.int/news-room/fact-sheets/detail/climate-change-and-health (accessed on 15 March 2020).
4. Regional Office for the Western Pacific World Health Organization. *Emergencies and Disasters*; Regional Office for the Western Pacific, World Health Organization: Manila, Philippines, 2005.
5. Bui, T.; Cho, S.; Sovereign, M. Negotiation issues in multinational humanitarian assistance/disaster relief. In *Proceedings of the 32nd Annual Hawaii International Conference on Systems Sciences, Maui, HI, USA, 5–8 January 1999*; HICSS-32. [CD-ROM]; Institute of Electrical and Electronics Engineers (IEEE): Piscataway Township, NJ, USA, 2003; p. 10.
6. Bathi, J.R.; Das, H.S. Vulnerability of Coastal Communities from Storm Surge and Flood Disasters. *Int. J. Environ. Res. Public Health* **2016**, *13*, 239. [CrossRef] [PubMed]
7. Davis, J.R.; Wilson, S.; Brock-Martin, A.; Glover, S.; Svendsen, E.R. The Impact of Disasters on Populations With Health and Health Care Disparities. *Disaster Med. Public Health Prep.* **2010**, *4*, 30–38. [CrossRef] [PubMed]
8. Braveman, P. What Are Health Disparities and Health Equity? We Need to Be Clear. *Public Health Rep.* **2014**, *129*, 5–8. [CrossRef] [PubMed]
9. Hsu, C.E.; Mas, F.S.; Jacobson, H.E.; Harris, A.M.; Hunt, V.I.; Nkhoma, E.T. Public health preparedness of health providers: Meeting the needs of diverse, rural communities. *J. Natl. Med. Assoc.* **2006**, *98*, 1784–1791.
10. Sharma, A.J.; Weiss, E.C.; Young, S.L.; Stephens, K.; Ratard, R.; Straif-Bourgeois, S.; Sokol, T.M.; Vranken, P.; Rubin, C.H. Chronic Disease and Related Conditions at Emergency Treatment Facilities in the New Orleans Area After Hurricane Katrina. *Disaster Med. Public Health Prep.* **2008**, *2*, 27–32. [CrossRef]
11. Hasegawa, A.; Ohira, T.; Maeda, M.; Yasumura, S.; Tanigawa, K. Emergency Responses and Health Consequences after the Fukushima Accident. *Clin. Oncol.* **2016**, *28*, 237–244. [CrossRef]
12. McCann, D.G. A Review of Hurricane Disaster Planning for the Elderly. *World Med. Health Policy* **2011**, *3*, 5–30. [CrossRef]
13. Pelling, M.; Uitto, J.I. Small Island developing states: Natural disaster vulnerability and global change. *Environ. Hazards* **2001**, *3*, 49–62.
14. Lamont-Doherty Earth Observatory Risk Analysis Reports over Half of World's Population Exposed to One or More Major Natural Hazards. Available online: http://www.earth.columbia.edu/news/2005/story03-29-05.html (accessed on 11 December 2019).
15. Kaohsiung County Office The Official List of survivors in Kaohsiung during the Typhoon Morakot. Available online: http://88taiwan.blogspot.tw/2009/08/0815.html (accessed on 11 April 2020).

16. National Science and Technology Center for Disaster Reduction, Disaster Survey and Analysis of Morakot Typhoon. *National Science and Technology Center for Disaster Reduction Anual Report, 2010*; National Science and Technology Center for Disaster Reduction: Taipei, Taiwan, 2010.
17. Hsieh, C.-Y.; Su, C.-C.; Shao, S.-C.; Sung, S.-F.; Lin, S.-J.; Yang, Y.-H.K.; Lai, E.C.-C. Taiwan's National Health Insurance Research Database: Past and future. *Clin. Epidemiol.* **2019**, *11*, 349–358. [CrossRef]
18. Lee, T.C.; Yang, C.L.; Wang, T.M. Population Aging and NHI Expenditures in Taiwan. *J. Popul. Stud.* **2011**, *43*, 1–35.
19. Center for Survey Research Academia Sinica Taiwan Social Change Survey. Available online: https://www2.ios.sinica.edu.tw/sc/en/home2.php (accessed on 10 January 2018).
20. The World Medical Association Annexe 2. WMA Declaration of Taipei on ethical considerations regarding health databases and biobanks. *J. Int. Bioethique Ethique Sci.* **2017**, *28*, 113–117. [CrossRef]
21. Aoki, T.; Fukumoto, Y.; Yasuda, S.; Sakata, Y.; Ito, K.; Takahashi, J.; Miyata, S.; Tsuji, I.; Shimokawa, H. The Great East Japan Earthquake Disaster and cardiovascular diseases. *Eur. Hear. J.* **2012**, *33*, 2796–2803. [CrossRef] [PubMed]
22. Aoki, T.; Takahashi, J.; Fukumoto, Y.; Yasuda, S.; Ito, K.; Miyata, S.; Shinozaki, T.; Inoue, K.; Yagi, T.; Komaru, T.; et al. Effect of the Great East Japan Earthquake on cardiovascular diseases—Report from the 10 hospitals in the disaster area. *Circ. J.* **2013**, *77*, 490–493. [CrossRef] [PubMed]
23. Swerdel, J.N.; Janevic, T.M.; Cosgrove, N.M.; Kostis, J.B. The Myocardial Infarction Data Acquisition System (MIDAS 24) Study Group the Effect of Hurricane Sandy on Cardiovascular Events in New Jersey. *J. Am. Hear. Assoc.* **2014**, *3*, 001354. [CrossRef]
24. Tsai, C.-H.; Lung, F.-W.; Wang, S.-Y. The 1999 Ji-Ji (Taiwan) Earthquake as a Trigger for Acute Myocardial Infarction. *J. Psychosom. Res.* **2004**, *45*, 477–482. [CrossRef]
25. Dedert, E.A.; Calhoun, P.S.; Watkins, L.L.; Sherwood, A.; Beckham, J.C. Posttraumatic Stress Disorder, Cardiovascular, and Metabolic Disease: A Review of the Evidence. *Ann. Behav. Med.* **2010**, *39*, 61–78. [CrossRef]
26. Edmondson, D.; Cohen, B.E. Posttraumatic stress disorder and cardiovascular disease. *Prog. Cardiovasc. Dis.* **2013**, *55*, 548–556. [CrossRef]
27. Onose, T.; Nochioka, K.; Sakata, Y.; Miura, M.; Tadaki, S.; Ushigome, R.; Yamauchi, T.; Sato, K.; Tsuji, K.; Abe, R.; et al. Predictors and Prognostic Impact of Post-Traumatic Stress Disorder After the Great East Japan Earthquake in Patients With Cardiovascular Disease. *Circ. J.* **2015**, *79*, 664–667. [CrossRef]
28. Lavie, C.J.; Gerber, T.C.; Lanier, W.L. Hurricane Katrina: The Infarcts beyond the Storm. *Disaster Med. Public Health Prep.* **2009**, *3*, 131–135. [CrossRef]
29. Kivimäki, M.; Steptoe, A. Effects of stress on the development and progression of cardiovascular disease. *Nat. Rev. Cardiol.* **2017**, *15*, 215–229. [CrossRef] [PubMed]
30. Peters, M.N.; Moscona, J.C.; Katz, M.J.; DeAndrade, K.B.; Quevedo, H.C.; Tiwari, S.; Burchett, A.R.; Turnage, T.A.; Singh, K.Y.; Fomunung, E.N.; et al. Natural Disasters and Myocardial Infarction: The Six Years After Hurricane Katrina. *Mayo Clin. Proc.* **2014**, *89*, 472–477. [CrossRef] [PubMed]
31. Epel, E.; Lin, J.; Wilhelm, F.H.; Wolkowitz, O.; Cawthon, R.; Adler, N.; Dolbier, C.; Mendes, W.; Blackburn, E. Cell aging in relation to stress arousal and cardiovascular disease risk factors. *Psychoneuroendocrinology* **2006**, *31*, 277–287. [CrossRef] [PubMed]
32. Glynn, L.; Buckley, B.; Reddan, N.; Newell, J.; Hinde, J.; Dinneen, S.F.; Murphy, A.W. Multimorbidity and risk among patients with established cardiovascular disease: A cohort study. *Br. J. Gen. Pr.* **2008**, *58*, 488–494. [CrossRef] [PubMed]
33. Lekoubou, A.; Ovbiagele, B. Prevalence and influence of chronic obstructive pulmonary disease on stroke outcomes in hospitalized stroke patients. *eNeurologicalSci* **2017**, *6*, 21–24. [CrossRef]
34. Yen, Y.-S.; Harnod, D.; Lin, C.-L.; Harnod, T.; Lin, C.-L. Long-Term Mortality and Medical Burden of Patients with Chronic Obstructive Pulmonary Disease with and without Subsequent Stroke Episodes. *Int. J. Environ. Res. Public Health* **2020**, *17*, 2550. [CrossRef]
35. Strand, L.B.; Tsai, M.K.; Wen, C.P.; Chang, S.-S.; Brumpton, B.M. Is having asthma associated with an increased risk of dying from cardiovascular disease? A prospective cohort study of 446 346 Taiwanese adults. *BMJ Open* **2018**, *8*, e019992. [CrossRef]

36. Sturgeon, K.M.; Deng, L.; Bluethmann, S.M.; Zhou, S.; Trifiletti, D.M.; Jiang, C.; Kelly, S.P.; Zaorsky, N.G. A population-based study of cardiovascular disease mortality risk in US cancer patients. *Eur. Heart J.* **2019**, *40*, 3889–3897. [CrossRef]
37. Kim, D.; Adejumo, A.C.; Yoo, E.R.; Iqbal, U.; Li, A.A.; Pham, E.A.; Cholankeril, G.; Glenn, J.S.; Ahmed, A. Trends in Mortality From Extrahepatic Complications in Patients with Chronic Liver Disease, From 2007 Through 2017. *Gastroenterology* **2019**, *157*, 1055–1066. [CrossRef]
38. Healthy People 2020. Disparities. Available online: https://www.healthypeople.gov/2020/about/foundation-health-measures/Disparities (accessed on 15 August 2020).
39. Basu, S.; Berkowitz, S.A.; Phillips, R.L.; Bitton, A.; Landon, B.E.; Phillips, R.S. Association of Primary Care Physician Supply With Population Mortality in the United States, 2005–2015. *JAMA Intern. Med.* **2019**, *179*, 506. [CrossRef]
40. Ford, E.S.; Mokdad, A.H.; Link, M.W.; Garvin, W.S.; McGuire, L.C.; Jiles, R.B.; Balluz, L.S.; B., J.R. Chronic disease in health emergencies: In the eye of the hurricane. *Prev. Chronic Dis.* **2006**, *3*, A46. [PubMed]
41. Cunningham, P.J.; Felland, L.E. Falling behind: Americans' access to medical care deteriorates, 2003–2007. *Track. Rep.* **2008**, *19*, 1–5.
42. Asaria, M.; Ali, S.; Doran, T.; Ferguson, B.; Fleetcroft, R.; Goddard, M.; Goldblatt, P.; Laudicella, M.; Raine, R.; Cookson, R. How a universal health system reduces inequalities: Lessons from England. *J. Epidemiol. Community Health* **2016**, *70*, 637–643. [CrossRef] [PubMed]
43. Marmot, M.; Friel, S.; Bell, R.; Houweling, T.A.J.; Taylor, S. Closing the gap in a generation: Health equity through action on the social determinants of health. *Lancet* **2008**, *372*, 1661–1669. [CrossRef]
44. Veugelers, P.; Yip, A.M. Socioeconomic disparities in health care use: Does universal coverage reduce inequalities in health? *J. Epidemiol. Community Health* **2003**, *57*, 424–428. [CrossRef]
45. Aitsi-Selmi, A.; Murray, V. The Sendai framework: Disaster risk reduction through a health lens. *Bull. World Health Organ.* **2015**, *93*, 362. [CrossRef]
46. Plough, A.; Fielding, J.E.; Chandra, A.; Williams, M.; Eisenman, D.; Wells, K.B.; Law, G.Y.; Fogleman, S.; Magana, A. Building community disaster resilience: Perspectives from a large urban county department of public health. *Am. J. Public Health* **2013**, *103*, 1190–1197. [CrossRef]
47. Ministry of the Interior. Toward a Sustainable Taiwan: Summary National Spatial Plan. Taiwan. Available online: https://www.cpami.gov.tw/filesys/file/rp6/rp1081203e.pdf (accessed on 15 August 2020).
48. United Nations. United Nations Sustainable Development Goals. Available online: https://sdgs.un.org/goals (accessed on 15 August 2020).
49. Ministry of the Interior. Disaster Prevention and Protection Act. Available online: https://law.moj.gov.tw/ENG/LawClass/LawAll.aspx?pcode=D0120014 (accessed on 15 August 2020).
50. Pan, Y.-J.; Yeh, L.-L.; Chan, H.-Y.; Chang, C.-K. Transformation of excess mortality in people with schizophrenia and bipolar disorder in Taiwan. *Psychol. Med.* **2017**, *47*, 2483–2493. [CrossRef]
51. Chiu, Y.-W.; Wu, C.-S.; Chen, P.-C.; Wei, Y.-C.; Hsu, L.-Y.; Wang, S.-H. Risk of acute mesenteric ischemia in patients with diabetes: A population-based cohort study in Taiwan. *Atherosclerosis* **2020**, *296*, 18–24. [CrossRef]
52. Kario, K. Disaster hypertension—Its characteristics, mechanism, and management. *Circ. J.* **2012**, *76*, 553–562. [CrossRef]
53. Messerli, F.H.; Panjrath, G.S. The J-Curve between Blood Pressure and Coronary Artery Disease or Essential Hypertension. *J. Am. Coll. Cardiol.* **2009**, *54*, 1827–1834. [CrossRef] [PubMed]
54. Zhou, N.; Xi, B.; Zhao, M.; Wang, L.; Veeranki, S.P. Uncontrolled hypertension increases risk of all-cause and cardiovascular disease mortality in US adults: The NHANES III Linked Mortality Study. *Sci. Rep.* **2018**, *8*, 9418. [CrossRef]
55. Shin, S.; Song, H.; Oh, S.-K.; Choi, K.E.; Kim, H.; Jang, S. Effect of antihypertensive medication adherence on hospitalization for cardiovascular disease and mortality in hypertensive patients. *Hypertens. Res.* **2013**, *36*, 1000–1005. [CrossRef]
56. Kim, S.; Shin, D.W.; Yun, J.M.; Hwang, Y.; Park, S.K.; Ko, Y.-J.; Cho, B.L. Medication Adherence and the Risk of Cardiovascular Mortality and Hospitalization Among Patients With Newly Prescribed Antihypertensive Medications. *Hypertension* **2016**, *67*, 506–512. [CrossRef] [PubMed]

57. Yang, Q.; Chang, A.; Ritchey, M.D.; Loustalot, F. Antihypertensive Medication Adherence and Risk of Cardiovascular Disease among Older Adults: A Population-Based Cohort Study. *J. Am. Hear. Assoc.* **2017**, *6*, 6. [CrossRef] [PubMed]
58. Bowling, C.B.; Davis, B.R.; Luciano, A.; Simpson, L.M.; Sloane, R.; Pieper, C.F.; Einhorn, P.T.; Oparil, S.; Muntner, P. Sustained blood pressure control and coronary heart disease, stroke, heart failure, and mortality: An observational analysis of ALLHAT. *J. Clin. Hypertens.* **2019**, *21*, 451–459. [CrossRef] [PubMed]

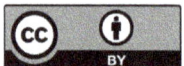

© 2020 by the authors. Licensee MDPI, Basel, Switzerland. This article is an open access article distributed under the terms and conditions of the Creative Commons Attribution (CC BY) license (http://creativecommons.org/licenses/by/4.0/).

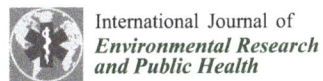 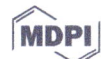

Article

The Mortality Risk and Socioeconomic Vulnerability Associated with High and Low Temperature in Hong Kong

Sida Liu [1,2], Emily Yang Ying Chan [1,2,*], William Bernard Goggins [2] and Zhe Huang [1,2]

1. Collaborating Centre for Oxford University and CUHK for Disaster and Medical Humanitarian Response (CCOUC), The Chinese University of Hong Kong, Hong Kong SAR, China; liusida2008@gmail.com (S.L.); huangzhe@cuhk.edu.hk (Z.H.)
2. JC School of Public Health and Primary Care, Faculty of Medicine, The Chinese University of Hong Kong, Hong Kong SAR, China; wgoggins@cuhk.edu.hk
* Correspondence: emily.chan@cuhk.edu.hk

Received: 31 July 2020; Accepted: 30 September 2020; Published: 7 October 2020

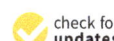

Abstract: (1) Background: The adverse health effect associated with extreme temperature has been extensively reported in the current literature. Some also found that temperature effect may vary among the population with different socioeconomic status (SES), but found inconsistent results. Previous studies on the socioeconomic vulnerability of temperature effect were mainly achieved by multi-city or country analysis, but the large heterogeneity between cities may introduce additional bias to the estimation. The linkage between death registry and census in Hong Kong allows us to perform a city-wide analysis in which the study population shares virtually the same cultural, lifestyle and policy environment. This study aims to examine and compare the high and low temperature on morality in Hong Kong, a city with a subtropical climate and address a key research question of whether the extreme high and low temperature disproportionally affects population with lower SES. (2) Methods: Poisson-generalized additive models and distributed-lagged nonlinear models were used to examine the association between daily mortality and daily mean temperature between 2007–2015 with other meteorological and confounding factors controlled. Death registry was linked with small area census and area-level median household income was used as the proxy for socioeconomic status. (3) Results: 362,957 deaths during the study period were included in the analysis. The minimum mortality temperature was found to be 28.9 °C (82nd percentile). With a subtropical climate, the low temperature has a stronger effect than the high temperature on non-accidental, cardiovascular, respiratory and cancer deaths in Hong Kong. The hot effect was more pronounced in the first few days, while cold effect tended to last up to three weeks. Significant heat effect was only observed in the lower SES groups, whilst the extreme low temperature was associated with significantly higher mortality risk across all SES groups. The older population were susceptible to extreme temperature, especially for cold. (4) Conclusions: This study raised the concern of cold-related health impact in the subtropical region. Compared with high temperature, low temperature may be considered a universal hazard to the entire population in Hong Kong rather than only disproportionally affecting people with lower SES. Future public health policy should reconsider the strategy at both individual and community levels to reduce temperature-related mortality.

Keywords: H-EDRM; climate change; extreme temperature; climate change; socioeconomic vulnerability; health disparities

1. Introduction

The adverse effect of extreme temperature on human health has been intensively reported during the last decade [1,2]. Epidemiological evidence shows that both high and low temperature were associated with increased mortality and morbidity in western, Asian and African countries [3–5]. With the effect of climate change, extreme weather events are expected to be more frequent and intensive in the future, which may impose a significant health burden in the years to come [6]. Previous studies have also identified that temperature may pose different health impact to population with different characteristics, some risk factors related to the vulnerability of extreme temperature include pre-existing diseases, housing, behavior as well as socioeconomic status (SES) [7–9].

The association between health inequities and socioeconomic disparities have been well established [10–12]. A number of research revealed that such disparities were also existed for health effect induced by temperature [13,14]. Current research has shown inconsistent results on whether socioeconomic disadvantages were associated with higher temperature-related health risk, especially for cold weather [7,8,14,15]. Previous studies of such kind were mainly conducted by city or country-level comparison [8,16,17]. This may be problematic since other confounding factors such as lifestyle, behavior, temperature-related policy and acclimation are difficult to properly controlled. An intra-city analysis has advantages to minimize the effect of other confounding factors. This was rarely conducted in previously due to methodological challenges that SES data are often absent in retrospective health-related data in most countries.

In Hong Kong, the mortality registry can be lined with area-level census data, which provide an opportunity to perform such city-wide analysis in which the study population shares virtually the same cultural, lifestyle and policy environment. Hong Kong is a developed metropolis with one of the largest income disparities in the world. The Gini coefficient was reported to be 0.539 for original and 0.473 for after social benefit transfer and it continues growing in the last two decades [18]. The large income disparity gap provides a good example with which to investigate the modifying effect of SES on temperature. Many mortality and morbidity related to extreme temperature are predictable and preventable [19]. As highlighted in UNISDR Sendai Framework and WHO health emergency disaster risk management (Health-EDRM), understanding the health risk and vulnerable population are priorities to reduce the exposure and adverse health consequences that are associated with disaster and environmental hazards [20]. In this study, we aimed to (1) examine and compare morality risk associated with high and low temperature in the subtropical city and (2) to address a key research question of whether the extreme high and low temperature disproportionally affects population with lower SES.

2. Materials and Methods

2.1. Environmental Data

Meteorological data including mean daily temperature, relative humidity and atmospheric pressure from 1 January 2007 to 31 December 2015 were obtained from Hong Kong Observatory, which is located at the center of the urban area. To adjust for the potential confounding effect of air pollution, daily mean air pollutant data including nitrogen dioxide (NO_2), Sulphur dioxide (SO_2), Ozone (O_3) and particulate matter less than 2.5 μm aerodynamic diameter ($PM_{2.5}$) of the same period were collected from the Hong Kong Environmental Protection Department. The daily air pollution variables were calculated by taking an average of ten general stations.

2.2. Mortality Data

The corresponding daily non-accidental mortality data were collected from the Hong Kong Census and Statistics Department for analysis. The data also contain the cause of death, gender and age for stratified analysis. Cause of death was also analyzed which classified according to International

Classification of Diseases, Tenth Revision (ICD-10) non-accidental (A00-T99, Z00-Z99), cardiovascular (I00-I99) and respiratory (J00-J98) diseases and cancer (C00-D48).

2.3. Socioeconomic Status Data

Several indictors have been chosen to reflect socioeconomic status (SES) in previous studies, including education, income, occupation, and race/ethnicity [7,14,21–23]. To further capture the multidimensional feature of SES, some studies used composite indices composed of multiple indicators to represent an individual's socioeconomic advantage [24–26]. However, many of those indices were not officially adopted by local government, and aggregating SES may introduce additional bias when interpreting. In this study, we used a signal measure indicator, the median monthly household income (MHI) of a deceased person's residential area, as a proxy to reflect the one's socioeconomic status (SES). Income is the most widely used SES indicator, which directly and indirectly affects access to goods and services for health. In the 2011 Hong Kong census, the territory of Hong Kong was divided into 289 small areas, which are also known as Tertiary Planning Units (TPUs). To minimize issues regarding privacy, TPUs with a population less than 1000 were merged into the nearby TPUs to form 209 TPU clusters. One TPU was intentionally excluded due to the entire population within the area being prisoners, and therefore 208 TPU clusters were included in the final analysis. All TPU clusters were then grouped into four levels using the quartering method according to its MHI (52 TPU clusters in each group, where 1 indicates the group with highest SES and 4 is the lowest SES group), to evaluate whether there were differences in the effect of temperature on all non-accidental and cause-specific mortality (Figure 1). Each death record was linked with an SES group code according to his/her residential area by the TPU code.

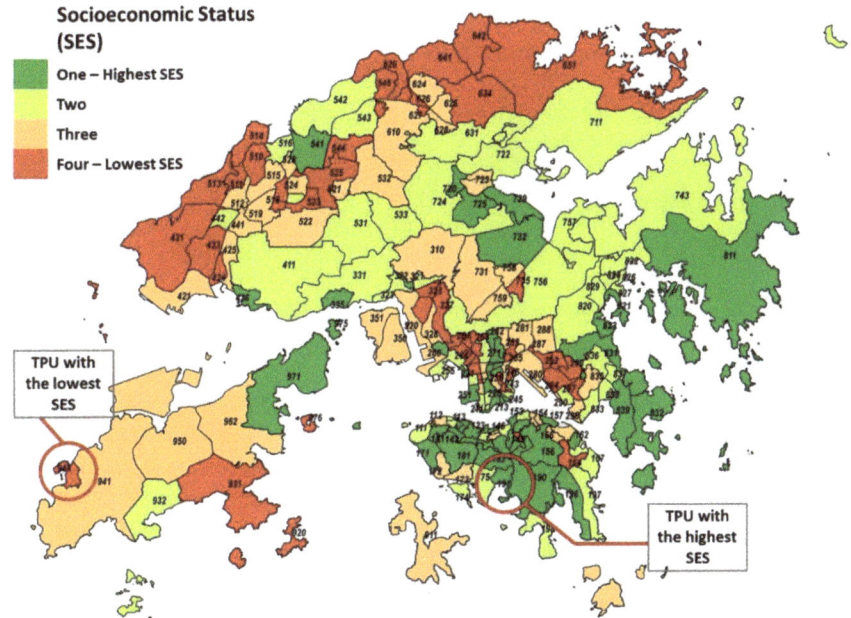

Figure 1. The geographical distribution of socioeconomic status (SES) groups by median monthly household income of tertiary planning units (TPUs) in Hong Kong, where One = highest SES, shown in green and Four = lowest SES, shown in red).

2.4. Statistical Analysis

Distributed lag linear and non-linear models (DLNM) were performed to determine the association between daily mortality and ambient temperature for each SES group. As daily mortality counts generally follow an overdispersed Poisson distribution, a distributed lag model with a quasi-Poisson regression was used to evaluate the health effect of heat and cold while adjusting for the temperature at different lag days. The model used the following formula:

$$\begin{aligned}\text{Log}[E(Y_t)] = {} & \alpha + cb(\text{Temp}_t) + ns(\text{Humidity}, df = 4) \\ & + ns(\text{Pressure}, df = 4) + ns(O_3, df = 4) \\ & + ns(SO_2, df = 4) + ns(NO_2, df = 4) + ns(PM_{2.5}, df = 4) + ns(\text{Time}, df = 9 \times 7) + \text{Dow}_t + \text{Holiday}_t\end{aligned}$$

where α is the intercept; cb is the crossbasis matrix built up with *dlnm*() package in R; ns(): smoothing function using a natural cubic spline. A quadratic B-spline with three internal knots placed at the 10th, 75th and 90th percentiles of temperature was used to model the exposure–response relationship and a natural cubic spline was fitted with three internal knots placed equally spaced in the log scale to model the lag–response association [27]. 4 degrees of freedom (df) were used for potentially confounding metalogical and air pollutant variables. The model uses a maximum lag period of 21 days to capture the long delay of effects of cold and to exclude deaths that were advanced by only a few days (harvesting effect) [28,29]. The long-term and seasonality effect was controlled using 7 df per year. Day of the week (Dow) and local public holidays were also adjusted in the model. The Akaike Information Criterion for quasi-Poisson (Q-AIC) values were used for the choice of the degree of freedom.

The relationship between temperature and mortality was summarized as the exposure–response curve of relative risk (RR) accumulated across all lags. Minimum mortality temperature (MMT), with its 95% confidence interval (95% CI), was calculated. RR for total death and each SES group were estimated. Subgroup analyses for gender, age group (0–65 years and 65 years above) and cause-specific death (cardiovascular, respiratory and cancer) were performed. The results show that the MMTs for each subgroup analysis were close to 27 °C, so that was chosen as the fixed reference temperature to compare the temperature effect on each SES groups. Modelling choices were tested by a sensitivity analysis using different degrees of freedom for temperature and long-term trends, and length of maximum lag period. All analyses were performed using R project for statistical computing (version 3.6) packages *dlnm* and *mgcv* [30,31].

3. Results

3.1. Data Description

Hong Kong is a subtropical city with hot summer and mild winter. The mean and median daily mean temperature during the study period were 23.5 °C and 24.7 °C, with a range between 8.4 and 32.4 °C, respectively (Table 1). As a coastal city, the relative humidity is relatively high, with a median of 79%. Overall, 362,957 non-accidental deaths were included in the analysis after excluding cases without a valid TPU code (1.34%). There were more deaths in the lower SES group than higher SES in Hong Kong, with daily mortality ranging from 0 to 26 cases in the highest SES group and 14 to 192 cases in the lowest one (Table 2). Figure 1 shows the distribution of the TPU cluster by SES groups, of which the highest cluster (Deep Water bay, HK$178,000 or US$22,960/month) has reported 20 times higher median household income compared to the lowest (Tai O, HK$8000 or US$1031/month), indicating a large SES disparity among districts in Hong Kong.

Table 1. Descriptive statistics of metalogical and air pollutant variables.

Variables	Mean	Min	Percentile					Max
			5th	25th	50th	75th	95th	
Mean Temperature (°C)	23.5	8.4	14.2	19.2	24.7	28.1	30.0	32.4
Mean Relative Humidity (%)	78.1	29.0	58.0	73.0	79.0	85.0	95.0	99.0
Atmospheric pressure (hPa)	1012.7	992.2	1002.6	1007.9	1012.7	1017.7	1023.1	1029.8
NO_2 ($\mu g/m^3$)	41.2	11.4	28.2	38.3	48.4	61	83.8	152.5
O_3 ($\mu g/m^3$)	51.2	4.9	13.6	21.7	36.9	56.1	85.4	139.3
SO_2 ($\mu g/m^3$)	13.9	3.2	5.6	8.4	11.8	16.9	28.9	80.6
$PM_{2.5}$ ($\mu g/m^3$)	31.4	4.9	9.2	15.8	27.5	42.5	67.5	138.5

Table 2. Descriptive statistics of daily mortality count in the study period.

SES Groups	Percentile							Total
	Min	5th	25th	50th	75th	95th	Max	
One—Highest SES	0	4	7	9	11	15	26	30,169
Two	3	10	14	18	21	26	38	63,808
Three	6	23	30	34	39	47	67	125,750
Four—Lowest SES	14	34	42	48	55	67	92	143,230
Total	31	86	99	109	120	143	192	362,957

3.2. Main Findings

As shown in Figure 2, the cumulative effect (lag 0–21) of cold posed a stronger effect on mortality when compared to heat with the reference temperature of 28.9 °C—the temperature with minimum mortality (MMT). When an extremely low temperature occurs (12.9 °C, 2.5th percentile of daily mean temperature), the mortality rate is almost 1.5 times higher compared to 27 °C. No significant overall heat was identified in the lag period of 0 to 21 days. For the lag–response effect, the hot effect tended to be more pronounced in the first 3 days with no harvesting effect. Meanwhile, the cold effect may last up to 3 weeks after the low temperature occurs (Figure 3). The cumulative cold effect in relative risk for lag 0–21 day was 1.463 (95% CI: 1.362, 1.571) and the heat effect for lag 0–3 days was 1.035 (95% CI: 1.011, 1.059) (Table 3). No overall clear harvesting effect in mortality was observed for both heat and cold effect.

For cause-specific temperature on mortality (Figure 4), the high temperature was found to be associated with significantly higher respiratory death, particularly among groups with the lower SES, whereas heat effect was not significant for cardiovascular deaths. On the other hand, the cold impact was significant for both cardiovascular and respiratory death and the effect was found to be generally higher in all SES groups. The results also suggested that the heat effect for respiratory death was higher than cardiovascular, whereas the cold effects were stronger for cardiovascular death than for respiratory death. The effect of cold temperature on cancer mortality was significant, although the effect size was much smaller than other causes. The cold effect on cancer deaths was found to be higher in lower SES groups, whereas the more affluent groups were not significantly affected. High temperature was found to be associated with increased mortality risk for cancer deaths.

Furthermore, the high temperature was associated with higher mortality risk among females than males, but no clear gender difference was observed for cold effect (Figure 5). Compared with the younger population, older individuals were generally associated with higher temperature-related mortality, especially for low temperature. Significantly higher cold-related mortality risk was observed in all SES groups, but heat-related mortality risk was only identified in the lowest SES group.

To compare the effect of high and low temperature among SES groups, the RR for each SES group were estimated (Figure 4). For non-accidental death, heat effect was found to be only significant in lower SES groups (Group Three: 1.039 (95% CI: 1.001, 1.078), Group Four: 1.040 (95% CI: 1.005, 1.076), while the cold effect was found to be significant across all SES groups (Figure 4).

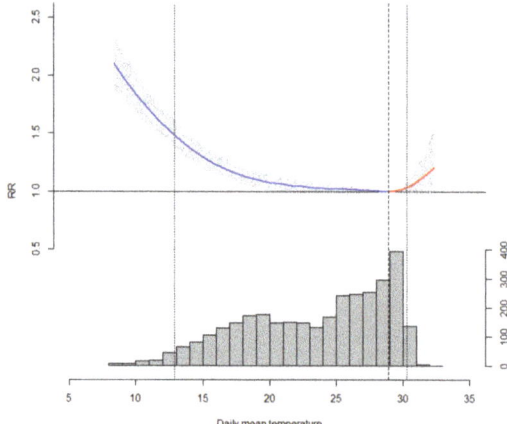

Figure 2. The cumulative effect (lag 0–21 days) of daily mean temperature on non-accidental mortality during 2007 and 2015 with the distribution of daily mean temperature at the bottom (number of days). The dashed in the middle indicates the minimum mortality temperature (28.9 °C) the two vertical lines on the sides indicates the 2.5th (12.9 °C) and 97.5th (30.3 °C) percentile of the daily temperature during study period.

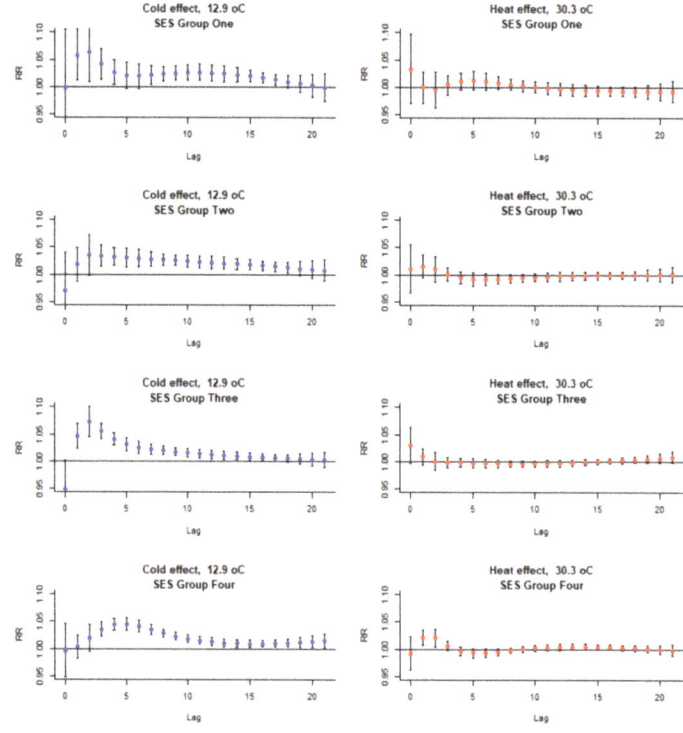

Figure 3. The Lag–response effect distribution during the 21 days lag period after exposed to a low (12.9 °C, 2.5th percentile) and high (30.3 °C, 97.5th percentile) temperature compared to reference temperature (27 °C).

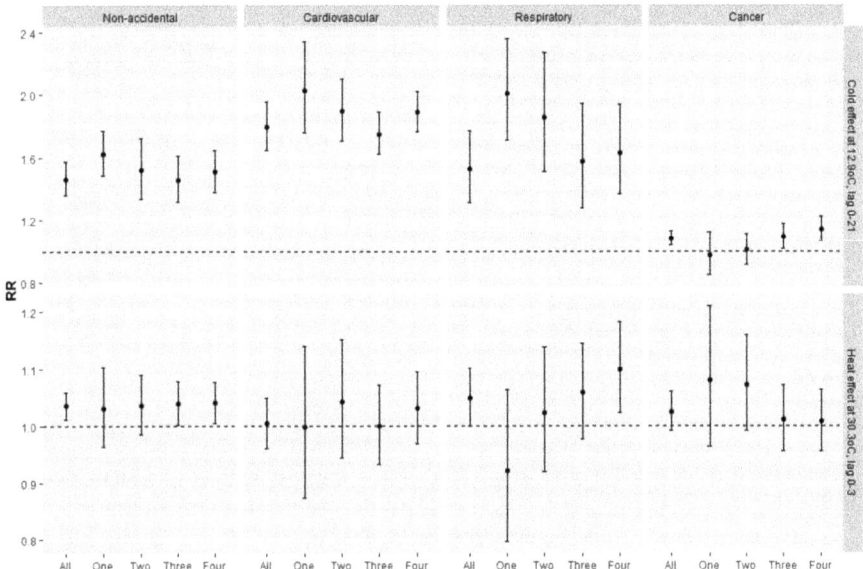

Figure 4. The cold (12.9 °C, 2.5th percentile at lag 0–21) and heat effect (30.3 °C, 97.5th percentile at lag 0–3) compared to 27 °C by cause of death and SES groups (where One = the highest SES, Four = lowest SES).

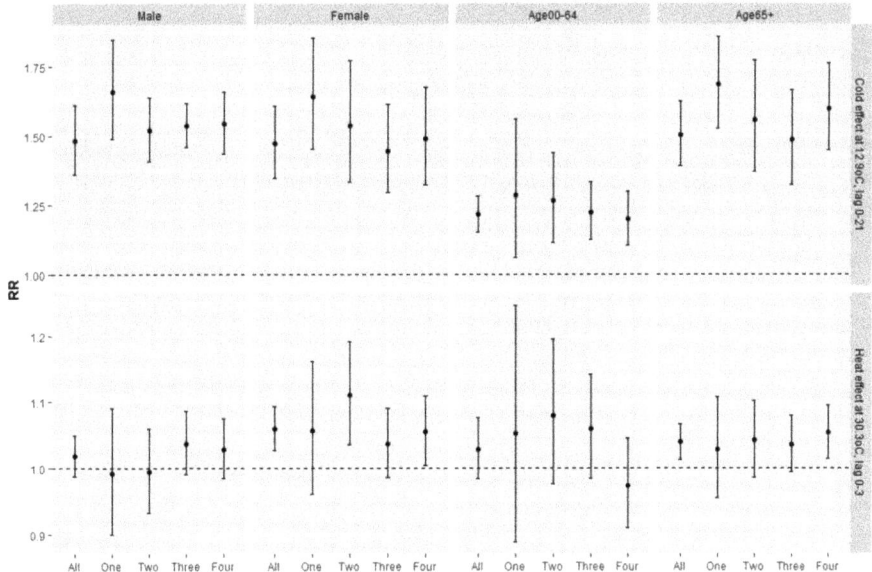

Figure 5. The cold (12.9 °C, 2.5th at lag 0–21) and heat effect (30.3 °C, 97.5th at lag 0–3) on non-accidental deaths compared to 27 °C by age, gender and SES groups where One = the highest SES, Four = the lowest SES.

Table 3. The relative risk (RR) for cold (12.9 °C, 2.5th percentile at lag 0–21) and heat effect (30.3 °C, 97.5th percentile at lag 0–3) compared to 27 °C with 95% confidence interval.

SES Group	Non-Accidental		Cardiovascular		Respiratory		Cancer	
	Cold	Heat	Cold	Heat	Cold	Heat	Cold	Heat
One	1.622 * (1.485, 1.771)	1.031 (0.964, 1.103)	2.026 * (1.755, 2.339)	0.998 (0.874, 1.140)	2.009 * (1.713, 2.356)	0.921 (0.797, 1.064)	0.976 (0.850, 1.121)	1.080 (0.964, 1.211)
Two	1.518 * (1.337, 1.723)	1.036 (0.985, 1.089)	1.893 * (1.707, 2.100)	1.043 (0.945, 1.152)	1.851 * (1.510, 2.268)	1.023 (0.920, 1.138)	1.009 (0.916, 1.111)	1.072 (0.991, 1.160)
Three	1.457 * (1.320, 1.607)	1.039 * (1.001, 1.078)	1.748 * (1.619, 1.888)	1.000 (0.933, 1.071)	1.575 * (1.278, 1.940)	1.058 (0.977, 1.145)	1.094 (1.018, 1.176)	1.012 (0.956, 1.071)
Four	1.506 * (1.378, 1.645)	1.040* (1.005, 1.076)	1.888 * (1.764, 2.019)	1.030 (0.969, 1.095)	1.626 * (1.364, 1.938)	1.099 * (1.022, 1.182)	1.142 * (1.068, 1.223)	1.008 (0.955, 1.064)
All	1.463 * (1.362, 1.571)	1.035 * (1.011, 1.059)	1.794 * (1.645, 1.955)	1.004 (0.961, 1.048)	1.525 * (1.312, 1.772)	1.049 * (0.999, 1.101)	1.081 * (1.037, 1.127)	1.025 (0.991, 1.060)

* Statistically significant at $\alpha \leq 0.05$.

4. Discussion

This study is the first study to investigate the SES-related disparities on the mortality risk associated with the high and low temperature in Hong Kong. A J-shape temperature–mortality association was identified for this subtropical urban metropolitan city. Results are consistent with previous studies, suggesting that the cold effect is stronger than heat effect in most populations across many countries [27,32,33], and in subtropical cities such as São Paulo [34], Guangzhou [29] and Taipei [27]. The finding provides supporting evidence to the hypothesis that population living in a warmer climate are more adapted to cope with high temperatures, and more susceptible to cold weather.

The minimum mortality temperature in Hong Kong was found to be 28.9 °C, at 82% percentile of the daily mean temperature in the study period, which was generally consistent with the finding from other studies conducted on population with similar climate [21]. One study examined the relationship between temperature and mortality in 66 Chinese communities found that the MMT was 27.4 °C in southern China, which is the highest compared to other regions in China [35]. Country-wide and worldwide studies found that the MMTs are usually higher in warmer regions [27,33,35,36]. Moreover, the MMT identified in this study was slightly higher than the mortality threshold (28.2 °C) reported in a previous local study [21] which used the data from 1998–2006. One assumption could be that the population are adopting the increasing temperature with the effect of climate change [3,37,38], leading to a slightly higher tolerance of hot weather. With the effect of climate change, some studies anticipated that heat-related mortality will increase and eventually compensate for the reduction in cold-related death after 2050 [39]. Other studies suggested that despite the fact that the cold burden will be reduced by the relative effect, heat-related death will remain high across the entire 21st century [40], and the net effect may be inconsistent and subject to local context [41,42], indicating that it is still too early to neglect the health impact of cold weather in the coming decades.

The climate in subtropical regions typically has a very hot summer and less harsh winter. Residents are usually acclimated to a high temperature, which was considered as an important reason why an overall insignificant effect of heat was observed in this study [29,43]. In Hong Kong, the air condition was commonly installed in almost all indoor areas and public transports. The actual exposure of the population could be substantially reduced. However, the study found that the 3-day cumulative heat effect was significantly higher among areas with lower SES, which was also reported in some local and international studies [21,44,45]. A possible reason may be due to the characteristics of housing. The buildings in low-income areas tend to have a higher proportion of old buildings with poor ventilation and insulation. Hong Kong is a city with the highest housing price in the world, and individuals who suffer from poverty usually live in subdivided or temporary dwellings [46]. Those dwellings are often small with poor ventilation, in which heat can be easily trapped inside.

This study found that the cold effect was significant across all SES groups for non-accidental, cardiovascular, respiratory and cancer death. The result also shows a counterintuitive pattern that communities with higher SES were associated with higher cold-related mortality risk, which despite the differences was not statistically significant. Although this kind of analysis was rarely conducted in previous studies, some reported similar results [15]. In Hong Kong, communities with lower SES tends to have higher living density and stronger urban heat island effect [47]. This may suggest that the urban heat island effect may have potential benefit against cold weather in highly urbanized populations, which has been reported recently elsewhere [48]. The universal impact of low temperature on mortality may also be due to the low prevalence of central heating. Despite the high air condition coverage in Hong Kong, most air conditioning devices do not have heating functions and buildings were not designed to restore heat.

A stronger cold effect was identified on cardiovascular than respiratory mortality, which was consistent with previous local and international studies [34,49]. Previous physiological studies suggested that exposure to low temperature may cause elevated blood pressure [50,51], blood viscosity [52], plasma cholesterol and the tendency of blood clot formation in the vessels [53]. Changes in those risk factors may subsequently increase the risk of cardiovascular death. When a high-temperature event occurs, the risk of respiratory death increases as the SES decreases and only individuals living in the lowest SES group were significantly associated with higher risk. A similar pattern was also generally observed for cardiovascular death, despite the effect for all SES groups not being statistically significant. Some earlier local and international studies indicated that the area with lower SES was disproportionally affected by a higher concentration of air pollutants [54,55] and may pose both short and long term adverse effects on health [56,57]. A US study also suggested that in a large city, the exposure of NO_2 concentration is significantly higher for individuals with lower household income [54]. A local study showed that areas with a high level of social deprivation were associated with higher exposure to $PM_{2.5}$ [24]. Furthermore, the effect on air pollution on mortality may also be modified by that temperature. Some studies found that an adverse effect of particulate matter on mortality is stronger under hotter weather in Chinese and European populations [58,59]. The disparity further supports that individuals living in a lower SES community had a higher relative risk after exposure to hot weather, especially for respiratory deaths. This study also identified that cold temperature was associated with significantly higher cancer mortality risk. Several recent studies suggested that cold temperature could be an independent risk factor for cancer [60]. Cold exposure may increase metabolic stress, may contribute to tumorigenesis and higher cancer deaths [61]. A study used data from 166 countries and found a positive association between cancer mortality rate and serum average total cholesterol, which could act as a mediator of cancer development [62]. Unlike other causes, a significant cold effect was only observed in groups with lower SES. higher deprivation and lower-income have been linked with higher cancer incidence and mortality rate due to inequalities on lifestyle, environmental factors and access to services [63,64]. However, the cold effect on cancer and the role of SES have been underreported in current literature, which may be a potential gap for future research.

Significantly higher cold-related mortality risk was found for both males and males, and gender difference was found to be minimum for cold effect. However, females were found to be more susceptible to high temperature. Such a pattern has also been found in a local study [21] and studies elsewhere [8,65]. Older age is a well-known factor associated with higher susceptibility to temperature-related mortality risk [8,29,66,67], and this study found no exception, especially for low temperatures. No clear intra-SES group heterogeneity was identified in both age groups for low temperature effect. However, older persons in the lower SES group were significantly associated with higher heat-related mortality risk, whilst high temperature only posed a very minimum effect to their counterparts in better-off groups. A UK study found that lower SES was associated with a higher uptake of protective measures when experiencing hot weather [68]. A local study indicated that low-income individuals did not have the same level of protective measures, and that some may face financial constraints and still have to work outdoors under hot weather [69]. However, a recent local study found that higher income and education level were not associated with a higher prevalence of protective behavior during cold weather, and vulnerable groups such as the older population commonly underestimated their health risk [70], which partially explained the universal cold effect across all SES groups.

In the UK and Spain, cold weather has been recognized as a major public health concern at the national level, even though the weather during the winter in the two countries is generally milder compared to many other European countries. Nevertheless, the health impact of cold weather has not received adequate attention in Hong Kong, and only limited public services are made available when low temperatures occur [71]. Future policy should consider establishing a holistic strategy to enhance the protective measures at both individual and community levels and reduce the mortality and morbidity associated with low temperature.

A limitation of this study, which is shared by many other researchers of this kind, is the selection of SES measures. The small area level SES may not directly reflect the SES at the individual level. Future multilevel studies with both small areas and individual measures should be conducted, to further understand the effect of SES on the association between temperature and adverse health outcome. Moreover, the actual temperature exposure may vary from person to person, and outdoor ambient temperature may not reflect the exposure if a person spends more of the time in the indoor environment. Some behavioral and physiological factors such as lifestyle and pre-existing diseases may not necessarily be associated with SES, but have also proven to be related to personal exposure and the outcome of extreme temperatures.

5. Conclusions

Despite the fact that Hong Kong has a milder winter climate, the overall cold effect was found to be much stronger and last for a longer period than the heat effect on mortality in Hong Kong. The subpopulation with lower SES is more vulnerable to high temperature, but low temperature universally affects the entire population across all SES groups in Hong Kong. A higher cold effect was observed in groups with the highest SES, despite the different was not statically significant. The heat island effect is a risk factor for heat-related deaths, but it may provide a protective effect during cold weather. This study raises the concern of the health effect of low temperature in subtropical regions, which should be recognized as an important public health issue at territory level. Strategies on mitigating the cold effect should not only focus on populations with lower SES; additional public services should be provided for different socioeconomic classes in Hong Kong.

Author Contributions: Conceptualization, S.L., E.Y.Y.C.; methodology, S.L. and W.B.G.; data analysis, S.L., Z.H., W.B.G.; writing—original draft preparation, S.L.; writing—review and editing, E.Y.Y.C., W.B.G., Z.H.; supervision, E.Y.Y.C. All authors have read and agreed to the published version of the manuscript.

Funding: This research received no external funding.

Acknowledgments: The authors would like to thank the Hong Kong Census and Statistics Department, the Hong Kong Observatory, and the Environmental Protection Department in Hong Kong for providing data for this study.

Conflicts of Interest: The authors declare no conflict of interest.

References

1. Song, X.; Wang, S.; Hu, Y.; Yue, M.; Zhang, T.; Liu, Y.; Tian, J.; Shang, K. Impact of ambient temperature on morbidity and mortality: An overview of reviews. *Sci. Total Environ.* **2017**, *586*, 241–254. [CrossRef]
2. Gronlund, C.J.; Sullivan, K.P.; Kefelegn, Y.; Cameron, L.; O'Neill, M.S. Climate change and temperature extremes: A review of heat- and cold-related morbidity and mortality concerns of municipalities. *Maturitas* **2018**, *114*, 54–59. [CrossRef]
3. Medina-Ramón, M.; Schwartz, J. Temperature, temperature extremes, and mortality: A study of acclimatisation and effect modification in 50 US cities. *Occup. Environ. Med.* **2007**, *64*, 827–833. [CrossRef]
4. Wang, X.; Li, G.; Liu, L.; Westerdahl, D.; Jin, X.; Pan, X. Effects of extreme temperatures on cause-specific cardiovascular mortality in China. *Int. J. Environ Res. Public Health* **2015**, *12*, 16136–16156. [CrossRef]
5. Amegah, A.K.; Rezza, G.; Jaakkola, J.J.K.K. Temperature-related morbidity and mortality in Sub-Saharan Africa: A systematic review of the empirical evidence. *Environ. Int.* **2016**, *91*, 133–149. [CrossRef]

6. Stocker, T.F.; Qin, D.; Plattner, G.K.; Tignor, M.M.B.; Allen, S.K.; Boschung, J.; Nauels, A.; Xia, Y.; Bex, V.; Midgley, P.M. *Climate Change 2013 the Physical Science Basis: Working Group I Contribution to the Fifth Assessment Report of the Intergovernmental Panel on Climate Change*; Cambridge University: New York, NY, USA, 2013; Volume 9781107057, ISBN 9781107415324.
7. O'Neill, M.S.; Zanobetti, A.; Schwartz, J. Modifiers of the temperature and mortality association in seven US cities. *Am. J. Epidemiol.* **2003**, *157*, 1074–1082. [CrossRef] [PubMed]
8. Huang, Z.; Lin, H.; Liu, Y.; Zhou, M.; Liu, T.; Xiao, J.; Zeng, W.; Li, X.; Zhang, Y.; Ebi, K.L.; et al. Individual-level and community-level effect modifiers of the temperature-mortality relationship in 66 Chinese communities. *BMJ Open* **2015**, *5*, e009172. [CrossRef] [PubMed]
9. Sun, S.; Tian, L.; Qiu, H.; Chan, K.P.; Tsang, H.; Tang, R.; Lee, R.S.Y.; Thach, T.Q.; Wong, C.M. The influence of pre-existing health conditions on short-term mortality risks of temperature: Evidence from a prospective Chinese elderly cohort in Hong Kong. *Environ. Res.* **2016**, *148*, 7–14. [CrossRef] [PubMed]
10. Bosma, H.; Van De Mheen, H.D.; Borsboom, G.J.J.M.; Mackenbach, J.P. Neighborhood socioeconomic status and all-cause mortality. *Am. J. Epidemiol.* **2001**, *153*, 363–371. [CrossRef]
11. Bethea, T.N.; Palmer, J.R.; Rosenberg, L.; Cozier, Y.C. Neighborhood Socioeconomic Status in Relation to All-Cause, Cancer, and Cardiovascular Mortality in the Black Women's Health Study. *Ethn. Dis.* **2016**, *26*, 157–164. [CrossRef]
12. Kim, D.; Glazier, R.H.; Zagorski, B.; Kawachi, I.; Oreopoulos, P. Neighbourhood socioeconomic position and risks of major chronic diseases and all-cause mortality: A quasi-experimental study. *BMJ Open* **2018**, *8*, 18793. [CrossRef] [PubMed]
13. Gouveia, N.; Hajat, S.; Armstrong, B. Socioeconomic differentials in the temperature–mortality relationship in São Paulo, Brazil. *Int. J. Epidemiol.* **2003**, *32*, 390–397. [CrossRef] [PubMed]
14. Marí-Dell'Olmo, M.; Tobías, A.; Gómez-Gutiérrez, A.; Rodríguez-Sanz, M.; García de Olalla, P.; Camprubí, E.; Gasparrini, A.; Borrell, C. Social inequalities in the association between temperature and mortality in a South European context. *Int. J. Public Health* **2019**, *64*, 27–37. [CrossRef] [PubMed]
15. Ma, W.; Chen, R.; Kan, H. Temperature-related mortality in 17 large Chinese cities: How heat and cold affect mortality in China. *Environ. Res.* **2014**, *134*, 127–133. [CrossRef] [PubMed]
16. Brooke Anderson, G.; Bell, M.L. Heat waves in the United States: Mortality risk during heat waves and effect modification by heat wave characteristics in 43 U.S. communities. *Environ. Health Perspect.* **2011**, *119*, 210–218. [CrossRef] [PubMed]
17. Basu, R.; Ostro, B.D. A multicounty analysis identifying the populations vulnerable to mortality associated with high ambient temperature in California. *Am. J. Epidemiol.* **2008**, *168*, 632–637. [CrossRef]
18. Hong Kong Census and Statistics Department. *2016 Population By-census: Thematic Report : Household Income Distribution in Hong Kong*; Hong Kong Census and Statistics Department: Hong Kong SAR, China, 2017.
19. Chalabi, Z.; Erens, B.; Hajat, S.; Heffernan, C.; Jones, L.; Mays, N.; Ritchie, B.; Wilkinson, P. *Evaluation of the Implementation and Health-Related Impacts of the Cold Weather Plan for England 2012 Final Report*; Policy Innovation Research Unit: London, UK, 2015.
20. WHO. *Health Emergency and Disaster Risk Management Framework*; WHO: Geneva, Switzerland, 2019.
21. Chan, E.Y.Y.; Goggins, W.B.; Kim, J.J.; Griffiths, S.M. A study of intracity variation of temperature-related mortality and socioeconomic status among the Chinese population in Hong Kong. *J. Epidemiol. Community Health* **2012**, *66*, 322–327. [CrossRef]
22. Ding, Z.; Li, L.; Wei, R.; Dong, W.; Guo, P.; Yang, S.; Liu, J.; Zhang, Q. Association of cold temperature and mortality and effect modification in the subtropical plateau monsoon climate of Yuxi, China. *Environ Res.* **2016**, *150*, 431–437. [CrossRef]
23. Aylin, P.; Morris, S.; Wakefield, J.; Grossinho, A.; Jarup, L.; Elliott, P. Temperature, housing, deprivation and their relationship to excess winter mortality in Great Britain, 1986–1996. *Int. J. Epidemiol.* **2001**, *30*, 1100–1108. [CrossRef]
24. Li, V.O.; Han, Y.; Lam, J.C.; Zhu, Y.; Bacon-Shone, J. Air pollution and environmental injustice: Are the socially deprived exposed to more $PM_{2.5}$ pollution in Hong Kong? *Environ. Sci. Policy* **2018**, *80*, 53–61. [CrossRef]
25. Wong, C.M.; Ou, C.Q.; Chan, K.P.; Chau, Y.K.; Thach, T.Q.; Yang, L.; Chung, R.Y.N.; Thomas, G.N.; Peiris, J.S.M.; Wong, T.W.; et al. The effects of air pollution on mortality in socially deprived urban areas in Hong Kong, China. *Environ Health Perspect.* **2008**, *116*, 1189–1194. [CrossRef] [PubMed]

26. Yu, W.; Vaneckova, P.; Mengersen, K.; Pan, X.; Tong, S. Is the association between temperature and mortality modified by age, gender and socioeconomic status? *Sci. Total Environ.* **2010**, *408*, 3513–3518. [CrossRef] [PubMed]
27. Gasparrini, A.; Guo, Y.; Hashizume, M.; Lavigne, E.; Zanobetti, A.; Schwartz, J.; Tobias, A.; Tong, S.; Rocklöv, J.; Forsberg, B.; et al. Mortality risk attributable to high and low ambient temperature: A multicountry observational study. *Lancet* **2015**, *386*, 369–375. [CrossRef]
28. Guo, Y.; Barnett, A.G.; Pan, X.; Yu, W.; Tong, S. The impact of temperature on mortality in Tianjin, china: A case-crossover design with a distributed lag nonlinear model. *Environ. Health Perspect.* **2011**, *119*, 1719–1725. [CrossRef]
29. Yang, J.; Ou, C.Q.; Ding, Y.; Zhou, Y.X.; Chen, P.Y. Daily temperature and mortality: A study of distributed lag non-linear effect and effect modification in Guangzhou. *Environ. Health A Glob. Access Sci. Source* **2012**, *11*, 63. [CrossRef]
30. Gasparrini, A. Modeling exposure-lag-response associations with distributed lag non-linear models. *Stat. Med.* **2014**, *33*, 881–899. [CrossRef]
31. Wood, S.N. *Generalized Additive Models: An Introduction with R*, 2nd ed.; CRC Press: Boca Raton, FL, USA, 2017; ISBN 9781498728348.
32. Anderson, B.G.; Bell, M.L. Weather-related mortality: How heat, cold, and heat waves affect mortality in the United States. *Epidemiology* **2009**, *20*, 205–213. [CrossRef]
33. Guo, Y.; Gasparrini, A.; Armstrong, B.; Li, S.; Tawatsupa, B.; Tobias, A.; Lavigne, E.; de Sousa Zanotti Stagliorio Coelho, M.; Leone, M.; Pan, X.; et al. Global variation in the effects of ambient temperature on mortality: A systematic evaluation. *Epidemiology* **2014**, *25*, 781–789. [CrossRef]
34. Son, J.Y.; Gouveia, N.; Bravo, M.A.; de Freitas, C.U.; Bell, M.L. The impact of temperature on mortality in a subtropical city: Effects of cold, heat, and heat waves in São Paulo, Brazil. *Int. J. Biometeorol.* **2016**, *60*, 113–121. [CrossRef]
35. Ma, W.; Wang, L.; Lin, H.; Liu, T.; Zhang, Y.; Rutherford, S.; Luo, Y.; Zeng, W.; Zhang, Y.; Wang, X.; et al. The temperature-mortality relationship in China: An analysis from 66 Chinese communities. *Environ. Res.* **2015**, *137*, 72–77. [CrossRef]
36. Iñiguez, C.; Ballester, F.; Ferrandiz, J.; Pérez-Hoyos, S.; Sáez, M.; López, A. Tempro-Emecas Relation between temperature and mortality in thirteen Spanish cities. *Int. J. Environ. Res. Public Health* **2010**, *7*, 3196–3210. [CrossRef] [PubMed]
37. Bobb, J.F.; Peng, R.D.; Bell, M.L.; Dominici, F. Heat-related mortality and adaptation to heat in the United States. *Environ. Health Perspect.* **2014**, *122*, 811–816. [CrossRef] [PubMed]
38. Barreca, A.; Clay, K.; Deschênes, O.; Greenstone, M.; Shapiro, J.S. Convergence in adaptation to climate change: Evidence from high temperatures and mortality, 1900–2004. *Am. Econ. Rev.* **2015**, *105*, 247–251. [CrossRef]
39. Ballester, J.; Robine, J.M.; Herrmann, F.R.; Rodó, X. Long-term projections and acclimatisation scenarios of temperature-related mortality in Europe. *Nat. Commun.* **2011**, *2*, 358. [CrossRef] [PubMed]
40. Hajat, S.; Vardoulakis, S.; Heaviside, C.; Eggen, B. Climate change effects on human health: Projections of temperature-related mortality for the UK during the 2020s, 2050s and 2080s. *J. Epidemiol. Community Health* **2014**, *68*, 641–648. [CrossRef]
41. Gasparrini, A.; Guo, Y.; Sera, F.; Vicedo-Cabrera, A.M.; Huber, V.; Tong, S.; de Sousa Zanotti Stagliorio Coelho, M.; Nascimento Saldiva, P.H.; Lavigne, E.; Matus Correa, P.; et al. Projections of temperature-related excess mortality under climate change scenarios. *Lancet Planet. Health* **2017**, *1*, e360–e367. [CrossRef]
42. Guo, Y.; Li, S.; Liu, D.L.; Chen, D.; Williams, G.; Tong, S. Projecting future temperature-related mortality in three largest Australian cities. *Environ. Pollut.* **2016**, *208*, 66–73. [CrossRef]
43. Wu, W.; Xiao, Y.; Li, G.; Zeng, W.; Lin, H.; Rutherford, S.; Xu, Y.; Luo, Y.; Xu, X.; Chu, C.; et al. Temperature-mortality relationship in four subtropical Chinese cities: A time-series study using a distributed lag non-linear model. *Sci. Total Environ.* **2013**, *449*, 355–362. [CrossRef]
44. Basu, R. High ambient temperature and mortality: A review of epidemiologic studies from 2001 to 2008. *Environ. Health Glob. Access Sci. Source* **2009**, *8*, 40. [CrossRef]
45. Madrigano, J.; Mittleman, M.A.; Baccarelli, A.; Goldberg, R.; Melly, S.; Von Klot, S.; Schwartz, J. Temperature, myocardial infarction, and mortality: Effect modification by individual-and area-level characteristics. *Epidemiology* **2013**, *24*, 439–446. [CrossRef]

46. Tim Wong, L. Tiny affordable housing in Hong Kong. *Indoor Built Environ.* **2018**, *27*, 1159–1161. [CrossRef]
47. Goggins, W.B.; Chan, E.Y.Y.Y.; Ng, E.; Ren, C.; Chen, L. Effect modification of the association between short-term meteorological factors and mortality by urban heat islands in Hong Kong. *PLoS ONE* **2012**, *7*, e38551. [CrossRef] [PubMed]
48. Yang, J.; Bou-Zeid, E. Should cities embrace their heat islands as shields from extreme cold? *J. Appl. Meteorol. Clim.* **2018**, *57*, 1309–1320. [CrossRef]
49. Goggins, W.B.; Chan, E.Y. A study of the short-term associations between hospital admissions and mortality from heart failure and meteorological variables in Hong Kong: Weather and heart failure in Hong Kong. *Int. J. Cardiol.* **2017**, *228*, 537–542. [CrossRef]
50. Shiue, I.; Shiue, M. Indoor temperature below 18 °C accounts for 9% population attributable risk for high blood pressure in Scotland. *Int. J. Cardiol.* **2014**, *171*, e1. [CrossRef]
51. Saeki, K.; Obayashi, K.; Iwamoto, J.; Tanaka, Y.; Tanaka, N.; Takata, S.; Kubo, H.; Okamoto, N.; Tomioka, K.; Nezu, S.; et al. Influence of room heating on ambulatory blood pressure in winter: A randomised controlled study. *J. Epidemiol. Community Health* **2013**, *67*, 484–490. [CrossRef]
52. Brown, H.K.; Simpson, A.J.; Murchison, J.T. The influence of meteorological variables on the development of deep venous thrombosis. *Thromb. Haemost.* **2009**, *102*, 676–682. [CrossRef]
53. Huynen, M.M.T.E.; Martens, P.; Schram, D.; Weijenberg, M.P.; Kunst, A.E. The impact of heat waves and cold spells on mortality rates in the Dutch population. *Environ. Health Perspect.* **2001**, *109*, 463–470. [CrossRef]
54. Clark, L.P.; Millet, D.B.; Marshall, J.D. National patterns in environmental injustice and inequality: Outdoor NO2 air pollution in the United States. *PLoS ONE* **2014**, *9*, e94431. [CrossRef]
55. Pearce, J.R.; Richardson, E.A.; Mitchell, R.J.; Shortt, N.K. Environmental justice and health: The implications of the socio-spatial distribution of multiple environmental deprivation for health inequalities in the United Kingdom. *Trans. Inst. Br. Geogr.* **2010**, *35*, 522–539. [CrossRef]
56. Hoek, G.; Krishnan, R.M.; Beelen, R.; Peters, A.; Ostro, B.; Brunekreef, B.; Kaufman, J.D. Long-term air pollution exposure and cardio-respiratory mortality: A review. *Environ. Health Glob. Access Sci. Source* **2013**, *12*, 43. [CrossRef] [PubMed]
57. Shang, Y.; Sun, Z.; Cao, J.; Wang, X.; Zhong, L.; Bi, X.; Li, H.; Liu, W.; Zhu, T.; Huang, W. Systematic review of Chinese studies of short-term exposure to air pollution and daily mortality. *Environ. Int.* **2013**, *54*, 100–111. [CrossRef] [PubMed]
58. Meng, X.; Zhang, Y.; Zhao, Z.; Duan, X.; Xu, X.; Kan, H. Temperature modifies the acute effect of particulate air pollution on mortality in eight Chinese cities. *Sci. Total Environ.* **2012**, *435–436*, 215–221. [CrossRef] [PubMed]
59. Stafoggia, M.; Schwartz, J.; Forastiere, F.; Perucci, C.A. Does temperature modify the association between air pollution and mortality? A multi-city case-crossover analysis in Italy. *Am. J. Epidemiol.* **2008**, *167*, 1476–1485. [CrossRef]
60. Sharma, A.; Sharma, T.; Panwar, M.S.; Sharma, D.; Bundel, R.; Hamilton, R.T.; Radosevich, J.A.; Mandal, C.C. Colder environments are associated with a greater cancer incidence in the female population of the United States. *Tumor Biol.* **2017**, *39*, 1–12. [CrossRef]
61. Sharma, A.; Verma, H.K.; Joshi, S.; Panwar, M.S.; Mandal, C.C. A link between cold environment and cancer. *Tumor Biol.* **2015**, *36*, 5953–5964. [CrossRef]
62. Bandyopadhayaya, S.; Ford, B.; Mandal, C.C. Cold-hearted: A case for cold stress in cancer risk. *J. Biol.* **2020**, *91*, 102608. [CrossRef]
63. Singh, G.K.; Jemal, A. Socioeconomic and Racial/Ethnic Disparities in Cancer Mortality, Incidence, and Survival in the United States, 1950-2014: Over Six Decades of Changing Patterns and Widening Inequalities. *J. Environ. Public Health* **2017**. [CrossRef]
64. Kim, C.W.; Lee, S.Y.; Moon, O.R. Inequalities in cancer incidence and mortality across income groups and policy implications in South Korea. *Public Health* **2008**, *122*, 229–236. [CrossRef]
65. Yang, J.; Yin, P.; Zhou, M.; Ou, C.Q.; Li, M.; Liu, Y.; Gao, J.; Chen, B.; Liu, J.; Bai, L.; et al. The effect of ambient temperature on diabetes mortality in China: A multi-city time series study. *Sci. Total Environ.* **2016**, *543*, 75–82. [CrossRef]
66. Li, J.; Xu, X.; Yang, J.; Liu, Z.; Xu, L.; Gao, J.; Liu, X.; Wu, H.; Wang, J.; Yu, J.; et al. Ambient high temperature and mortality in Jinan, China: A study of heat thresholds and vulnerable populations. *Environ. Res.* **2017**, *156*, 657–664. [CrossRef]

67. Onozuka, D.; Hagihara, A. Variation in vulnerability to extreme-temperature-related mortality in Japan: A 40-year time-series analysis. *Environ. Res.* **2015**, *140*, 177–184. [CrossRef] [PubMed]
68. Khare, S.; Hajat, S.; Kovats, S.; Lefevre, C.E.; De Bruin, W.B.; Dessai, S.; Bone, A. Heat protection behaviour in the UK: Results of an online survey after the 2013 heatwave. *BMC Public Health* **2015**, *15*, 878. [CrossRef] [PubMed]
69. Lee, W.K.M. Women and Retirement Planning: Towards the "Feminization of Poverty" in an Aging Hong Kong. *J. Women Aging* **2003**, *15*, 31–53. [CrossRef] [PubMed]
70. Lam, H.C.Y.; Huang, Z.; Liu, S.; Guo, C.; Goggins, W.B.; Chan, E.Y.Y. Personal cold protection behaviour and its associated factors in 2016/17 cold days in Hong Kong: A two-year cohort telephone survey study. *Int. J. Environ. Res. Public Health* **2020**, *17*, 1672. [CrossRef]
71. Hong Kong Home Affairs Department Public Services–Emergency Relief Services. Available online: https://www.had.gov.hk/en/public_services/emergency_services/emergency.htm (accessed on 26 July 2020).

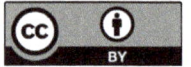

© 2020 by the authors. Licensee MDPI, Basel, Switzerland. This article is an open access article distributed under the terms and conditions of the Creative Commons Attribution (CC BY) license (http://creativecommons.org/licenses/by/4.0/).